Diagnostic Radiology

Editor

ANGELA J. MAROLF

VETERINARY CLINICS OF NORTH AMERICA: SMALL ANIMAL PRACTICE

www.vetsmall.theclinics.com

May 2016 • Volume 46 • Number 3

ELSEVIER

1600 John F. Kennedy Boulevard • Suite 1800 • Philadelphia, Pennsylvania, 19103-2899
http://www.vetsmall.theclinics.com

**VETERINARY CLINICS OF NORTH AMERICA: SMALL ANIMAL PRACTICE Volume 46, Number 3
May 2016 ISSN 0195-5616, ISBN-13: 978-0-323-44488-0**

Editor: Patrick Manley
Developmental Editor: Meredith Clinton

Veterinary Clinics of North America: Small Animal Practice (ISSN 0195-5616) is published bimonthly by Elsevier Inc., 360 Park Avenue South, New York, NY 10010-1710. Months of issue are January, March, May, July, September, and November. Business and Editorial Offices: 1600 John F. Kennedy Blvd., Ste. 1800, Philadelphia, PA 19103-2899. Customer Service Office: 3251 Riverport Lane, Maryland Heights, MO 63043. Periodicals postage paid at New York, NY and additional mailing offices. Subscription prices are $310.00 per year (domestic individuals), $564.00 per year (domestic institutions), $100.00 per year (domestic students/residents), $410.00 per year (Canadian individuals), $701.00 per year (Canadian institutions), $455.00 per year (international individuals), $701.00 per year (international institutions), and $220.00 per year (international and Canadian students/residents). To receive student/resident rate, orders must be accompanied by name of affiliated institution, date of term, and the *signature* of program/residency coordinator on institution letterhead. Orders will be billed at individual rate until proof of status is received. Foreign air speed delivery is included in all *Clinics* subscription prices. All prices are subject to change without notice. **POSTMASTER:** Send address changes to *Veterinary Clinics of North America: Small Animal Practice*, Elsevier Health Sciences Division, Subscription Customer Service, 3251 Riverport Lane, Maryland Heights, MO 63043. Customer Service (orders, claims, online, change of address): Elsevier Periodicals Customer Service, Elsevier Health Sciences Division Subscription **Customer Service 3251 Riverport Lane Maryland Heights, MO 63043. Tel: 1-800-654-2452 (U.S. and Canada); 314-447-8871 (outside U.S. and Canada). Fax: 314-447-8029. E-mail: journalscustomerservice-usa@elsevier.com (for print support); journalsonlinesupport-usa@elsevier.com (for online support).**

Reprints. For copies of 100 or more of articles in this publication, please contact the Commercial Reprints Department, Elsevier Inc., 360 Park Avenue South, New York, NY 10010-1710. Tel.: 212-633-3874; Fax: 212-633-3820; E-mail: reprints@elsevier.com.

Veterinary Clinics of North America: Small Animal Practice is also published in Japanese by Inter Zoo Publishing Co., Ltd., Aoyama Crystal-Bldg 5F, 3-5-12 Kitaaoyama, Minato-ku, Tokyo 107-0061, Japan.

Veterinary Clinics of North America: Small Animal Practice is covered in *Current Contents/Agriculture, Biology and Environmental Sciences, Science Citation Index, ASCA, MEDLINE/PubMed (Index Medicus), Excerpta Medica,* and *BIOSIS.*

Contributors

EDITOR

ANGELA J. MAROLF, DVM
Diplomate, American College of Veterinary Radiology; Associate Professor of Radiology, Department of Environmental and Radiological Health Sciences, College of Veterinary Medicine and Biomedical Sciences, Colorado State University, Fort Collins, Colorado

AUTHORS

ELIZABETH A. BALLEGEER, BS, DVM
Diplomate, American College of Veterinary Radiology; Assistant Professor, Diagnostic Imaging, Department of Small Animal Clinical Sciences, College of Veterinary Medicine, Michigan State University, East Lansing, Michigan

ALLYSON C. BERENT, DVM
Diplomate, American College of Veterinary Internal Medicine; Director, Interventional Endoscopy; Staff Veterinarian Internal Medicine, Department of Interventional Radiology and Endoscopy, The Animal Medical Center, New York, New York

CRISTI R. COOK, DVM, MS
Diplomate, American College of Veterinary Radiology; Assistant Research Professor, Comparative Orthopaedic Laboratory, Veterinary Health Center, University of Missouri, Columbia, Missouri

WILLIAM T.N. CULP, VMD
Diplomate, American College of Veterinary Surgeons; ACVS Founding Fellow of Surgical Oncology; Assistant Professor, Department of Surgical and Radiological Sciences, University of California-Davis, School of Veterinary Medicine, Davis, California

LISA J. FORREST, VMD
Diplomate, American College of Veterinary Radiology (Radiology, Radiation Oncology); Professor, Department of Surgical Sciences, University of Wisconsin-Madison School of Veterinary Medicine, Madison, Wisconsin

PATRICK GAVIN, DVM, PhD
Diplomate, American College of Veterinary Radiology (Radiation Oncology); Professor Emeritus, Department of Veterinary Medicine, Washington State University, Pullman, Washington; CEO, Chief Radiologist, MRVets, P.C., Sagle, Idaho

MARTHA MOON LARSON, DVM, MS
Diplomate, American College of Veterinary Radiology; Department of Small Animal Clinical Sciences, Virginia-Maryland College of Veterinary Medicine, Blacksburg, Virginia

ANGELA J. MAROLF, DVM
Diplomate, American College of Veterinary Radiology; Associate Professor of Radiology, Department of Environmental and Radiological Health Sciences, College of Veterinary Medicine and Biomedical Sciences, Colorado State University, Fort Collins, Colorado

ELISSA K. RANDALL, DVM, MS
Diplomate, American College of Veterinary Radiology; Associate Professor, Department of Environmental and Radiological Health Sciences, Veterinary Teaching Hospital, Colorado State University, Fort Collins, Colorado

JAIME E. SAGE, DVM, MS
Diplomate, American College of Veterinary Radiology; Radiologist, MRVets, P.C., Austin, Texas

BRIAN A. SCANSEN, DVM, MS
Diplomate, American College of Veterinary Internal Medicine (Cardiology); Associate Professor, Department of Clinical Sciences, College of Veterinary Medicine & Biomedical Sciences, Colorado State University, Fort Collins, Colorado

Contents

Musculoskeletal ultrasound is a rapidly growing field within veterinary medicine. Ultrasound for musculoskeletal disorders has been commonly used in equine and human medicine and is becoming more commonly performed in small animal patients due to the increase in the recognition of soft tissue injuries. Ultrasound is widely available and cost-effective, but it is technically difficult to learn. Advantages of musculoskeletal ultrasound are the opposite limb is commonly used for comparison to evaluate symmetry of the tendinous structures and the ease of repeat examinations to assess healing. The article discusses the major areas of shoulder, stifle, iliopsoas, gastrocnemius, and musculoskeletal basics.

Computed tomography (CT) has specific uses in veterinary species' appendicular musculoskeletal system. Parameters for acquisition of images, interpretation limitations, as well as published information regarding its use in small animals are reviewed.

MRI has the unique ability to detect abnormal fluid content, and is unparalleled in its role of detection, diagnosis, prognosis, treatment planning and follow-up evaluation of musculoskeletal disease. MRI in companion animals should be considered in the following circumstances: a definitive diagnosis cannot be made on radiographs, a patient is unresponsive to medical or surgical therapy, prognostic information is desired, assessing surgical margins and traumatic and/or infectious joint and bone disease, ruling out subtle developmental or early aggressive bone lesions. The MRI features of common disorders affecting the shoulder, elbow, stifle, carpal, and tarsal joints are included in this article.

 Video content accompanies this article at http://www.vetsmall. theclinics.com

Ultrasound is an extremely valuable diagnostic modality for the diagnosis of hepatobiliary and pancreatic disease. Normal appearance and normal variations are important to understand to avoid misinterpretation. Although

MRI and computed tomographic (CT) imaging are becoming more common in the diagnosis of hepatobiliary and pancreatic disorders in small animals. With the advent of multislice CT scanners, sedated examinations in veterinary patients are feasible, which is increasing the use of this imaging modality. CT and MRI provide additional information for dogs and cats with hepatobiliary and pancreatic diseases because of lack of superimposition of structures, operator dependence, and through intravenous contrast administration. This added value provides more information for diagnosis, prognosis, and surgical planning.

Computed tomography (CT) imaging has become the mainstay of oncology, providing accurate tumor staging and follow-up imaging to monitor treatment response. Presurgical evaluation of tumors is becoming commonplace and guides surgeons as to the extent and whether complete tumor resection is possible. CT imaging plays a crucial role in radiotherapy treatment planning. CT imaging in oncology has become ubiquitous in veterinary medicine because of increased availability of this imaging modality. This article focuses on CT cancer staging in veterinary oncology, CT imaging for surgical planning, and advances in CT simulation for radiation therapy planning.

PET/CT is an advanced imaging modality that is becoming more commonly used in veterinary medicine. It is most commonly used to image patients with cancer, and the most frequently used radiopharmaceutical is F-18 FDG. F-18 FDG is a glucose analog that highlights areas of increased glucose metabolism on the PET images. CT images provide excellent anatomic depiction and aid in interpretation of the PET data. Many types of cancer are hypermetabolic on PET/CT scans, but normal structures and areas of inflammation are also hypermetabolic, so knowledge of normal imaging and cytologic or histopathologic evaluation of lesions is essential.

The breadth of small animal diseases that can now be treated by a minimally invasive, transcatheter approach continues to expand. Interventional radiology is the field of medicine that affects a therapeutic outcome via minimally invasive catheterization of peripheral blood vessels or body orifices guided by imaging. The intent of this article is to provide an overview of the equipment required for interventional radiology in veterinary medicine with a discussion of technical uses in diseases of dogs and cats.

William T.N. Culp

The approach to the treatment of cancer in veterinary patients is constantly evolving. Whenever possible, surgery is pursued because it provides the greatest opportunity for tumor control and may result in a cure. Other cancer treatments, such as chemotherapy and radiation therapy, are commonplace in veterinary medicine, and the data outlining treatment regimens are growing rapidly. An absence of treatment options for veterinary cancer patients has historically existed for some tumors. Interventional oncology options have opened the door to the potential for better therapeutic response and improved patient quality of life.

Allyson C. Berent

Minimally invasive treatment options using interventional radiology and interventional endoscopy for urologic disease have become more common over the past decade in veterinary medicine. Urinary tract obstructions and urinary incontinence are the most common reasons for urinary interventions. Ureteral obstructions are underdiagnosed and a common clinical problem in veterinary medicine. Ureteral obstructions should be considered an emergency, and decompression should be performed as quickly as possible. Diagnostic imaging is the mainstay in diagnosing a ureteral obstruction and has changed in the last few years, with ultrasound and radiographs being the most sensitive tools in making this diagnosis preoperatively.

VETERINARY CLINICS OF NORTH AMERICA: SMALL ANIMAL PRACTICE

RELATED INTEREST

Veterinary Clinics of North America: Food Animal Practice
March 2016, Volume 32, Issue 1
Update on Ruminant Ultrasound
Sébastien Buczinski, *Editor*

THE CLINICS ARE NOW AVAILABLE ONLINE!
Access your subscription at:
www.theclinics.com

Preface

Diagnostic Radiology

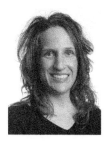

Angela J. Marolf, DVM, DACVR
Editor

This issue of *Veterinary Clinics of North America: Small Animal Practice* describes new imaging techniques and interpretive methods in the diagnosis of important diseases. Advancements in diagnostic imaging are happening at a rapid pace, and the information gained from these developments is furthering our diagnostic capabilities and improving outcomes for veterinary patients.

It is not possible to include the full array of diagnostic imaging in one issue. Subsequently, this issue focuses on some expanding areas of imaging in small animal veterinary medicine. These topics include musculoskeletal imaging, hepatobiliary and pancreatic imaging, oncologic imaging, and last, interventional radiologic techniques. With interventional radiology's use of fluoroscopy, therapeutic procedures can be performed noninvasively, decreasing morbidity and recovery time for veterinary patients. Computed tomography (CT), MRI, PET-CT, and ultrasound imaging are being utilized in new ways to provide more accurate diagnoses and treatment options. These advancements in imaging are refining and expanding the role of diagnostic imaging in veterinary medicine today.

I selected authors with imaging expertise and understanding of the clinical applicability of their topic. I would like to sincerely thank the contributing authors for their efforts, skills, and time in writing pertinent and clinically applicable articles for this issue. I would also like to thank all of the individuals who have mentored and assisted me throughout my career as a veterinary radiologist.

Vet Clin Small Anim 46 (2016) ix–x
http://dx.doi.org/10.1016/j.cvsm.2016.02.006
0195-5616/16/$ – see front matter © 2016 Published by Elsevier Inc.

vetsmall.theclinics.com

I am also very grateful to Patrick Manley, for his invitation to be a guest editor for this issue, and Meredith Clinton and the Elsevier staff, for their efforts and assistance in its publication.

Angela J. Marolf, DVM, DACVR
Department of Environmental and Radiological Health Sciences
College of Veterinary Medicine
and Biomedical Sciences
Colorado State University
300 West Drake Road
Fort Collins, CO 80523-1620, USA

E-mail address:
angela.marolf@colostate.edu

Ultrasound Imaging of the Musculoskeletal System

Cristi R. Cook, DVM, MS

KEYWORDS

- Musculoskeletal • Ultrasonography • Canine • Shoulder • Stifle • Iliopsoas

KEY POINTS

- Imaging of the shoulder includes the supraspinatus, infraspinatus, biceps, and subscapularis tendons and medial glenohumeral ligament.
- Stifle imaging should include the quadriceps tendon, patellar ligament, cranial joint space, medial and lateral menisci, and the cruciate ligaments.
- Ultrasound imaging of tendons and ligaments needs to maintain the transducer perpendicular to the structure to avoid anisotropy, an off-axis artifact in musculoskeletal imaging.
- Evaluation of the tendon should include the tendon to the musculotendinous junction and a portion of the muscle in the area of interest.

Musculoskeletal ultrasound is a rapidly growing field within the veterinary caseload. Ultrasound for musculoskeletal disorders has been commonly used in equine and human medicine and is becoming more commonly performed in small animal patients because of the increase in the recognition of soft tissue injuries. The use of ultrasound in small animal practice is highly dependent on the experience of the ultrasonographer, the ultrasound machine, and the knowledge of the anatomy. As with other areas, ultrasound availability, rapidness of the procedure, ease and capability of repeat examinations, and inexpensive cost are all advantages of the use of ultrasound over other advanced imaging modalities. Another advantage of musculoskeletal ultrasound is the opposite limb is commonly used for comparison to evaluate symmetry of the tendinous structures. This comparison can be difficult when the orthopedic disease is bilateral, but the ultrasonographic findings are often not exactly the same; therefore, asymmetrical findings within the tendon between each limb are significant. The use of ultrasound does not negate the use of radiography and is viewed as a complementary modality for orthopedic injuries. Diagnostic ultrasound can be performed in the awake or lightly sedated patient and uncommonly necessitates the use of general anesthesia.

The author has nothing to disclose.
Comparative Orthopaedic Laboratory, Veterinary Health Center, University of Missouri, 1600 East Rollins Street, Columbia, MO 65201, USA
E-mail address: CookCR@Missouri.edu

Vet Clin Small Anim 46 (2016) 355–371
http://dx.doi.org/10.1016/j.cvsm.2015.12.001
0195-5616/16/$ – see front matter © 2016 Elsevier Inc. All rights reserved.

Diagnostic ultrasound is commonly used to assess healing of musculotendinous injuries through repeat examinations.

TECHNIQUE AND EQUIPMENT

The area of interest should be clipped of hair, followed by an application of isopropyl alcohol and coupling gel to get direct contact and avoid artifact formation. Musculoskeletal ultrasound requires the use of high-resolution, linear transducers to evaluate superficial structures of the musculoskeletal system. The transducers most beneficial for musculoskeletal imaging are within the range of 8 to 15 MHz. The transducer footprint should be small to medium length to maintain good contact with these structures and in proper alignment. Curvilinear or sector transducers can be used, but caution needs to be taken as these probes will lead to artifacts produced by the curved surface of the probe. It is important when performing ultrasounds of tendons and ligaments to have the ultrasound beam perpendicular to the area of interest. The fibers of the tendons and ligaments will become hypoechoic when the angle of the tendon is no longer perpendicular to the ultrasound beam and is referred to as anisotropy or off-axis artifact (**Fig. 1**).[1–3]

ULTRASONOGRAPHIC ANATOMY

The structures commonly evaluated with musculoskeletal ultrasound include tendon, ligament, muscle, and bone. Bone has a hyperechoic, smooth surface with distal acoustic shadowing deep to the bone, due to the reflection of the ultrasound beam back to the transducer. Ultrasound can be helpful with evaluating osseous structures for early osteomyelitis, fungal osteomyelitis, osseous neoplasias (primary, metastatic, or lymphoma reticular), and fracture healing. The subtle signs of early osteomyelitis include a focal area of hypoechoic fluid along the smooth surface of the bone caused by subperiosteal edema. As osteomyelitis progresses, the irregular osseous surface is seen typically without cortical disruptions (**Fig. 2**). This irregular osseous surface could be similar to osseous neoplasias, but neoplasia will commonly have cortical disruptions, and a soft tissue component is commonly visualized adjacent to this, whether intramedullary or superficial (**Fig. 3**).

Another common tool for bone ultrasound is the acquisition of fine-needle aspirates or core biopsies. The ultrasound can be used to guide the needle into the margins of

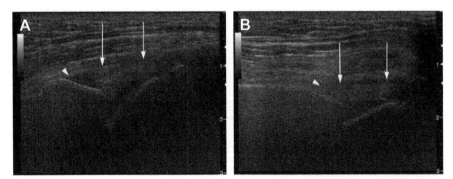

Fig. 1. Off-axis artifact of the biceps tendon (BT). Arrows identify the biceps tendon. Note the hypoechoic BT at the origin on the scapula (*arrowhead*) (*A*). The BT tendon fibers are visible (*B*).

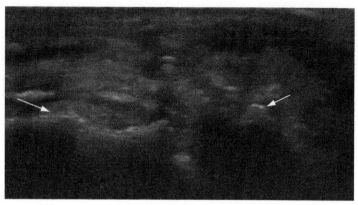

Fig. 2. Osteomyelitis with irregular cortical surface of the long bone (*arrows*).

the cortical disruption as well as the soft tissue component of the tumor for cytologic examination. The same would be true with core biopsies for histopathologic analysis. The best area for sampling the osseous neoplasias would be within the soft tissue mass or the osseous margins, not in the center of the lesion where there could be areas of hemorrhage and necrosis.

When muscle ultrasound is performed, it is important to be longitudinal to the muscle belly of interest. The ultrasonographic appearance of normal muscle has a hyperechoic surface due to the epimysium and fascial tissue surrounding the muscle. Most of the muscle is hypoechoic, with longitudinal hyperechoic, fine striations on longitudinal imaging and multifocal, pinpoint hyperechogenicities on transverse imaging through the muscle (**Fig. 4**A).[4–6] These striations represent the connective tissue between each muscle fascicle. Common muscle disorders include trauma with disruption of the fibers, which can be partial to complete disruption (see **Fig. 4**B).

Ultrasonographic evaluation of masses can be performed to identify the difference between hemorrhage, abscesses, and soft tissue neoplasias. Acute hemorrhage will

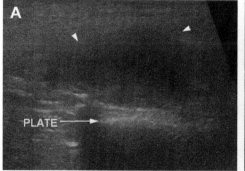
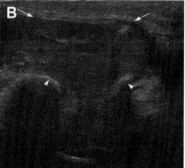

Fig. 3. Soft tissue mass (*arrowheads*) adjacent to a bone plate (*A*). Cortical disruption (*arrowheads*) with a soft tissue mass (*arrows*). Synovial cell sarcoma (*B*).

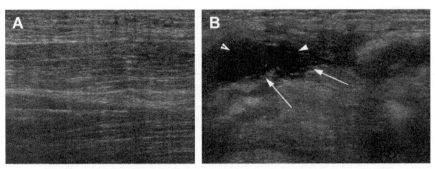

Fig. 4. Normal muscle (*A*). Semimembranosis muscle tear. Note the hypoechoic hemorrhage (*arrowheads*) and retraction of the torn muscle fibers (*arrows*) (*B*).

be hypoechoic, commonly ill-defined margins and will regress over time.[7] Cellulitis appears as hypoechoic interdigitations between the muscle fibers (**Fig. 5**). Organized abscesses will have a thickened hyperechoic wall with hypoechoic to hyperechoic fluid centrally and may have distal acoustic enhancement. Soft tissue neoplasias of the muscle and tendon have ill-defined margins, a mixed echogenicity throughout the mass with or without areas of hypoechoic hemorrhage and necrosis. Soft tissue neoplasias cannot be accurately differentiated from benign neoplasias or other diseases such as hemorrhage.[8]

A normal tendon/ligament appears as a fine, thin structure with hyperechoic parallel fibers within the ligament. The tendons can be followed to the musculotendinous junction and will be of varying lengths depending on which tendon is being evaluated. Several tendons such as the biceps or carpal flexor tendons will have a small amount of hypoechoic fluid seen superficial to them and within the tendon sheath. Abnormal tendons will be hypoechoic with disruption of the fibers and thickening of the tendon in the acute phase. Whereas, the tendon in the chronic phase will be normal to hyperechoic in appearance, narrowed, reorganization or realignment of the tendon fibers and may have dystrophic mineralization within the area of the injury.

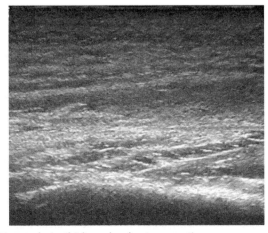

Fig. 5. Cellulitis. Hyperechoic, thickened, subcutaneous tissues.

SHOULDER

Orthopedic injuries of the shoulder are common in a wide variety of canine and feline patients. Shoulder injuries are commonly seen in working dogs and may be difficult to diagnose on radiography alone. Acute and chronic injuries are seen within the shoulder and will vary on their appearance in both radiography and ultrasound. The structures of the shoulder that are commonly evaluated include the supraspinatus, infraspinatus, and biceps tendons/muscles. Other structures with less common injuries include teres minor and major as well as deltoid and pectoral muscles or tendons. The medial aspect of the shoulder is difficult to evaluate with ultrasound, although the use of a hockey-stick probe can be used to evaluate the medial glenohumeral ligament and subscapularis tendons, depending on the experience of the ultrasonographer (**Fig. 6**). In order to evaluate the medial shoulder, sedation is recommended.

The normal supraspinatus muscle is seen cranial to the spine of the scapula with a central hyperechoic tendon. The supraspinatus tendon within the muscle has a typical appearance with long, parallel fibers. As the supraspinatus tendon crosses the scapulohumeral joint, it becomes hypoechoic and triangular in appearance on long axis as it becomes fibrocartilage before its insertion on the medial aspect of the greater tubercle of the proximal humerus (**Fig. 7**).[5,6,9,10] To the author's knowledge, this is the only tendon within the body of the canine or feline patient that has this insertion configuration and appearance.

The normal infraspinatus muscle is caudal to the spine of the scapula with a tendon that lies more eccentric, toward the spine of the scapula, within the muscle. The infraspinatus tendon crosses the scapulohumeral joint and inserts within a depression along the lateral aspect of the proximal humeral cortex (**Fig. 8**). Caudodistal to the infraspinatus insertion, the teres minor attaches as a flat, hyperechoic tendon (**Fig. 9**).[5,6,9,10] These tendons have the typical appearance at insertion sites with the tendon fibers directly attaching to the cortex of the bone.

The biceps tendon originates at the supraglenoid tubercle and extends distal across the joint. The biceps tendon sheath is an extension of the joint capsule and has a thin (<1 mm) rim of hypoechoic fluid surrounding the tendon. The tendon continues distally to the level of the musculotendinous junction. Near the musculotendinous junction,

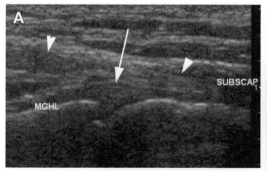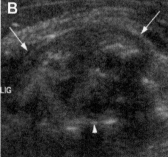

Fig. 6. Medial shoulder, normal. The subscapularis tendon is seen deep to the arrowheads. The arrow identifies the medial surface of the medial glenohumeral ligament (MGHL) (*A*). Medial shoulder instability due to subscapularis tendon tear and medial glenohumeral ligament tears and hypertrophy (*arrows*). Arrowhead identifies the medial scapular surface (*B*). LIG, ligament on image; MGHL, medial glenohumeral ligament; SUBSCAP, subscapularis.

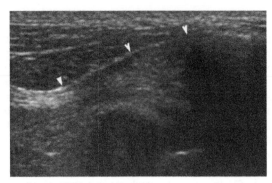

Fig. 7. Normal supraspinatus (SST) (*arrowheads*).

there may be a small outpocketing of fluid, which is considered a normal structure at this location and is commonly referred to as the biceps bursa.[5,6,10,11] On transverse images, the biceps tendon is seen within the bicipital groove between the greater and lesser tubercles. Evaluation of the relationship between the supraspinatus and biceps tendon is necessary because biceps injuries can be either primary or secondary to supraspinatus abnormality.[12]

Supraspinatus abnormalities are common in the canine patient. The supraspinatus tendinopathy is a generic description for abnormalities associated with overuse injuries. Degenerative disorders of the canine supraspinatus tendon are also identified, including calcifying tendinitis or tendinosis (microtears with dystrophic mineralization) or tears, partial or complete (**Fig. 10**A, B). Injuries of the supraspinatus can occur at any level within the muscle or tendon, with the most common injury occurring at the insertion along the greater tubercle. Supraspinatus tendonopathy can appear as a thickened, mottled structure at the point of insertion with or without irregular mineralization at the insertion or within the fibrous portion of the tendon. Insertional irregularity of the bone is often thought to be a result of partial tear of the supraspinatus insertion. Uncommonly, complete tears or avulsions of the supraspinatus tendon are identified (**Fig. 11**).[12]

Infraspinatus tendon injuries are occasionally identified at the musculotendinous junction as well as at the insertion. Infraspinatus tendon injuries will have a similar appearance to the insertion of the supraspinatus as an irregular osseous surface

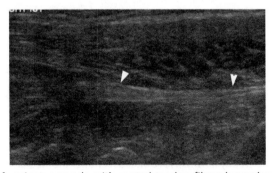

Fig. 8. Normal infraspinatus muscle with central tendon fibers (*arrowheads*).

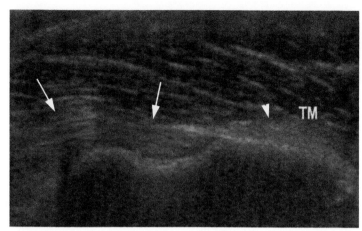

Fig. 9. Normal infraspinatus tendon (*arrows*) with the caudodistal teres minor insertion (TM). (*Arrowhead*, teres minor tendon.)

with thickening of the tendon insertion site (**Fig. 12**). Contracture of the supraspinatus or infraspinatus muscles can occur and will often appear as hyperechoic musculature or narrowing of the respective tendon. If the contracture is unilateral, comparative views of the respective muscles are useful in identifying early signs of this disorder.

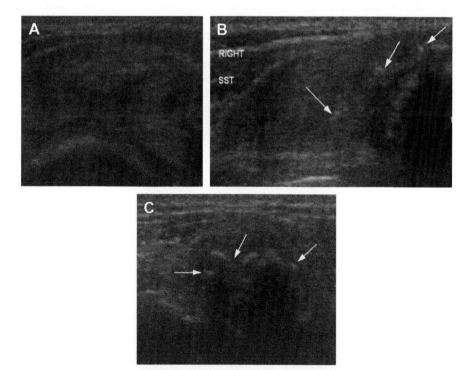

Fig. 10. Supraspinatus tendon (SST) proliferation with mottled tendon and fiber disruption (*A*); SST mineralization (*arrows*) (*B*); transverse axis of the SST with mineralization (*arrows*) with calcifying tendinopathy (*C*).

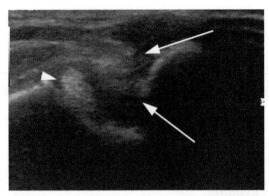

Fig. 11. Complete tear of the SST. Thickened joint capsule is seen (*arrows*) with a partial tear of the SST and displacement of the biceps tendon (BT) (*arrowhead*).

Biceps tendon injuries can either be primary or secondary.[12–14] An ultrasonographically normal biceps tendon with fluid accumulation surrounding it may be identified in cases of the supraspinatus tendinopathy and impingement or medial shoulder instability. Occasionally, the biceps tendon sheath will be thickened with hyperechoic tissue or hyperechoic fluid surrounding it, which is more common in biceps tenosynovitis. The biceps tendon can have mottled hypoechoic foci within the tendon as a result of this inflammation and degradation of the biceps tendon over a period of time (**Fig. 13**A). Dystrophic mineralization within the biceps tendon can also be seen. Biceps tendon tears can be identified with ultrasound and are generally classified as interstitial, partial, or complete tears. The interstitial tears will appear as focal hypoechoic areas with focal enlargement and deviation of the fibers. There is no disruption of the fibers with this type of tear. A partial tear of the tendon would appear similar to this with visualization of fiber disruption. Partial tendon tears can occur anywhere within the tendon, but are commonly seen at the origin (see **Fig. 13**B). A complete biceps tendon tear would be identified as a lack of visualization of the tendon in the biceps groove and can commonly be seen retracted in the distal aspect of the tendon sheath (see **Fig. 13**C).[5,11–13,15]

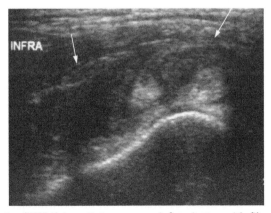

Fig. 12. Infraspinatus (INFRA) tear. Heterogenous infraspinatus with fiber loss (*arrows*).

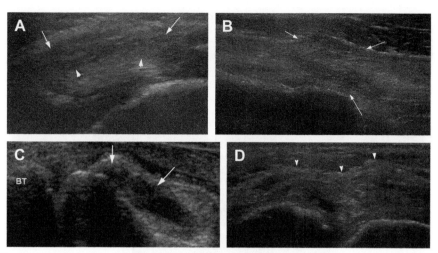

Fig. 13. Tenosynovitis with thickening of the tendon sheath (*arrows*). Biceps tendon (*arrowheads*) (*A*); partial tear of the biceps tendon (*arrows*) (*B*); complete tear of the biceps tendon with retraction distal within the sheath (*arrows*) (*C*); thickening of the joint capsule with undulation of the capsule during range of motion due to an adhesion (*arrowheads*) (*D*).

Adhesions of the biceps tendon to the tendon sheath or joint capsule can be identified as hyperechoic thickened areas, most commonly at the proximal margin of the tendon sheath and origin of the biceps tendon (see **Fig. 13**D). Dynamic ultrasound of the biceps tendon can be performed to evaluate for adhesions. A normal biceps tendon will glide in the opposite direction of the joint capsule/tendon sheath. With an adhesion, a hyperechoic tag may be identified between the joint capsule or tendon sheath and the biceps tendon surface or may appear as bunching of either the joint capsule or the biceps tendon as the forelimb is put through a range of motion.

The shoulder joint is occasionally evaluated for osteochondral defects. The humeral head is a convex hyperechoic curvilinear line with a thin hypoechoic layer representing cartilage (**Fig. 14**A). These osteochondral defects are most common within the caudal humeral head and will appear as irregular surfaces to the hyperechoic osseous margin (see **Fig. 14**B). Osteochondral flaps or joint mice can be identified within the joint space and appear as hyperechoic, usually flat-appearing structures within the caudal joint pouch or within the tendon sheath. Care should be taken to differentiate a free-floating or adherent flap from dystrophic mineralization, gas, or osseous fragments, such as avulsions of the tendon. Occasionally, an osteochondral flap can be identified with fluid dissecting between the cartilage flap and bone surface and will appear as a double or multiple hyperechoic linear surface (see **Fig. 14**C).[11,16–18]

STIFLE

Ultrasound of the stifle joint is a common procedure depending on the experience of the ultrasonographer. The structures of the stifle joint that can be identified include the patellar ligament and tendon, cranial joint space, including the infrapatellar fat pad, synovium and cranial cruciate ligament, and both the medial and the lateral menisci.[19–21] The patellar tendon and ligament injuries will appear similar to what is identified in the shoulder as hypoechoic areas within the tendon or ligament. The patellar ligament can appear as a thickened, hypoechoic area within the ligament

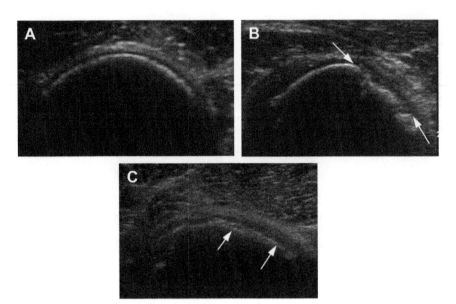

Fig. 14. Normal humeral head (A). Osteochondrosis with a defect in the caudal humeral head (arrows) (B). Osteochondritis dissecans with a double hyperechoic line representing the cartilage flap (arrows) (C).

and can be associated with hypertrophy secondary to change in biomechanical stress, desmitis, or partial tear, including interstitial. The hypertrophy and desmitis are similar in appearance ultrasonographically and can be differentiated by pain, which is associated with the desmitis. The hypertrophy of the patellar ligament will regress in 4 to 8 weeks, following a procedure that changes the biomechanical stresses of the patellar ligament (examples include tibial plateau leveling osteotomy or tibial tuberosity advancement).[22,23]

Partial tears of the patellar ligament can be identified with trauma with or without avulsions and occasionally are iatrogenic, usually associated with orthopedic implants inserted through the distal aspect of the ligament during surgical procedure.

The menisci can be identified with ultrasound as hyperechoic, triangular structures along the medial and lateral aspects of the joint (**Fig. 15**A). Because of the "C" shape of the meniscus, thorough evaluation of the cranial, central, and caudal portions of the menisci should be evaluated.[19–21] To completely evaluate the meniscus, the medial collateral ligament is identified ultrasonographically, which would be an anatomic landmark for the central aspect of the medial meniscus. To evaluate the cranial aspect of the meniscus, the transducer is placed cranial to the medial collateral ligament and angled slightly caudally to evaluate the cranial portion of the meniscal structure. To fully evaluate the caudal portion of the meniscus, the transducer is moved caudal to the collateral ligament and angled cranially to evaluate the caudal portion. The medial and caudal aspects of the meniscus are the most common locations of meniscal tears.

Four abnormal characteristics have been identified with ultrasound to diagnose meniscal abnormalities. These abnormal characteristics include (1) fluid accumulation surrounding the meniscus; (2) change in the meniscal echogenicity, mottled or hypo-echoic; (3) change in the meniscal shape (see **Fig. 15**B); and (4) displacement of the meniscus from its normal location (see **Fig. 15**C). Displacement is only identified when a displaced bucket handle tear of the meniscus is the cause.[24] The lateral

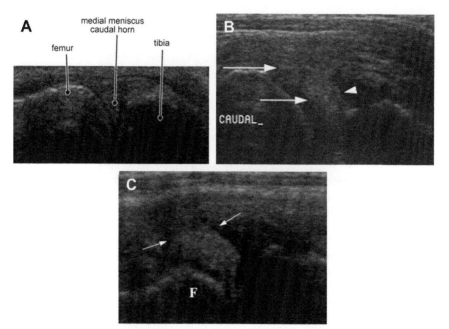

Fig. 15. Normal meniscus. The normal, triangular appearance of the medial meniscus with the surface at the level of the femoral and tibial cortex (*A*). Abnormal shape of the meniscus (*arrows*) with flattening of the tibial side of the triangular meniscus (*arrowhead*) (*B*). Bucket handle meniscal tear. Abaxial displacement of the meniscus (*arrows*) from the alignment of the femoral (F) and tibial cortical surface (*C*).

meniscus varies more in its ability to be visualized in individual patients. Often, the fibular head interferes with the visualization of the central and caudal portion of the lateral meniscus.

The cranial cruciate ligament is difficult to evaluate with ultrasound because the ligament is off axis to the surface of the joint, resulting in anisotropy and nonvisualization of the ligament margins and fibers. The distal insertion of the cruciate ligament can occasionally be identified as a hypoechoic structure with a hyperechoic surface, which is the connective tissue or periligamentous structure. Occasionally, a cruciate tear can be identified when the tear is at the distal aspect of the ligament and the ligament fibers are retracted. These tears will be identified as irregular soft tissue structures in the region of the cruciate attachment site as well as synovial thickening in chronic disease **(Fig. 16).**[19,25,26] Several ultrasonographers have attempted to increase the visualization of the cranial cruciate ligament by infusing fluid into the joint; this improved visualization of the cranial cruciate ligament, but was not considered a useful clinical tool.[27]

GASTROCNEMIUS

The common calcaneal tendon is considered the combination of 5 tendons (superficial digital flexor tendon, gastrocnemius, and the combined tendon of the semimembranosis, semitendinosis, and gracilis) inserting onto the calcaneus and distal extremity.[5,6,28] Injuries of the gastrocnemius can occur anywhere along the muscles or tendons, but commonly occur between the musculotendinous junction and insertion

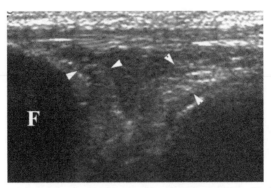

Fig. 16. Thickening of the synovium (*arrowheads*) within the cranial stifle joint secondary to a chronic cranial cruciate ligament rupture. F, femur.

to the calcaneus. During the ultrasound, careful evaluation of the region for concurrent superficial digital extensor tendon injuries is important. The superficial digital tendon proximally is deep to the other tendons and becomes the superficial tendon approximately at the distal diaphyseal level of the tibia. The superficial digital flexor tendon travels distal to the calcaneus with insertion sites at the lateral and medial surface of the tuber calcaneus and continues distally to the phalanges.[28]

Tendon ruptures are common injuries seen in veterinary medicine. These injuries may include lacerations or avulsion injuries. Degenerative injuries to the tendon can also be seen with diabetes or steroid administration, resulting in a variety of tears and dystrophic mineralization (**Fig. 17**).[14,29,30] Occasionally, luxation of the superficial digital flexor tendon can be seen with a retinacular tear (**Fig. 18**). A retinacular tear can be diagnosed on ultrasound because the superficial digital flexor tendon will commonly luxate from the groove as the normal transducer pressure is placed on the tendon.

As with the shoulder joint, ultrasound of tarsal osteochondral lesions can be identified, depending on the location of the lesion. Advanced imaging is typically not necessary, because osteochondral lesions are easily diagnosed with orthogonal radiographs and a skyline tarsal view. The irregular margins of the talus with hyperechoic synovial thickening and hypoechoic effusion are commonly identified in these cases.

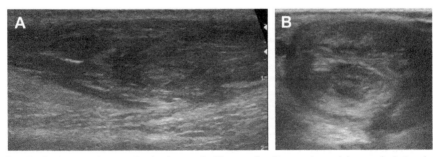

Fig. 17. Gastrocnemius tear in the long axis. The tendon is an enlarged, hypoechoic tendon with loss of normal fiber pattern (*A*). Gastrocnemius tendon tear in transverse axis. Focal hypoechoic defects within the enlarged, mottled tendon (*B*).

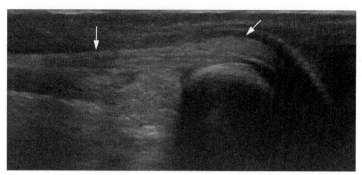

Fig. 18. Superficial digital flexor tendon (*arrows*) with effusion.

ILIOPSOAS/HIP

The iliopsoas musculature arises from the transverse processes of L2 and L3 ventral aspect of the L4 through 7 vertebral bodies. The iliopsoas muscle is a fusion of the psoas major and iliacus muscles. The iliacus muscle arises from the ventral surface of the ilium. The 2 combined muscles insert on the lesser trochanter of the femur **(Fig. 19**A).[9,31] The iliopsoas is commonly referred to as the "spring" of the pelvic limbs. Common causes of these injuries include slipping or splay leg injury to the pelvic limb, jumping out of a vehicle, or repetitive stress injury during training/working. The injuries to the iliopsoas are commonly seen at the musculotendinous junction and distal to the

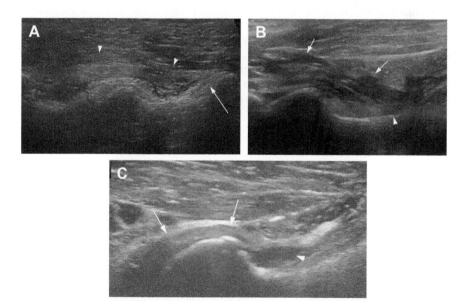

Fig. 19. Normal iliopsoas tendon (*arrowheads*). Arrow indicates insertion of the tendon (*A*). Thickened iliopsoas tendon with hypoechoic interdigitations (*arrows*) within the tendon representing partial tears proximal to the lesser trochanter (*arrowhead*) (*B*). The coxofemoral joint effusion (*arrowhead*) is identified with thickening of the joint capsule (*arrows*) and mild femoral head remodeling (*C*).

insertion on the lesser trochanter. Iliopsoas injuries are diagnosed with ultrasound as a thickened, hypoechoic tendon, usually between the musculotendinous junction and lesser trochanteric insertion.[32–34] There may be separation of the parallel fibers or partial to complete tendon fiber disruption (see **Fig. 19**B). Avulsions of the iliopsoas can also be identified with a mineralized fragment of the lesser trochanter and retraction of the tendon from its fragment bed.

The coxofemoral joint should concurrently be evaluated with the iliopsoas during the ultrasound procedure. Commonly increased volume of fluid within the coxofemoral joint is identified on ultrasound with or without thickening of the joint capsule and irregularities of the osseous margins. Ultrasound of the coxofemoral joint can be useful in the evaluation of hip laxity, osteoarthrosis, hip dysplasia, and avascular necrosis of the femoral head (see **Fig. 19**C).[35–37]

MISCELLANEOUS MUSCULOSKELETAL STRUCTURES

Diagnostic ultrasound of the elbow can be performed, depending on the caseload. Common abnormalities of the elbow include triceps tendon, biceps brachii insertional tendinopathy, and medial coronoid disease.[5,6] The triceps and biceps insertional injuries appear similar to other tendon injuries as hypoechoic, thickened tendons with disruption of fibers with or without avulsions, partial or complete. The medial coronoid disease can be identified as an irregular osseous surface of the medial coronoid, proliferation of the medial coronoid process, or a distinct fragment and fragment bed of the medial coronoid process. Secondary changes of the elbow can also be identified as an irregular osseous surface of the medial epicondyle as well as thickening of the soft tissue structures adjacent to the medial joint, collateral ligament, and anconeal process.[38–42]

Ultrasound of the carpal canal, which includes the digital flexor tendons and median nerve, has been described.[43] The tendon injuries appear similar to other tendinous injuries. Fluid accumulation within the tendon sheaths can be visualized as well as retinacular tears.

Ultrasound of other joints can also be performed with general guidelines for abnormalities, including thickening of the joint capsule; irregular, thickened, hyperechoic synovium; and increased joint fluid volume. Comparison to the contralateral limb is often performed in the joints that are not commonly imaged with ultrasound.

SUMMARY

Musculoskeletal diagnostic ultrasound is a useful modality to identifying both osseous and soft tissue injuries. Although the shoulder is the most common joint and tendon evaluated, almost any other joint or tendon can be imaged. The same characteristics of canine ultrasound would also apply to feline musculoskeletal ultrasound, although the structures would be smaller. Musculoskeletal ultrasound can be limited by the depth of the structure, overlying osseous structures, and experience of the ultrasonographer. The basics of ultrasound are the same, and just like anatomy is important in other areas of ultrasonography, it is critically important in musculoskeletal system. Also, knowledge of the common, and sometimes uncommon, musculoskeletal disorders is vital. Once the anatomy and knowledge of the disorders are learned, the procedures are easily performed, are quick and less expensive than other more expensive modalities, and also have the benefit of the ease of follow-up examinations, allowing assessment of healing and monitoring the injury during rehabilitation and following the patient's return to function.

REFERENCES

1. Crass JR, van de Vegte GL, Harkavy LA. Tendon echogenicity: ex vivo study. Radiology 1988;167:499–501.
2. Garcia T, Hornof WJ, Insana MF. On the ultrasound properties of tendon. Ultrasound Med Biol 2003;29:1787–97.
3. Jamadar DA, Jacobson JA, Caoili EM, et al. Musculoskeletal sonography technique: focused versus comprehensive evaluation. AJR Am J Roentgenol 2008; 190:5–9.
4. Kramer M, Gerwing M, Hach V, et al. Sonography of the musculoskeletal system in dogs and cats. Vet Radiol Ultrasound 1997;38:139–49.
5. Kramer M, d'Anjou M. Musculoskeletal system. In: Kramer M, d'Anjou M, editors. Atlas of small animal ultrasonography. Ames (MO): Blackwell Publishing; 2008. p. 465–510.
6. Zwingenberger A, Benigni L, Lamb CR. Musculoskeletal system. In: Mattoon JS, Nyland TG, editors. Small animal diagnostic ultrasound. 3rd edition. St Louis (MO): Elsevier Saunders; 2015. p. 517–40.
7. Giovagnorio F, Andreoli C, De Cicco M. The echographic and computed tomographic assessment of "spontaneous" hematomas of the abdominal wall. Radiol Med 1997;94(5):481–5.
8. Doyle AJ, Miller MV, French JG. Ultrasound of soft-tissue masses: pitfalls in interpretation. Australas Radiol 2000;44(3):462–4.
9. Hermanson JW. The muscular system. In: Evans HE, de Lahunta A, editors. Miller's anatomy of the dog. 4th edition. St Louis (MO): Elsevier Saunders; 2013. p. 185–280.
10. Samii VF, Long CD. Musculoskeletal system. In: Nyland TG, Mattoon JS, editors. Small animal diagnostic ultrasound. 2nd edition. Philadelphia: W. B. Saunders Co; 2002. p. 267–84.
11. Long CD, Nyland TG. Ultrasonographic evaluation of the canine shoulder. Vet Radiol Ultrasound 1999;40(4):372–9.
12. Canapp SO, Kirby K. Disorders of the canine forelimb: veterinary diagnosis and treatment. In: Zink MC, Van Dyke JB, editors. Canine sports medicine and rehabilitation. Ames (IA): Wiley-Blackwell; 2013. p. 223–49.
13. Kramer M, Gerwing M, Sheppard C, et al. Ultrasonography for the diagnosis of diseases of the tendon and tendon sheath of the biceps brachii muscle. Vet Surg 2001;30(1):64–71.
14. Rivers BJ, Walter PA, Kramek B, et al. Sonographic findings in canine common calcaneal tendon injury. Vet Comp Orthop Traumatol 1997;10:45–53.
15. Rivers B, Wallace L, Johnston GR. Biceps tenosynovitis in the dog: radiographic and sonographic findings. Vet Comp Orthop Traumatol 1992;5:51–7.
16. Wall CR, Cook CR, Cook JL. Diagnostic sensitivity of radiography, ultrasonography, and magnetic resonance imaging for detecting shoulder osteochondrosis/osteochondritis dissecans in dogs. Vet Radiol Ultrasound 2015;56(1):3–11.
17. Vandevelde B, Van Ryssen B, Saunders JH, et al. Comparison of the ultrasonographic appearance of osteochondrosis lesions in the canine shoulder with radiography, arthrography, and arthroscopy. Vet Radiol Ultrasound 2006;47(2): 174–84.
18. Piórek A, Adamiak Z. Ultrasonography of the canine shoulder joint and its pathological changes. Pol J Vet Sci 2010;13(1):193–200.
19. Reed AL, Payne JT, Constantinescu GM. Ultrasonographic anatomy of the normal canine stifle. Vet Radiol Ultrasound 1995;36:315–21.

20. Marino DJ, Loughin CA. Diagnostic imaging of the canine stifle: a review. Vet Surg 2010;39(3):284–95.
21. Kramer M, Stengel H, Gerwing M, et al. Sonography of the canine stifle. Vet Radiol Ultrasound 1999;40(3):282–93.
22. Mattern KL, Berry CR, Peck JN, et al. Radiographic and ultrasonographic evaluation of the patellar ligament following tibial plateau leveling osteotomy. Vet Radiol Ultrasound 2006;47(2):185–91.
23. Kühn K, Ohlerth S, Makara M, et al. Radiographic and ultrasonographic evaluation of the patellar ligament following tibial tuberosity advancement. Vet Radiol Ultrasound 2011;52(4):466–71.
24. Mahn MM, Cook JL, Cook CR, et al. Arthroscopic verification of ultrasonographic diagnosis of meniscal pathology in dogs. Vet Surg 2005;34(4):318–23.
25. Gnudi G, Bertoni G. Echographic examination of the stifle joint affected by cranial cruciate ligament rupture in the dog. Vet Radiol Ultrasound 2001;42(3):266–70.
26. Arnault F, Cauvin E, Viguier E, et al. Diagnostic value of ultrasonography to assess stifle lesions in dogs after cranial cruciate ligament rupture: 13 cases. Vet Comp Orthop Traumatol 2009;22(6):479–85.
27. Seong Y, Eom K, Lee H, et al. Ultrasonographic evaluation of cranial cruciate ligament rupture via dynamic intra-articular saline injection. Vet Radiol Ultrasound 2005;46(1):80–2.
28. Lamb CR, Duvernois A. Ultrasonographic anatomy of the normal canine calcaneal tendon. Vet Radiol Ultrasound 2005;46(4):326–30.
29. Kramer M, Gerwing M, Michele U, et al. Ultrasonographic examination of injuries to the Achilles tendon in dogs and cats. J Small Anim Pract 2001;42(11):531–5.
30. Caine A, Agthe P, Posch B, et al. Sonography of the soft tissue structures of the canine tarsus. Vet Radiol Ultrasound 2009;50(3):304–8.
31. Cannon MS, Puchalski SM. Ultrasonographic evaluation of normal canine iliopsoas muscle. Vet Radiol Ultrasound 2008;49(4):378–82.
32. Breur GJ, Blevins WE. Traumatic injury of the iliopsoas muscle in three dogs. J Am Vet Med Assoc 1997;210(11):1631–4.
33. Nielsen C, Pluhar GE. Diagnosis and treatment of hind limb muscle strain injuries in 22 dogs. Vet Comp Orthop Traumatol 2004;18:247–53.
34. Lotsikas PJ, Canapp SO, Dyce J, et al. Disorders of the pelvic limb: diagnosis and treatment. In: Zink MC, Van Dyke JB, editors. Canine sports medicine and rehabilitation. Ames (IA): Wiley-Blackwell; 2013. p. 267–95.
35. Greshake RJ, Ackerman N. Ultrasound evaluation of the coxofemoral joints of the canine neonate. Vet Radiol Ultrasound 1993;34:99–104.
36. Lonsdale R, Todhunter R, Yeager A, et al. Ultrasound assessment of femoral head epiphyseal mineralization and subluxation in labrador retrievers. Vet Radiol Ultrasound 1998;39:595.
37. O'Brien RT, Dueland RT, Adams WC, et al. Dynamic ultrasonographic measurement of passive coxofemoral joint laxity in puppies. J Am Anim Hosp Assoc 1997;33:275–81.
38. Knox VW, Sehgal CM, Wood AK. Correlation of ultrasonographic observations with anatomic features and radiography of the elbow joint in dogs. Am J Vet Res 2003;64:721–6.
39. Lamb C, Wong K. Ultrasonographic anatomy of the canine elbow. Vet Radiol Ultrasound 2005;46:319–25.
40. Seyrek-Intas D, Michele U, Tacke S, et al. Accuracy of ultrasonography in detecting fragmentation of the medial coronoid process in dogs. J Am Vet Med Assoc 2009;234(4):480–5.

41. Cook CR, Cook JL. Diagnostic imaging of canine elbow dysplasia: a review. Vet Surg 2009;38:144–53.
42. Michele U, Gerwing M, Kramer M, et al. Pathologic sonographical findings in the canine elbow. Vet Radiol Ultrasound 1999;40:559.
43. Turan E, Ozsunar Y, Yildirim IG. Ultrasonographic examination of the carpal canal in dogs. J Vet Sci 2009;10(1):77–80.

Computed Tomography of the Musculoskeletal System

Elizabeth A. Ballegeer, BS, DVM

KEYWORDS

- Computed tomography • Appendicular • Musculoskeletal • Shoulder • Hip
- Elbow • Foot

KEY POINTS

- Musculoskeletal computed tomography (CT) is mostly useful for diagnosing bony abnormalities, although with added contrast it may be sensitive for some soft tissue lesions.
- Musculoskeletal CT is much more sensitive than radiography for detecting abnormalities to areas superimposed on planar images.
- The ability of CT to obtain images and 3-dimensional (3D) reconstruction of the imaged part leads to a better understanding of the complexity and precise configuration of abnormalities.
- The scientific literature is focused primarily on the canine species and joint abnormalities. Brief synopses of what is available are presented.
- Imaging should always be interpreted with the patient's clinical presentation in mind; the contralateral limb often provides a good comparison for interpretation.

INTRODUCTION

Computed tomography (also known as CT or CaT scanning) is an imaging modality that is of increasing availability, usefulness, and ease of use for the modern-day veterinarian. What was once only available in veterinary referral institutions of higher learning is more commonplace. Briefly, CT uses the differential absorption of x-rays by tissues to mathematically create a 2-dimensional matrix with pixels of differing greys dependent upon that absorption, to give cross-sectional information about

The author has nothing to disclose.
Diagnostic Imaging, Department of Small Animal Clinical Sciences, College of Veterinary Medicine, Michigan State University, 736 Wilson Road, D211 Sm An Clin Sci, East Lansing, MI 48824, USA
E-mail address: ballegee@cvm.msu.edu

the third dimension of an object. Radiographs did and do project the information of all of the structures in an object, superimposed into a single planar image, and, therefore, decrease the conspicuity of each individual structure. By slicing through an object, this superimposition is removed, and the third dimension of data reconstructs a much more conspicuous image. This imaging has progressed from its first medical application in 1971 with long acquisition times and largely pixelated images,[1] to extraordinarily detailed small-pixeled matrices acquired in fractions of seconds.

Among the most impactful developments in CT were the invention of slip-ring technology, which allowed helical and not single-slice/axial (much slower) data acquisition, and multislice scanners, which allow acquisition of multiple rows of data simultaneously. The most recent developments involve software that facilitates further computational manipulations to the raw data, which allows reconstruction into 3-dimensional (3D) models capable of showing specific internal or surface structures, is able to be rotated or sliced as the operator desires, and can be modified experimentally to mimic traumatic and physiologic events, or operative procedures.[2,3]

The usefulness of CT for large body cavities and the axial skeleton is indisputable. Its rapid acquisition of images allows the ability to breath-hold or hyperventilate and respiratory pause for intrathoracic structures or cranial abdominal structures affected by the motion of respiration, the ability to obtain images from suboptimally positioned, perhaps unanesthetized or critically ill patients,[4,5] or those animals that will be subsequently continuing to very long surgical procedures under the same anesthetic event, and need the shortest time allocated to their imaging as possible. The radiation dose received by the patient is substantially greater with CT than radiography[6]; thus, in humans with greater life-time cumulative DNA damage from this ionizing radiation, the benefit must be weighed against the risk of possible carcinogenesis. The short life span and relative lack of procedures performed on veterinary patients makes this less of a concern, but should be taken into account if a patient is receiving repeated CT scans. Whole-body scanning protocols exist for small animal patients,[7] but as a screening tool are usually discouraged in humans.

For veterinary applications, the use of CT for the appendicular skeleton is still developing. The relative paucity of veterinary patients compared with human subjects indicates that caution must be used in interpreting the validity of fledgling techniques in studies, or may be loosely adapted from techniques in use for humans, requiring perhaps reduced skepticism. The published data presented in compiled form here are presented with these caveats in mind.

For ease of referencing, the appendicular skeleton will be divided into its component joints, first in an anatomic manner, then in terms of what has been done and what can be interpreted about that particular joint. The bulk of the literature presented regards canine patients, although a specific section is included regarding oncologic changes specifically, and both feline patients and applications not confined to a joint will occupy their own section.

General guidelines for performing musculoskeletal CT

- In general, CT requires minimal movement to avoid streaking artifact (**Fig. 1**). This blurs the margins of the image, reduces symmetry useful for interpretation, and is scanner/technique dependent. In other words, the patient only needs to be still for the amount of time it takes that body part to pass through the gantry. This may be achieved through general anesthesia, particularly if very unnatural positions or manipulations are needed to the body part, or may be achieved with a heavy sedative protocol that produces sufficient stillness, such as alpha-2 adrenergic agonists. This is, of course, dependent on the physiologic status of the

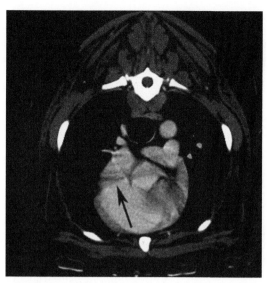

Fig. 1. The black lines radiating from surfaces/edges represent streaking from motion, most conspicuous where the black arrow is. Although this is a heart rather than a musculoskeletal structure, it is a common place to have this artifact, because cardiac motion can only be gated with acquisition of computed tomography scans, and not stopped.

patient. The part in question can usually be imaged again if the patient happens to move during acquisition, but at the cost of higher dose exposure.

- The long axis of the body part is best imaged along the Z-axis, or perpendicular to the gantry.[8] This reduces the cross-sectional area of the part the x-rays need to pass through, and also reduces streaking artifact that may occur when high attenuating parts, such as a long bone, are arranged parallel to the projecting ray. Whenever possible, additional high attenuating objects (eg, metal leads [**Fig. 2**], axial body cavities, the skull) should not be included at the same cross-sectional level in the gantry as the imaged body part.
- Intravenous iodinated contrast is not always necessary for musculoskeletal applications. Unless a vascular component to the soft tissues of the body part needs to be highlighted, such as with neoplasia, abscessation, suspected loss of vascularity, or specific vascular malformations, abnormalities to bones specifically do not require iodinated enhancement.
- As an alternative to intravenous contrast, consider contrast injected into draining tracts to explore their full extent (fistulogram). Small communications with important cavities such as joint spaces are much easier to interpret without the superimposition of radiography.
- Musculoskeletal imaging is usually detail oriented, thus lower pitch, higher mÅ, sometimes axial acquisition parameters are desirable. A reduction in signal-to-noise ratio occurs with thinner and smaller field of view slices, and so should be chose with the size of the patient in mind. The processing algorithm of reconstruction should be tailored to the desired results. Bone or high-pass filter algorithms produce a more edge-enhanced look to images, but can enhance artifact related to the "noise" of the image. Detail or low-pass filter algorithms may instead be used to better see contrast enhancement,[9] or take away the jaggedness of bone margins, as for a 3D reconstruction (**Fig. 3**).

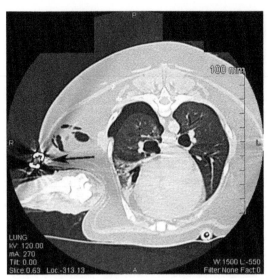

Fig. 2. Note the fluid line plastic control piece outside this imaged pneumothorax with significant streaking, enhanced by the lung window and level, adjacent to the body part, and depicted by the black arrow.

- Positioning aids are very useful for musculoskeletal imaging, but should be radiolucent (**Fig. 4**). Tape is also exceedingly useful during positioning of a sessile patient.

APPLICATIONS
Shoulder

Three-dimensional imaging is providing more information on the shoulder than was previously obtained with planar or surface imaging techniques. As expected, given

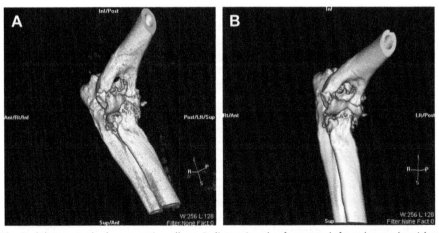

Fig. 3. (*A*) A severely degenerative elbow 3-dimensional reformatted, from bone algorithm processed data. Note the jaggedness and apparent discontinuity of the edges of the reconstruction. (*B*) The elbow, reformatted in a soft tissue algorithm, which tends to smooth edges rather than edge enhance, and does not enhance artifactual noise to the same degree. Ant, anterior; Inf, inferior; Lft, left; Post, posterior; Rt, right; Sup, superior.

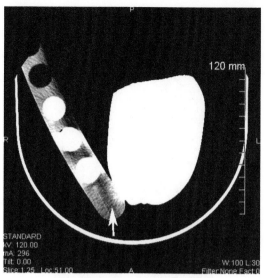

Fig. 4. A sandbag, viewed on soft tissue, and not a bone window. Note the defects in attenuation along its edge and edge of the adjacent phantom (*white arrow*).

CT remains based on differences in x-ray attenuation, which is in turn based on the physical properties of the tissues they pass through, it is best used to diagnose bony abnormalities. The bones of the shoulder articulate at the glenohumeral joint, which is a highly mobile, ball and socket, simple synovial joint. The articulating surfaces should have dense, smooth, and compact subchondral bone, with uniformly coarser underlying trabecular bone. It is important to recognize that significant abduction of the limb can be obtained at this joint,[10] especially under sedation or anesthesia, without disruption of the supporting soft tissues of the medial shoulder joint (**Fig. 5**), and that the clavicle lies medial to the greater tubercle and has variable amounts of mineralization and size extent, more so in cats than dogs (**Fig. 6**).

The positioning of the limb should also be taken into consideration, given that the resulting images are interpreted in planes slicing through the humerus and scapula. These slices may be able to be manipulated using reformatting, but depending on the user's viewing software, may be limited to the original and 2 direct orthogonal planes from the original conformation, and their relationship to each other cannot be manipulated. Mild controversy exists regarding imaging the shoulder in extended or flexed positioning, mostly with regard to MRI of the shoulder,[11] but arguably should be done consistently within the parameters of what the interpreter is used to seeing. Perpendicularity to the gantry is also strongly recommended to avoid the appearance of distortion.

When imaging the limbs for abnormality, it is often confusing to interpret changes to 1 limb or joint only. However, equally challenging is the ability to position the limbs perfectly straight and identically positioned within the gantry in a single view. For this reason, the author suggests positioning the limbs the same in pitch, roll, and yaw directions (**Fig. 7**), worrying about the Z direction later, which is the most difficult to achieve, and reformatting after acquisition so that the area of interest is the same for each limb. This may also be achieved by scanning with identical positioning of the

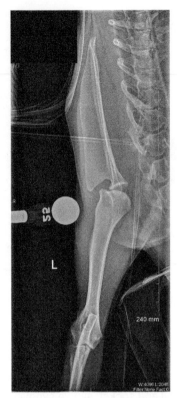

Fig. 5. Although this is a craniocaudally positioned radiograph and not a computed tomography scan, note the large amount of opening obtainable at the medial aspect of the glenohumeral joint in this normal shoulder. The large opaque ball next to it is used to calibrate measurements, used by the orthopedic surgeons.

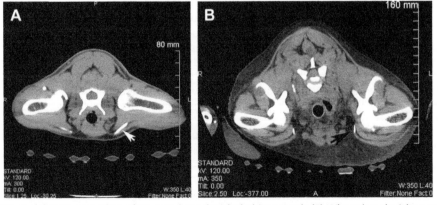

Fig. 6. (*A*) Transverse slice of a normal cat clavicle (*white arrow*). (*B*) When dog clavicles are seen, they are often small, linear structures (*black arrow*).

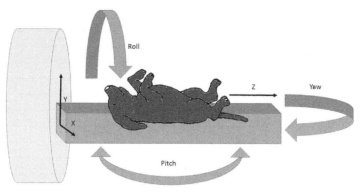

Fig. 7. A schematic representing a canine patient lying in dorsal recumbency on the computed tomography table, who will be moved in the Z-direction into and through the gantry, and the rotational directional terms of pitch, roll, and yaw applying to a horizontally positioned object, often used by pilots.

opposing limbs, in separate events. In either case, providing both limbs or joints for interpretation will make interpreting the study easier for the interpreter, and complete from an extent of disease characterization, for the patient.

Beginning developmentally, physeal closure times should be taken into consideration, mostly pertaining to possibly nondisplaced Salter–Harris type fractures through physeal planes, or delayed closure, which may point to a more systemic problem. There are 2 physes surrounding the glenohumeral joint, and their closure times are provided in **Table 1**,[12] for both dogs and cats.

Another developmental disease that usually has subtle subchondral and medullary bone changes is osteochondrosis (-itis), which may or may not have mineralization of a cartilage flap lending the term dissecans to the end, or osteochondral defect. This disease is a developmental failure of the enchondral ossification process, which leads secondarily to defects of articular surface including the cartilage, as well as subchondral bone. The bone surrounding the cartilage that has failed to mineralize often has additional sclerosis surrounding it, presumptively from inflammation and pressure from intervening joint fluid.[12] A retrospective study by Lande and colleagues[13] in 2014 described the prevalence of osteochondral defects of immature dogs receiving CT of the shoulder as 30% of shoulders in 41% of dogs. As expected, these were mostly osteochondral defect lesions located in the classic described location of the caudal humeral head, but they also described a 6-month-old Labrador with bilateral glenoid cavity defects. A surprising number of these immature dogs also had supraspinatus enthesopathy (4 pf 64 joints; **Fig. 8**), 3 without concurrent additional pathology.

There are a number of bony conditions described in the shoulder that have not specifically been characterized on CT. Congenitally, glenoid dysplasia with associated shoulder luxation is somewhat predisposed in toy breeds of dogs.[14] Another developmental condition that has been described as usually incidental, but possibly painful if the fragment is mobile, is incomplete ossification of the caudal glenoid cavity (**Fig. 9**). Rochat[15] has also described an emerging cause of shoulder lameness to be mineralization of the infraspinatus bursa, but has not described its imaged appearance in detail. Synovial osteochondromatosis, or synovial chondrometaplasia, has a classic radiographic appearance of multiple mineralized, rounded bodies within the joint space and is common in the shoulder, but again, has not been specifically described

Table 1
Dog and cat physeal closure times

Bone	Dog Range (Average)	Cat Range
Scapula		
Tuber scapulae	117–210 (186)	112
Humerus		
Proximal epiphysis	273–465 (375)	547–730
Medial to lateral condyle	187	98
Medial epicondyle	187–240 (216)	112–126
Radius		
Proximal epiphysis	136–330 (256)	196
Distal epiphysis	136–510 (318)	406–616
Ulna		
Olecranon tuber	161–450 (256)	266–364
Distal epiphysis	217–450 (308)	406–700
*Anconeal process	140–168	—
Carpus		
Intermediate	101	—
Radial	101	—
Central	110	—
Epiphysis of accessory	113–180 (135)	112–226
Metacarpus		
Proximal epiphysis of 1	145	—
Distal epiphyses of 2–5	165–240 (200)	203–280
Phalanges		
Prox		
Proximal epiphysis of 1	141	—
Proximal epiphyses of 2–5	131–224 (186)	126–154
Middle		
Proximal epiphyses of 2–5	131–224 (183)	112–140
Sesamoids	—	140
Os coxae		
Ilium	101–124 (112)	—
Ischium	101–124 (112)	—
Pubis	101–124 (112)	—
Acetabulum	101–124 (112)	—
Tuber ischii	292	—
Femur		
Femoral head	129–540 (320)	210–280
Greater trochanter	129–540 (320)	196–252
Lesser trochanter	129–360 (209)	238–308
Distal epiphysis	136–392 (330)	378–532
Tibia		
Condyles	143–413 (322)	350–532
Tibial tuberosity	143–435 (249)	350–532
Distal epiphysis	136–495 (313)	280–364
Medial malleolus	138	—

(continued on next page)

Table 1 (continued)		
Bone	**Dog Range (Average)**	**Cat Range**
Fibula		
Proximal epiphysis	136–360 (297)	378–504
Distal epiphysis	136–496 (288)	280–392
Tarsus		
Calcaneus	152–166 (159)	210–364
Third and fourth	101	—
Metatarsus		
Distal epiphyses of 2–5	165–270 (217)	224–308
Phalanges		
Prox		
Proximal epiphyses of 2–5	161–210 (187)	126–168
Middle		
Proximal epiphyses of 2–5	161–210 (187)	126–154

* Indicates that not all dog breeds have a physis in this location.

with CT. Less common mineralized conditions that may be able to be diagnosed from CT include metastatic calcification of soft tissues in general, resulting from an increased calcium phosphorus product, and chondrocalcinosis or "pseudogout," mineralization of the articular cartilage seen in racing Greyhounds.[14]

In the glenohumeral joint (or shoulder), the arguably most relevant and hard to diagnose significant changes are to the soft tissue supporting structures, although secondary changes to the periarticular bones or tissue dystrophic mineralization may be present to increase the inherent contrast of the tissues. If this mineralization is not present, it may be difficult to discern the soft tissue structures from one another.

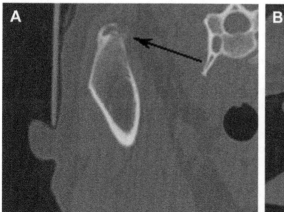
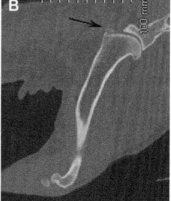

Fig. 8. Supraspinatus insertional enthesopathy in a dog, imaged in (A) dorsal and (B) sagittally reformatted planes. The black arrow depicts the irregular region of bony proliferation along the proximal aspect of the greater tubercle.

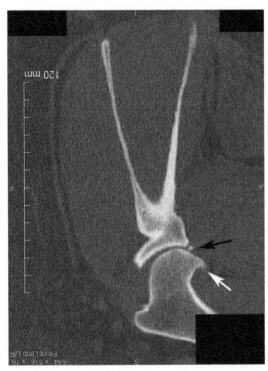

Fig. 9. A separate center of ossification along the caudal glenoid (*black arrow*) in patient with waxing and waning chronic lameness, although an osteophyte indicating osteoarthritis of the shoulder is also seen (*white arrow*), as is intertubercular groove proliferation from biceps tenosynovitis (*white asterisk*), making the significance of the lesion unknown.

However, the muscular structures have been anatomically described as conspicuous from one another on CT by da Silva and colleagues[16] in 2013. The addition of an extended limb position CT arthrogram, with injection of iodinated contrast at 60 to 80 mg I/mL concentrations aided in the identification of tendinous and ligamentous structures. The commonly affected soft tissue structures of the shoulder, in debatable order of decreasing commonality, are the biceps tendon, supraspinatus tendon, medial joint compartment instability including the medial glenohumeral "ligament" and the subscapularis tendon, infraspinatus tendon, and complete disruption of the joint capsule including lateral glenohumeral "ligament" disruption.[17] Again, the CT diagnosis of these conditions is often a result of mineralization (**Fig. 10**) or the addition of an aiding injected iodinated contrast. Brachial plexus or cervical nerve root abnormalities cause lameness and pain localized to the shoulder and can be highly debilitating, but unless a gross mass is present, may also be difficult to discern on CT, especially without contrast enhancement (**Fig. 11**).

Elbow

The overwhelming bulk of the literature available for small animal musculoskeletal CT pertains to the canine elbow joints, containing the humeroulnar and humeroradial joints. This is in part owing to the difficulty and lack of conspicuity in interpreting small superimposed bony structures on planar radiographs, such as the commonly affected medial coronoid process. The elbow consists of a composite, synovial hinge joint, in

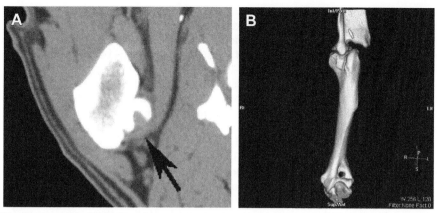

Fig. 10. An agility patient with severe mineralization in the intertubercular groove of the humerus from biceps tenosynovitis, almost resembling contrast injection into the tendon sheath during an arthrogram, in (A) dorsal plane, with black arrow denoting proliferation and the central divot of the tendon, and (B) 3-dimensional volume rendering. Ant, anterior; Inf, inferior; Lft, left; Post, posterior; Rt, right; Sup, superior.

which the humeroradial joint primarily functions to bear the weight of the thoracic limb, and the humeroulnar joint functions to escort the flexion and extension of the limb. A small amount of rotation (pronation and supination) of the antebrachium is achieved at the radioulnar joint, which plays a much lesser role in pathologic conditions of the elbow, although it is relevant to congruency or incongruency.

The humeral condyle consists of 2 portions, the aptly named capitulum on the lateral side, which articulates with the radial head, and the medial trochlea, which provides more of the hingelike portion of the joint, articulating at the ulnar notch. Pertaining to the already provided physeal closure information (see **Table 1**), the ossification of

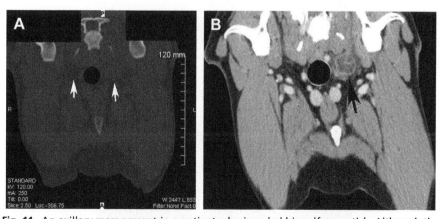

Fig. 11. An axillary mass present in a patient who impaled himself on a stick. Although the window and level are different, they are designed to simulate a window/level one may be using to look at images, and (A) noting the asymmetry of the soft tissues (*white arrows*), but they are not conspicuously different, until (B) contrast is given, causing rim enhancement of the abscess (*black arrow*), and the window and level are changed to maximize this conspicuity.

the 2 portions should occur at roughly 187 days (6 months) of age. A predisposition to humeral condylar fractures in Spaniel dogs led to the realization that this could be congenitally affected in these breeds. Incomplete ossification of the humeral condyle has been established as the formation of a fissure in the cartilage between these 2 portions (**Fig. 12**) that delays or precludes its normal ossification process, whether it be developmental[18,19] or a condylar stress fracture.[20] Although in small numbers this condition has been described in the Rottweiler[21] and Labrador Retrievers,[22] its preponderance is for Spaniel dogs. This was reported in 2012 by Moores and colleagues[19] because only 14% prevalent in 50 English Springer Spaniels at large, but 19 of 20 dogs in a retrospective study of incomplete ossification of the humeral condyle on CT were spaniels, mostly Springer Spaniels, but also a Cocker Spaniel and Cavalier King Charles Spaniel. Of dogs with the condition, 95% had it bilaterally. This in turn leads to condylar fractures obtained during times of no trauma or normal everyday levels of activity, usually lateral condyle/capitulum, or "Y" fractures, involving extension through both medial and lateral epicondylar bone to the supracondylar foramen.[12] Although a plausible correlation between this and medial coronoid process disease was not proposed in either study, both reported a high number of concurrence, at 26%[23] and 44%[19] of the elbows examined. This included fragmentation, fissures, osteophyte formation, hyperattenuation or hypoattenuation, or "irregular" shape in both studies.

Although indisputably important developmentally, incomplete ossification of the humeral condyle is not included as one of the disorders aggregated into the category of

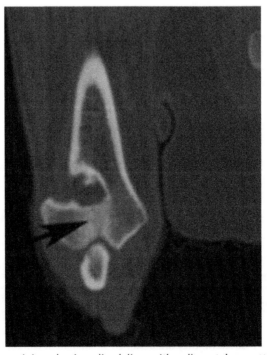

Fig. 12. A faint remaining demineralized line with adjacent hyperattenuation remains between the trochlea and the capitulum of the humeral condyle (*black arrow*) in this 9-year-old American Cocker Spaniel, who presented for a condylar fracture of the contralateral elbow.

elbow dysplasia, which as a broad classification is considered a developmental condition. Conditions included are ununited anconeal process, osteochondrosis (-itis) dissecans of the trochlea/medial portion of the humeral condyle, medial coronoid process disease, and elbow incongruity. Each of these conditions is best judged in different reconstruction planes, with medial coronoid process and radial incisure changes seen best in transverse plane, medial humeral condylar changes best in dorsal plane, and incongruity best in sagittal plane.[24]

Elbow dysplasia is long assumed to have a least a partial genetic link, and thus is undesirable for the purposes of breeding and progeny. Current screening programs for elbow dysplasia changes have been based on a very specific, although insensitive method of observing an extreme flexed lateral radiographic projection of the elbows, looking only for a bump of bone present on the cranioproximal aspect of the anconeal process to classify an elbow as dysplastic or not. This is undoubtedly a site where osteoproliferation occurs with osteoarthritis, and is more sensitively indicative of elbow dysplasia in conjunction with additional easily interpreted causes of elbow dysplasia, such as medial humeral condylar osteochondrosis, ununited anconeal process, or very obvious elbow incongruence, most accurately diagnosed on multiple orthogonal radiographic projections. It has been proven, however, that a certain subset of dogs has a normal anatomic variation bump (**Fig. 13**) in the region of the olecranon ligament and synovial attachments, in absence of other CT changes suggestive of elbow dysplasia.[25,26] This argues that those dogs with the bump but no lameness and no additional radiographic changes could benefit from being classified with additional CT or arthroscopic imaging.

The least described of dysplastic conditions on CT, perhaps because it is usually radiographically apparent on planar films, is an ununited anconeal process. Strangely, this secondary center of ossification only exists in some breeds of dog, with the majority being large breeds, and a predilection for lack of ossification within Labrador Retrievers, Rottweilers, and German Shepherd Dogs. The smallest breed described with this condition was the Pomeranian,[27] with the majority being over 30 lb in weight.[28] Similar to the fusion of the humeral condyle, the diagnosis of delayed closure can

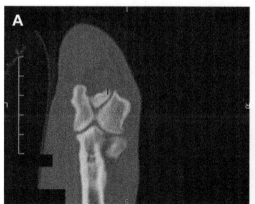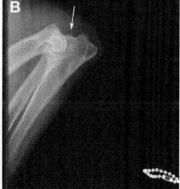

Fig. 13. (*A*) A dorsal reformatted image of a nonlame 3-year-old Golden Retriever with no additional changes noted in the elbow, and an asymmetrical bump (*black line* measuring its height) on the proximolateral surface of the anconeal process, which is (*B*) clearly visible on radiographs (*white arrow*), and would cause the Orthopedic Foundation for Animals to say she is dysplastic.

be made after 6 months of age,[29] although the appearance of a secondary center of ossification and ununited anconeal process was been described as more cranially located to the normal fissure seen with ununited anconeal process.[28] In 2012, Gasch and colleagues[29] described both complete and incomplete fissures (**Fig. 14**) of ununited anconeal process on CT, with cystic and hyperattenuating regions not expected in the regular ossification process. The disease was not always bilateral, in fact slightly more often (5 of 9 dogs) unilateral, but often associated with other classes of elbow dysplasia. In order of commonality these were medial coronoid process disease, medial humeral condylar "changes," including both erosions and osteochondrosis lesions, and radioulnar incongruency. These authors concluded that when a ununited anconeal process was visualized, the patient should receive a CT examination to fully classify these concurrent changes.

It is perhaps technically easiest to group both osteochondrosis of the trochlea/ medial portion of the humeral condyle and secondary cartilage erosions ("kissing" lesions) owing to fragmented medial coronoid process into a single group of erosions of the medial compartment of the elbow. This classification by Coppieters and colleagues[30] in 2015 approaches the full-thickness cartilage loss with subchondral bone exposure, as an endpoint problem rather than from an etiology standpoint, and has been further characterized as a more prevalent problem in dogs greater than 6 years of age.[31] It has been suggested these 2 subclassifications may be distinguishable from one another by the presence of subchondral hyperattenuation or hypoattenuation in adjacent bone surfaces of the adjacent radius or ulna in

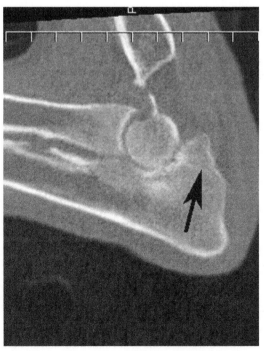

Fig. 14. The anconeal process is separated from the remaining proximal ulna by a faint linear lucency (*black arrow*) in this 6-year-old Newfoundland elbow. Note the highly irregular proximal surface of the process from degeneration.

osteochondrosis.[32,33] Regardless of etiology, however, CT is excellent at depiction of the subchondral bone changes of flattening or concavity at the articular surface and surrounding hyperattenuation (**Fig. 15**), owing to the soft tissue nature of cartilage and similarity of joint fluid attenuation; it is much worse at depicting just cartilage lesions. An arthroscopic study of medial humeral condylar osteochondrosis only obtained the final diagnosis from CT in 4 of 10 elbows.[34] In a study done on cadaver dogs, erosion of the cartilage was the only finding in 6 of 236 elbows,[35] which would normally not be visible with CT. The addition of contrast arthrography correlated the CT measured thickness of normal articular cartilage with histopathologic thickness well,[36] but did not delve into the realm of focal cartilage loss and its visualization as used for humans.[37] For this reason, and the correlation of poor prognosis with severe loss of articular cartilage, surgeons consider arthroscopy as the gold standard for diagnosis of cartilage lesions[30] rather than CT.

Medial coronoid process fragmentation is a definitive sign of elbow disease, that is, inarguable, and with at least a small degree of displacement, recognizable on CT (**Fig. 16**). This often happens in conjunction with the other causes of elbow dysplasia or pathology, or on its own with little additional changes.[38] What is less clear and confounds the interpretation of the published literature regarding CT, is the classification of additional "diseased" states. This includes fissures (see Pitfalls), hypoattenuating regions in the process (**Fig. 17**), abnormal shape (**Fig. 18**), and perhaps the least well-characterized hyperattenuating bone of the medulla of the process (**Fig. 19**) or the subtrochlear notch.

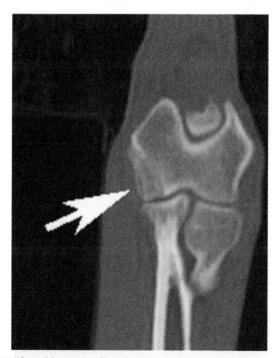

Fig. 15. Lucency with mild surrounding hyperattenuation (*white arrow*) in the medial portion of the humeral condyle (capitulum). This 7-year-old English Setter also had a fragmented medial coronoid process, making differentiation between osteochondrosis and an erosive "kissing" lesion difficult.

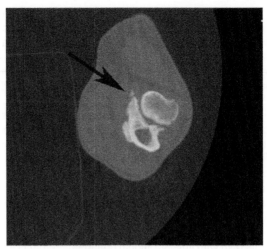

Fig. 16. A separate fragment (*black arrow*) is seen cranial to the body of the medial coronoid process on this transverse image of an elbow with significant surrounding hyperattenuation and osteophyte formation.

- Fissures are suspected to be nondisplaced fragments, but are often confounded by the addition of streaking artifact, artifactual noise of the reconstruction algorithm, orientation to the surrounding straight margins of the ulna, or a combination of the 3 (**Fig. 20**). Nevertheless, these are well-described in the literature, as narrow or faint lucent lines incompletely separating the medial coronoid process,

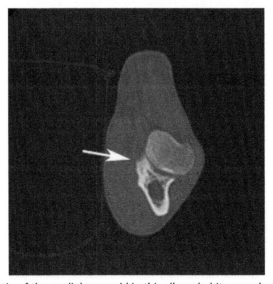

Fig. 17. Note the tip of the medial coronoid in this elbow (*white arrow*), which is hypoattenuating to the remaining process, and to normal bone. This is an area with chondromalacia-type change.

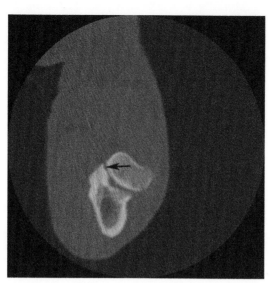

Fig. 18. This medial coronoid process tip has a divot (*black arrow*) at its radial articulation, leading it to look like a hook. The medial margin is also more undulating than most coronoids. This was a 5-year-old Rottweiler, and this same configuration was noted in another Rottweiler elbow.

in 43% of stable fissures that were observed at arthroscopy.[38] The possibility of these artifact and recognition of such as confounding, has led to a personal decrease in the use of this as an end diagnosis, as the level of experience of this author increases.

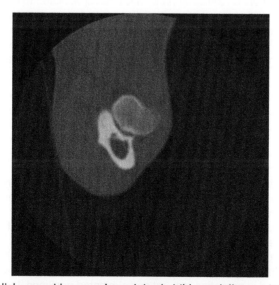

Fig. 19. This medial coronoid process has minimal visible medullary cavity, and has similar attenuation centrally as it does in the cortex. This Golden Retriever was 4 years old, and had no other signs of osteoarthritis in the elbow.

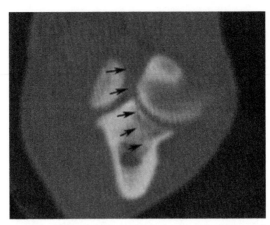

Fig. 20. A thin linear line continues in a sagittal plane across the proximal portion of this medial coronoid, but on close examination, the line continues into the tissues outside the bone as well (*black arrows*), identifying it as enhanced noise, and not a fissure. Sometimes it is not this obvious.

- Abnormal shape of the process has been described as a sign of diseased state,[25,38–40] but is less precisely defined. Blunting,[40] blurring,[39] misshapen,[38] and irregular margination[25] have all been used in the description.
- Hypoattenuation within the process bone itself is correlated to the presence of demineralized bone, similar to chondromalacia,[31] which may have a correlation to altered weight-bearing of the ulnar notch,[41] with[25] or without[42] the use of CT osteoabsorptiometry to normalize patient and scanner parameters. In each of these studies, those with medial coronoid process fragments had decreased significantly the attenuation of the coronoid process bone.
- Hyperattenuation, on the other hand, has been speculated to be associated with increasingly brittle bone that may predispose the process to fragmentation,[25,40] but is more often described in the subchondral bone of the trochlear notch.[38,39,41] Unfortunately, this area has also been proven to increase significantly in mineral density as a dog ages, unrelated to the disease status of the elbow.[43]

Elbow incongruity, particularly in its more mild degrees, has a controversial ability to be assessed with different CT manipulations, measurement methods, and variable threshold of diseased versus nondiseased state, based on the literature one refers to regarding this particular classification. It is reportedly highly influenced by positioning,[44] weight-loading,[45] presence of an arthroscope,[46] and the method of reconstruction.[47–49]

Earlier techniques of measuring incongruence involved either a dorsal, sagittal,[50] or obliqued sagittal reformatted image,[51] and measuring various distances between the radioulnar articulation at different levels[50] (**Fig. 21**), or the humeroulnar and humeroradial joints[51] (**Fig. 22**). These 2 techniques resulted in very different outcomes, with Gemmill and colleagues[52] concluding their method was correlated with fragmented medial coronoid processes and Kramer and associates[50] claiming it was not. However, when the limb was positioned in 135° of extension to simulate weight-bearing stance, and imaged in pronation, neutral and supinated positions, the House and colleagues[44] method measurements were highly inconsistent and varied from 38% to 505%. Additional loading to the limb by Burton and colleagues[45] suggested pronation

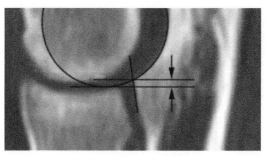

Fig. 21. Demonstration of the 2 measurements made by on sagittal reformatted images between the humeroradial and humeroulnar joint. (*From* Kramer A, Holsworth IG, Wisner ER, et al. Computed tomographic evaluation of canine radioulnar incongruence in vivo. Vet Surg 2006;35(1):27; with permission.)

occurs during weight loading, indicating this may be more appropriate for positioning during imaging. For the myriad of reasons listed, different techniques are being sought that vary less and are more reproducible in vivo.

Although the 3D reconstruction process may seem complex and limited to academic venues, many diagnostic imaging and communications in medicine (DICOM) imaging programs used to view CT studies are now including 3D reconstruction tools, including the open source–based OsiriX, but this requires hardware with high processing power and large amounts of RAM to create these reconstructions in a timely fashion.[53] These 3D models are also useful for gaining a better spatial understanding of rotational and angular limb deformities, common in the antebrachium, and creation of sterolithographic models (or 3D printing) that allow for preoperative manipulations of the limb,[54,55] or fitting orthopedic implants.[3] This printing technology is also decreasing in price and increasing in availability, currently ranging in price from $650 to $3000; however, it requires the input of spooled polymer material for object construction that is an added cost.

The last area within the literature of diagnostic importance within the elbow is the medial humeral epicondyle, in the region of the origin of the antebrachial flexor muscles. De Bakker and colleagues in Belgium have written multiple publications regarding this location, stating the changes to this surface can be concomitant with other elbow pathologies, but should not be confused with them. These authors maintain that primary flexor enthesopathy should be considered as a significant cause of lameness, although the diagnosis is based on positive findings in multiple imaging modalities such as radiography, ultrasonography, MRI, scintigraphy, and arthroscopy,[56–58] rather than more gold standard histopathologic changes. CT changes are described as irregular, cortically thickened or sclerotic epicondyle, thickened flexor muscles with variable contrast enhancement, and/or the presence of a separate mineral attenuating body adjacent to the epicondyle[56] (**Fig. 23**). It is believed that all the previous terms used to describe this condition, including ununited medial humeral epicondyle, osteochondrosis, separate center of ossification, traumatic avulsion, or dystrophic calcification of the flexor muscle origins, and a bony "spur" formed at the caudal aspect of the medial epicondyle are all part of this disease process.[57]

Carpus, Manus, and Pes

In contrast with the elbow, little is published regarding CT of the carpus. The carpus is a complex, multiarthrodal collection of cuboidal bones with a large number of

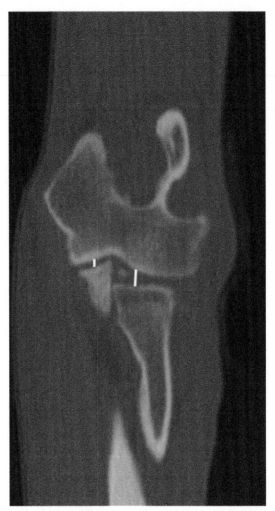

Fig. 22. A dorsally reformatted elbow of an 8-month-old Golden Retriever incongruent elbow measured in the style of Gemmill and colleagues.[52] Note the radius is too short, with secondary fragmentation of the coronoid, and a fragment seen in the humeroradial joint. The white lines represent the humeroulnar joint distance (*left*) and humeroradial joint distance (*right*).

intercarpal ligaments and communicating synovial joints. The joint is divided into surfaces of the antebrachiocarpal joint, middle carpal joint, carpometacarpal joint, and intercarpal joints. The carpus functions as a ginglymus, with flexion, extension, and a milder amount of lateral movement.[59] The antebrachiocarpal joint provides 70% of the motion of the carpus,[60] although the middle carpal joint contributes more of the remaining motion than the carpometacarpal joint. The joint capsule itself has palmar and dorsal thickenings that also provide support to the joint and are fused to the free surfaces of the bones. On the palmar surface, this is called the flexor retinaculum. The carpus does not have continuous collateral ligaments that span all of the carpal joints, but instead has short intercarpal and collateral ligaments spanning directly adjacent joints.[59]

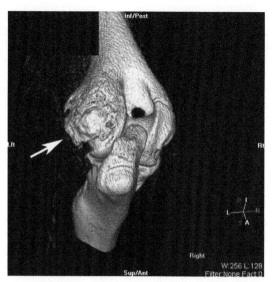

Fig. 23. The white arrow denotes a partially separate piece of bone at the medial humeral epicondyle, in a 7-year-old English Setter, as seen in a volume-rendered image from caudal. Note part of the jagged appearance originates from bone algorithm processed data for reconstruction. Ant, anterior; Inf, inferior; Lft, left; Post, posterior; Rt, right; Sup, superior.

The scope of this article does not allow for a full review of all these anatomic details, but the ability to discern all the separate surfaces and bones of the carpus on CT slices or reconstructions, instead of trying to interpret them superimposed over one another on radiographs, at various angles and with many superimposed Mach lines, is invaluable (**Fig. 24**). Fractures that require multiple specialized obliquities and skyline views are especially "easy" to discern, although reformatting in different

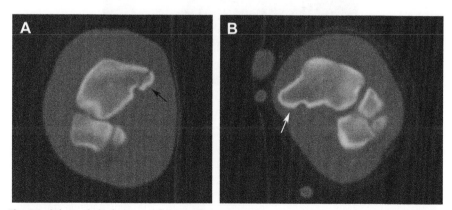

Fig. 24. (*A*) A subtle fracture of the radiointermediate carpal bone (*black arrow*) that had little chance of being imaged tangentially with radiographs, in a Bernese Mountain Dog who came in with a Monteggia fracture of the same limb. (*B*) The normal side is provided for comparison (*white arrow* pointing to process without fracture). This may not have changed therapy, but may have confounded surgeons when the dog remained slightly lame after its elbow fracture was fixed.

planes or the ability to 3D reconstruct the bones is a big part of this (**Fig. 25**). Again, imaging both carpi for an anatomic reference and individual variation is recommended. This usefulness and not the specifics of CT findings, was mentioned by Fitzpatrick[61] in his proceedings on the carpal and metacarpal injuries of working dogs, at the European Society of Veterinary Orthopedics and Traumatology in 2008. It must be noted, however, that the carpal hypertextension injuries, described by Fitzpatrick often require stressed radiographic projections that do not lend themselves well to the cross-sectional planes available for CT. Although the limb can be stressed and the patient reimaged, the slices generated may be highly confusing, because they cut through multiple normally adjacent structures in different planes. For laxity ligamentous and tendinous injuries specifically, therefore, CT changes on images obtained in a normal, axial plane would then need to be correlated with a very accurate orthopedic examination.

The manus and pes, other than the increased presence of the first digit on the forelimb and its high rate of variability, are very similar anatomically, thus will be addressed in the same section. Each metacarpophalangeal or metatarsophalangeal joint is a separate synovial entity with collateral ligaments, has a pair of palmar or plantar sesamoid connected by an intersesamoidean ligament, and to the metacarpals/tarsal and proximal phalanges by lateral, medial, and distal sesamoidean ligaments, and a smaller dorsal sesamoid associated with common (manus) or long (pes) digital extensor tendons. With the thought of spread of inflammation, infection, or neoplasia between soft tissue spaces and myofascial compartments, these were described by Ober and colleagues[62] in 2010 in the canine manus. By injecting a mixture of iodinated contrast and ink, 13 soft tissue compartments and 5 myofascial compartments were identified and interdigital spaces defined[63] (**Fig. 26**) that could assist in surgical

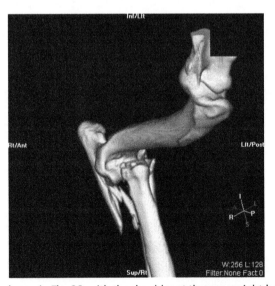

Fig. 25. The same dog as in **Fig. 26**, with the shoulder at the upper right-hand corner of the picture, and the antebrachium down. This is the comminuted, complex fracture of the elbow in a 3-dimensional volume rendering, which can be rotated, or the window and level changed so the surface soft tissues show. Some programs also allow the ability to make some soft tissues lucent while others retain their opacity. Ant, anterior; Inf, inferior; Lft, left; Post, posterior; Rt, right; Sup, superior.

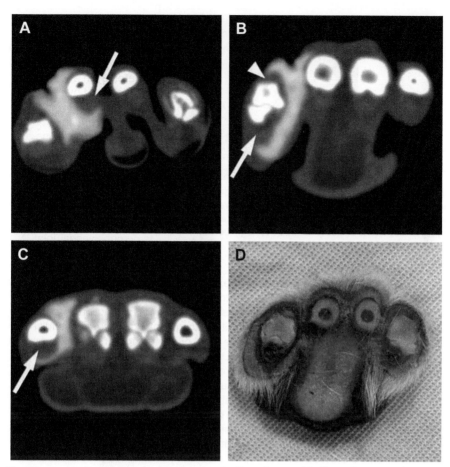

Fig. 26. A mixed injection of ink for anatomic dissection, and iodinated contrast for transverse computed tomography slices of the normal dog manus, showing contrast wrapping around deep digital flexor tendons (*white arrows*) and a long digital extensor tendon (*arrowhead*), to simulate planes in which infection may spread. (*A–D*) Different levels of cross-sections through the manus. (*From* Ober CP, Jones JC, Larson MM, et al. Modeling of the spread of infection in the interdigital spaces of the manus in limbs from clinically normal dogs. Am J Vet Res 2010;71(3):270; with permission.)

exploration and reduction of morbidity of such, and prediction of foreign body migration, or the aforementioned pathologic spread of disease. The pinnacle of these projects was identifying non–contrast-enhanced CT as the best imaging modality among ultrasonography, CT, and MRI to depict wooden foreign bodies, although slightly more hindered at the level of the metacarpal pad.[64] These were revealed mostly by the presence of gas within them, seen as a hypoattenuating linear or cylindrical structure (**Fig. 27**), although interpreting care should be taken if intrafascial air is also present, mimicking a foreign body.

Coxofemoral Joints

As could be predicted from the focus of most of the elbow literature, the vast majority of CT publications on the coxofemoral joint regard laxity or secondary changes from

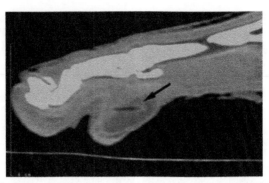

Fig. 27. A sagittally reformatted image of a dog manus with a wood foreign body (*black arrow*) in the metacarpal pad, seen as a thick-walled lucency. (*From* Ober CP, Jones JC, Larson MM, et al. Comparison of ultrasound, computed tomography, and magnetic resonance imaging in detection of acute wooden foreign bodies in the canine manus. Vet Radiol Ultrasound 2008;49(5):413; with permission.)

hip dysplasia, although a smaller number exist on other topics. The hip is a ball and socket synovial joint, with extensive study done on the anatomy, genetics, kinematics, and osteoarthritis of the joint. Not only does the bony structure of the acetabular cup and femoral head determine the functionality of the joint, but the numerous ligamentous structures, such as the ligament of the head of the femur, transverse acetabular ligament, and an accessory ligament within the acetabular notch,[65] as well as the joint capsule itself, have huge bearing on its ability to remain well-articulated. Again, because these latter structures are soft tissues, most of the imaging literature focuses on the bones, bone density, and measureable congruency of the joint.

Hip laxity is a quick measureable that can determine the phenotype, if not strictly the underlying genotype, of a young patient being considered for siring the next generation of individuals, or a working dog at the brink of his extensive training. As screening tests, in the United States the most widely accepted radiographic techniques are the hip-extended view with internal rotation of the stifles, and the Penn hip procedure, which qualitatively evaluates the degree of laxity during distraction, and the accuracy of fit on compression. Laxity is reported in terms of a distraction index (DI) and reported in the context of all other database individuals of the same breed as the imaged patient rather than a quantitative "normal" value. The DI is calculated by dividing the distance of the center of the femoral head to the center of the acetabular socket by the radius of the femoral head.[66] A number of different parameters other than the DI, such as the Norberg angle, were used to evaluate laxity on radiographs but are less universally accepted than the DI.

Initial CT techniques involved positioning patients in a simulated weight-bearing stance on their stifles, using a measureable termed dorsolateral subluxation, comparing it with the DI, and assessing that radiographs and CT are roughly similar and predictive of laxity,[67] but did not prove that the weight-bearing stance was better at assessing laxity than standard positioning. In fact, this was proven a poor predictor of hip dysplasia in 2009.[68] A plethora of other parameters are used on a number of CT studies of canine with hip dysplasia,[69,70] but all of these parameters are related to the radiographic parameter of the DI as a gold standard, rather than proving their worth as a superior method of measurement.

More with regard to acetabular shape than laxity, but also using the DI as a reference for CT, in 2010 Dueland and colleagues[71] determined that cautery fusion of the pubic symphysis before 17 weeks of age can increase acetabular ventroversion and decrease laxity in dogs identified at risk for hip dysplasia very early in life, with angles formed between both dorsal and ventral rims of the acetabulum (acetabular angle), and between the femoral neck and dorsal rim of the acetabulum (dorsal acetabular rim angle [DARA]; **Fig. 28**). Slightly earlier in 2005, however, it was determined the acetabular angle is affected significantly by pelvic tilt and selection of the slice on which to do the measurements, whereas the DARA is not affected. For this reason, it seems that the DARA is a better choice, with as consistent a pelvic tilt as can be accomplished, placing dogs in sternal recumbency in a trough, with legs extended and abducted, and a rolled towel placed under the abdomen.[8] Normal DARA angles are defined at less than 15%, with slightly increased angles (indicating "shallower" acetabulum) at 15% to 20%.[72] Because this measurement is performed more easily in cross-section than radiographs, which require a challenging radiographic projection,[73] this may be the usefulness of CT of the hips over the DI laxity measurement that can be obtained on radiographs.

The femoral head shape, volume, and mineral density with relation to hip dysplasia have received research attention as well. Most of these parameters apply to very young animals, and thus would need to be done as a very early screening test. A flattening of the capital physis in the perifoveal region at 32 weeks of age was positively correlated with subluxation with use of CT (**Fig. 29**), but not as early as 14 weeks,[74] to identify dogs at risk for cartilage damage, and to preemptively do corrective surgery such as triple pelvic osteotomy. Similarly, the same group proved the bone mineral density of these same hips with greater subluxation had a more laterally located density of higher magnitude than lesser subluxed hips. The use of these findings is slightly questionable, because the subluxation was seen at the same time as the flattening of change of mineralization—at 32 weeks—but was speculated owing to altered weight-bearing during chronic subluxation during development. The density was also proven to progress in concert with osteoarthritic changes to the joint as the patient aged.[75] Slightly more

A **B**

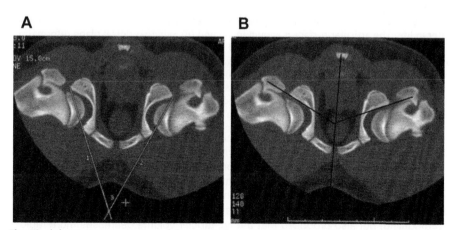

Fig. 28. (*A*) A transverse image of the pelvis demonstrating measuring the acetabular angle as the rims of both acetabulae and the angle where they intersect. This is significantly affected by position and slice selection. (*B*) The dorsal acetabular rim angle (DARA) calculation on the same image. However, the shape of the acetabulum should not be changed by positioning. The larger obtuse angle minus 90° equals the DARA. (*From* Dueland RT, Adams WM, Patricelli AJ, et al. Canine hip dysplasia treated by juvenile pubic symphysiodesis. Part I: 2 year results of computed tomography and distraction index. Vet Comp Orthop Traumatol 2010;23(5):307; with permission.)

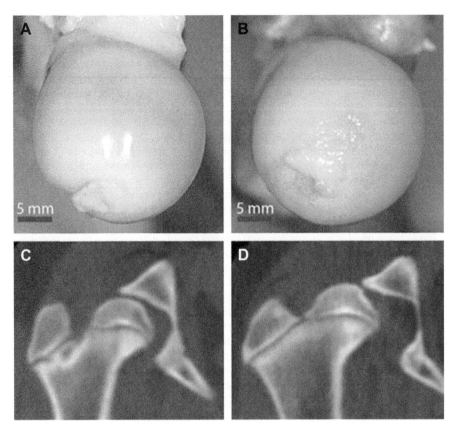

Fig. 29. Flattening of the perifoveal area of a patient of 32 weeks of age, either normal (*A*) and (*C*), or with a perifoveal flattening that correlated with subluxation and degeneration later in life, The articular surface is shown in (*A*) and (*B*), whereas dorsal plane reformatted computed tomography images are in (*C*) and (*D*). (*A* and *B*: *From* Vanden Berg-Foels WS, Todhunter RJ, Schwager SJ, et al. Effect of early postnatal body weight on femoral head ossification onset and hip osteoarthritis in a canine model of developmental dysplasia of the hip. Pediatr Res 2006;60:549–54; with permission. *C* and *D*: *From* Vanden Berg-Foels WS, Schwager SJ, Todhunter RJ, et al. Femoral head bone mineral density patterns may identify hips at risk of degeneration. Ann Biomed Eng 2011;39(1):76; with permission.)

useful as a predictor of disease was the significantly decreased bone mineral density in dogs younger than 14 weeks that later became more lax, although this parameter would require extensive mathematical computations to obtain these density scores.[76]

Somewhat intuitively, D'Amico and colleagues[77] proved that a ratio of femoral head volume within the acetabulum, when compared with either the femoral head or acetabular volume, decreased over time and with increasing osteoarthritis with CT 3D modeling, but also proposed that the acetabular volume decreases more rapidly in those hips with worse laxity, between 16 and 32 weeks of age.

More indirectly related to dysplasia and technically challenging is the assessment of total hip replacement with CT, owing to the high metal content of the majority of hip implants, and the resulting large, often obscuring metal artifact (see Pearls, Pitfalls, and Variants). Regardless of this artifact, CT has been used frequently in humans for assessing the presence of lysis surrounding implants that may indicate imminent implant failure, given that these implants have a life span much shorter than the life span of their patients, less of an issue in canine patients. Instead of taking implants out that have lytic lesions adjacent to them, they place a bone allograft in the lytic lesions, and thus buy more life for the implant. Identifying the lytic lesion as soon as possible becomes paramount, and CT with 2 applied algorithms designed to remove streaking artifact and enable volumetric measurements by segmenting and classifying images based on their statistical properties.[78] In 2009, Cook and colleagues[79] used this enhanced ability to see around metallic implants in dogs with periacetabular surgically created lesions used as a model for humans, determining the optimal ratio of bone allograft to bone morphogenic protein to inject and induce new bone generation in the periimplant gaps. Again, however, the practice of revising hip implants is less applicable in canine patients, the suppression of large metal artifacts is exceedingly useful in patients with implants and reassessment of healing or implant failure, regardless of location (**Fig. 30**).

Stifle

The majority of injury to the canine stifle involves soft tissue injury; thus, it should be expected that slightly less usefulness of CT in the stifle has been established. The stifle joint is another synovial joint, but is a condylar joint containing cartilaginous menisci, encompassing the femoropatellar joint, between the caudal aspect of the patella and the femoral trochlea, with the patella held in place by the patellar tendon. The 3 sacs of the canine stifle joint communicate freely, and encompass a complex of ligaments connecting the bones to one another, menisci to the bones and one another,[59] and are often involved in traumatic injury to the stifle.

Such huge morbidity and expenditure is involved with canine stifle disease, particularly with cranial cruciate ligament injury, CT morphometry has been used to try and predict those individuals that may damage their cranial cruciate. The tibial plateau angle and femoral anteversion angle were correlated most significantly with predisposition (unaffected limbs in patients with cruciate rupture in the contralateral stifle) for rupture in Labrador Retrievers, as compared with normal stifles,[80] and were further defined within the dogs with unilateral disease as steeper in the affected limb but not in the unaffected limb. This latter study also identified distal tibial torsion as a predisposing factor for disease, proving rotational deformity in either the proximal or distal portion of the tibia alters pressures on the ligament.[81] The steeper tibial plateau angle is the basis for two of the currently most used surgical procedures designed to alter this angle, the tibial plateau osteotomy and the tibial tuberosity advancement.

By again adding positive contrast to the joint, attempts to identify the more CT inconspicuous soft tissue injuries were attempted by multiple groups. Samii and colleagues[82] concluded in 2009 that the contrast, of the concentration 150 mg I/mL, injected to distension of the joint, aided in detection of cruciate ligament ruptures, but not meniscal tears. When this was further defined to surgically induced partial tears in Korea by Han and colleagues,[83] a cross-sectional area of the ligament significantly correlated with the damage. This may prove slightly more useful than the more obvious complete tears with a positive cranial drawer or tibial thrust on examination, and more obvious radiographic changes as compared with partial injuries, in reducing morbidity of unnecessary stifle surgery.

Patellar luxation is another common malady of the stifle joint. A tibial tuberosity hypoattenuating region was identified as a hyaline cartilage core on histopathology and significantly positively associated with medial patellar luxation in smaller, younger dogs as compared with those without the cartilage, and negatively correlated with cranial cruciate ligament disease[84] (**Fig. 31**). Parameters of the femoral trochlear deepness, laterality of the patellar tendon, patellar tendon length, and a parameter

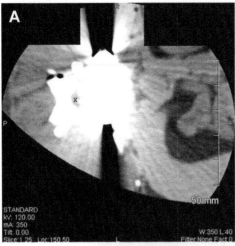
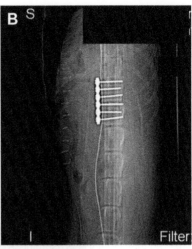
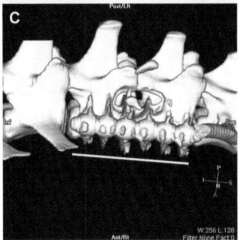

Fig. 30. A dog with destabilization after a spinal window was created in the laminae at surgery for debulking of an intramedullary tumor. (*A*) In a soft tissue window designed to see the spinal cord, note the adjacent metal causes effacement of all but a small area, denoted by the black *x*. (*B*) The scout is provided to show the actual configuration of the plate. (*C*) On volume rendering (3-dimensional) after artifact reduction. Note what the remaining artifact does to the shape of the plate for the span of the white line, but the bone window is visible adjacent to it, rather than effaced.

termed the quadriceps angle (**Fig. 32**) evaluated preoperative risk factors for medial patellar luxation, and also evaluated their improvement after the common surgical corrections of femoral trochleoplasty and tibial tuberosity transposition. This both validates the procedures as well as provides a means for predicting the postoperative recurrence of the luxation.[85] Lateral patellar luxation is not currently addressed in the literature, likely owing to decreased incidence, compared with medial.

Isolated case studies describing synovial osteochondromatosis in a stifle joint[86] and chronic long digital extensor tendon avulsion[87] provide reference for these particular, less common diseases of the stifle, although they do not differ significantly from their known radiographic appearances (**Fig. 33**).

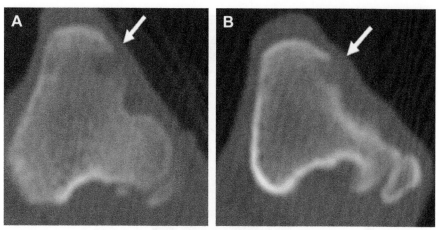

Fig. 31. (*A, B*) The white arrows depict 2 similar hypoattenuating areas in 2 different dogs, with islands of hyaline cartilage imaged on subsequently necropsied cadavers. These were positively correlated with medial patellar luxation, although most were small dogs, who were perhaps predisposed to that disease entity, anyway. (*From* Paek M, Engiles JB, Mai W. Prevalence, association with stifle conditions, and histopathologic characteristics of tibial tuberosity radiolucencies in dogs. Vet Radiol Ultrasound 2013;54(5):456; with permission.)

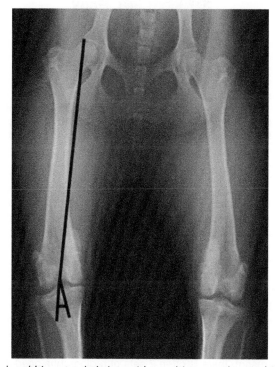

Fig. 32. A ventrodorsal hip extended view with quadriceps angle, an objective measure of the degree of femoral varus that may predispose a patient to medial patellar luxation demonstrated with crossing of femoral and tibial axes. Note the medial location of both patellae on this radiograph. (*From* Towle HA, Griffon DJ, Thomas MW, et al. Pre- and post-operative radiographic and computed tomographic evaluation of dogs with medial patellar luxation. Vet Surg 2005;34(3):267; with permission.)

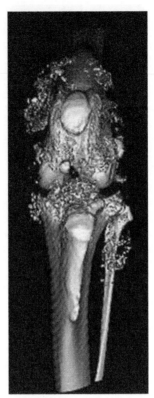

Fig. 33. A 3-dimensional volume rendering in a bone window provides a global look at the extent of multiple separate mineral bodies in the synovium, representative of synovial osteochrondromatosis. (*From* Smith TJ, Baltzer WI, Löhr C, et al. Primary synovial osteochon-dromatosis of the stifle in an English Mastiff. Vet Comp Orthop Traumatol 2012;25(2):162; with permission.)

The usefulness of CT for the stifle is likely minimal for cranial cruciate ligament disease, because the surgical intervention will likely be the same stemming from orthopedic examination and/or radiographs, but it may be warranted to evaluate predisposing factors for cruciate disease, medial patellar luxation, postoperative parameters of medial patellar luxation surgical procedures, as well as the more obvious and nonspecific usefulness for definition of complex or ill-defined fractures.

Although the tibia is a portion of both the stifle and tarsal joints, mention of a study of tibial torsion will be included here, as a measure of the degree of difference between the flexor and extensor planes of the stifle and tarsus in relation to each other, in a "roll" direction (see **Fig. 7**), or around the long axis of the crus. This is relevant for developmental abnormalities involving the tibia, which often provide extensive difficulty in obtaining radiographs that are straightly positioned at both joints. In cases where torsion is present, there is often 2 sets of radiographs needed, to tangentially project through each joint separately. By slicing through the tibia transversely in 2005, Aper and colleagues[88] identified the axes of proximal and distal aspects of the tibia, are were able to accurately measure the divergence between the two. This was performed on axial slices and proximal and distal axes based on anatomic landmarks, mostly related to the tibial condyles and the cranial and caudal surfaces of the distal tibia. This determined that measurement of these axes on CT is accurate compared with photographic measurement, but not try to establish a normal reference to compare to adult humans, who have an approximately 20% external tibial torsion.

Tarsus

The tarsus is similar to the carpus in its arrangement of multiple bones arranged in multiple joint rows, and a large number of connecting intertarsal ligaments. The joint is arranged in slightly less linear rows than the carpus, with the tarsocrural joint proximally, proximal and distal intertarsal joints (which does not traverse the fourth tarsal bone), and the tarsometatarsal joint, but also contains intertarsal joints. Also similar to the carpus, this allows for flexion, extension, and an even milder amount of lateral movement, 80% of which is located at the tarsocrural joint.[60] The trochlea of the talus interdigitates with the ridges of the cochlea of the distal tibia, and functions here as a hinge joint. Similar to the carpus joint capsule itself, it has dorsal and plantar surface thickenings that also provide support to the joint and are fused to the free surfaces of the bones, most notable in the hind limb at the extensor retinaculum. Lateral and collateral ligaments, in contrast with the carpus, have multiple components, some of which span multiple rows of tarsal bones.[59]

The 2 main points of pathology of the tarsus described in CT literature involve bony abnormalities as expected. The first of these chronologically in the life span of the dog is osteochrondrosis (-itis), which occurs most commonly in the trochlear ridges of the talus (**Fig. 34**). In a study of medial trochlear ridge lesions by Gielen and colleagues,[89] comparison of the size of lesions causing clinical lameness versus contralateral nonclinical lesions was significantly different, and associated with more joint thickening and osteoarthritis, as would be expected. Similar characteristics of articular surface defects, surrounding hyperattenuating bone of the talus, secondary osteophyte production, and soft tissue thickening to other osteochondrosis lesions were included, but no mention of the variably seen separate mineral attenuating bodies, representing

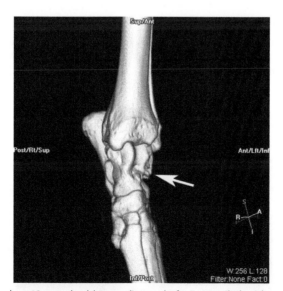

Fig. 34. Surprisingly, a 10-month-old Boxer (instead of a Rottweiler) with extensive subchondral bone erosions indicate of lateral trochlea ridge osteochondrosis (-itis), noted by the white arrow. Ant, anterior; Inf, inferior; Lft, left; Post, posterior; Rt, right; Sup, superior.

fragmented and ossified cartilage flaps. This same group did describe separate fragments, and quantified them in a study comparing the characteristics of lateral trochlear ridge osteochondrosis (-itis) seen more commonly in Rottweilers, versus medial trochlear ridge lesions. It was determined that not only do lateral trochlea ridge lesions get imaged earlier in life, they were significantly larger with a shorter duration of lameness before presentation.[90]

The second described bony abnormality regards a common racing injury seen Greyhound dogs, namely, central tarsal bone remodeling and subsequent fractures. Horses and human athletes also experience stress fractures of the cuboidal bones that undergo cyclical loading, although horses' lesions are more often within the third and radial carpal bones of the carpus.[91] Johnson and colleagues[92] described the remodeling in terms of bone mineral density obtained with CT in 2000, revealing increased density in the right (inside leg) central tarsal bones of Greyhounds that race counterclockwise as compared with the left (outside leg), that decreased with time after the dog retired from racing. This was taken further by Bergh and colleagues[93] in 2012 to describe that fractured central tarsal bones had significantly greater bone mineral density in the dorsal and midbody central tarsal bone, predisposing the bone to fracture owing to suggested increased brittleness, as compared with the nonfractured ones. Again, even although cartilage damage is associated significantly with these injuries,[91] specific disclaimer regarding this was presented by Johnson, because soft tissues defects are not optimal for CT techniques.[92]

The usefulness of CT for subtle or complex fracture of the tarsus remains the same as the carpus, where a large number of complex-shaped cuboidal bones and joint surfaces confound interpretation of linear lucencies on radiographs (**Fig. 35**). This complexity was stressed specifically in the feline tarsus by Benlloch-Gonzalez and colleagues,[2] because CT was particularly useful in selecting very narrow bone corridors (1.5–2 mm diameter and 15–18 mm length) for placement of screws for plate implants, relevant to both fractures or tarsal arthrodesis. These locations are demonstrated in **Fig. 36**.

Oncology Applications

Again, the focus of the literature regarding CT appearance of neoplasms is mostly centered on imaging the skeleton, rather than soft tissues. However, the inherent contrast of fatty-based tumors can make CT useful, and the addition of iodinated

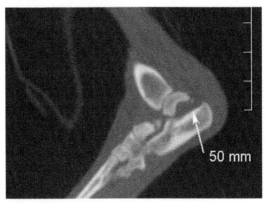

50 mm

Fig. 35. A small fracture of the caudal portion of the talus is a comminution likely to be missed on radiographs, in a sagittal reformatted view.

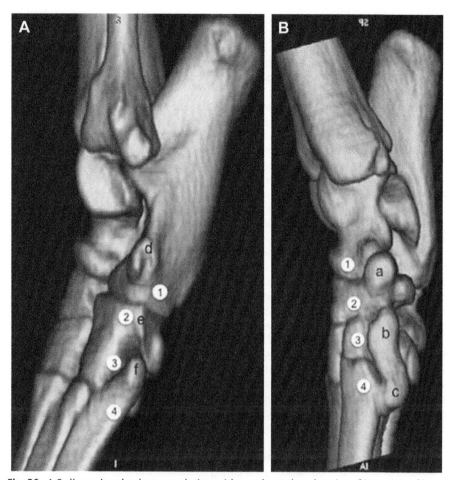

Fig. 36. A 3-dimensional volume rendering with numbers placed at site of insertion of bone screws (*A*) laterally; 1, talocalcaneal corridor; 2, centroquartal corridor; 3, distal tarsal corridor; 4, metatarsal corridor; d, peroneal tubercle of the calcaneus; e, tuberosity of fourth tarsal bone; f, plantarolateral ridge of metatarsal bone V, and (*B*) medially; 1, talocalcaneal corridor; 2, centroquartal corridor; 3, distal tarsal corridor; 4, metatarsal corridor; a, proximomedial process of the central tarsal bone; b, first tarsal bone; c, metatarsal bone I, in the tarsus of cats, as determined with "bone corridors" defined with computed tomography sections. (*From* Benlloch-Gonzalez M, Grapperon-Mathis M, Bouvy B. Computed tomography assisted determination of optimal insertion points and bone corridors for transverse implant placement in the feline tarsus and metatarsus. Vet Comp Orthop Traumatol 2014;27(6):444; with permission.)

contrast can make the inconspicuous or barely conspicuous soft tissue tumor visible, because of relative vascular changes, be they enhanced or a lack thereof, centrally. These vascular enhancing areas are often used to determine margins of soft tissue neoplasms for surgical planning, but need to incorporate considerations for inflammation associated either primarily with the tumor, or secondary to previous treatment.[94]

When reviewing the characteristics of primary bone tumors, the characteristics of osteosarcoma on CT do not vary significantly from those seen on radiography. Both lysis and hyperattenuating medullary regions are seen, as well as palisading periosteal reaction (perpendicular to the long axis of the bone), indistinct margins, cortical lysis, and long zones of transition from diseased to normal status. Other sarcomas within the bone cavity (chondrosarcoma, fibrosarcoma, hemangiosarcoma) do not differ significantly from osteosarcoma. Claims that CT is better than radiographs at distinguishing aggressive lesions between neoplasia and osteomyelitis are not discovered. However, CT becomes especially helpful in cases of parosteal osteosarcoma, in which subtle regions of cortical lysis adjacent to a tumor can help increase suspicion of malignancy, as opposed to benign juxtacortical tumors such as osteochondromas, or in their multifocal form, multiple cartilaginous exostoses, usually seen in young growing animals.[95] These neoplasms have the ability to transform into malignancies later in life, but more commonly in the cat than the dog.[96] Well-defined margins are the radiographic hallmark of more benign lesions.[97] However, malignancies that can have this appearance, such as multiple myeloma or lymphoma, or other benign tumors are not specifically described for CT appearance.

The accuracy of CT for determining osteosarcoma lesion size was undertaken with the intent of defining margins for limb-sparing excision surgery by Karnik and colleagues[98] in 2012. CT overestimated the extent of the tumor in the majority of cases, by a mean of 1.8% (SD 15%) either by assessing periosteal or intramedullary/endosteal proliferation, or by observing contrast enhancement. The best predictor in this series was intramedullary endosteal changes. However, 30% of the dogs were underestimated on CT, of up to 47.4%; the majority of these underestimations were based on contrast enhancement. When staging osteosarcomas with different modalities, Oblak and colleagues[7] proved that whole body CT was not as sensitive as bone scan with 99mTc-methylene diphosphonate, but detected more pulmonary metastatic lesions than thoracic radiographs (6 of 14 dogs negative on radiographs). It was hypothesized that whole body CT scans generate too many images for surveys, are often thicker slices with volume averaging, and thus both human and imaging error contribute to missing lesions.

Infiltrative lipomas have been characterized on CT, as well. The full extent of disease is difficult to determine on radiographs owing to summation that can be removed in CT, and has been determined to adequately identify margins for radiation therapy.[99] Specifically describing the characteristics of these tumors, most do not contrast enhance, most have well-defined margins, with a smaller number with ill-defined margins, all had evidence of muscular infiltration (**Fig. 37**), and many contact bony structures but do not affect them.[100]

Vignoli and colleagues[101] have published 2 differently focused articles on imaging of musculoskeletal tumors. In the first, the authors describe free-hand CT-guided biopsies of bone lesions, using contrast enhancement to choose viable sites without large vessels, receiving diagnostic samples in 100% of core biopsies, and 83.3% of fine needle aspirates. The second described muscular metastases, a site often not considered when staging. These metastatic lesions resembled generation from a single implanted cell as it does in other tissues (round to ovoid, well-demarcated), and were often located one the trunk of the body, in paraspinal muscles, thoracic wall, surrounding the scapula or shoulder, and abdominal wall muscles, although a small number had hindlimb metastases. With a rough split in commonality between sarcomas and carcinomas.[102] This was suggested to be owing to inappropriate environment for propagation of tumor cells within skeletal muscles owing to inappropriate local pH, contraction of muscles, or collection of muscular metabolites such as lactic acid.[103]

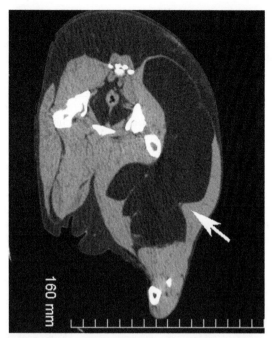

Fig. 37. A large lobular fat attenuating object (*white arrow*) has well-defined margins, but is definitively within a muscle belly, given its location directly adjacent to and wrapping around the femur, and identifying it as an intramuscular lipoma.

Feline Musculoskeletal Diseases

Although veterinarians are regularly taught and exposed to the fact that cats are not small dogs, there is a relative paucity of literature regarding cats, particularly as pertains to musculoskeletal CT. Anecdotally, there is a mild fear among imagers of the "lame cat," because it seems that radiographs do not often reflect changes expected to accompany lameness in canine patients. Particular attention to the literature regarding cats and conditions that may not occur frequently in dogs is provided.

Injection site–associated sarcomas have been well-documented in felines, and may be associated with a number of different injectates and nonabsorbable suture material that causes an aberrant response to a chronic inflammatory process.[104–107] Naturally, they have been singled out to describe on CT, but did not have specific distinguishing characteristics from other sarcomas. The "classic" sarcoma appearance that was also described in these masses is the linear peripheral extensions into surrounding musculature, but only defined as "frequently" seen, and abnormal fat was also noted around many of these masses, having linear or nodular hyperattenuating foci suggestive of the inciting inflammation.[108]

Benign calcifications of soft tissues can be in characteristic locations of cats, such as synovial osteochondromatosis[109] or multiple cartilaginous exostoses.[96] One such cat with a less prevalent disease process was described, with a disorder of fibrosis of and heterotopic bone formation within connective tissue, termed fibrodysplasia ossifican progressiva, characterized by linear islands of mineral along the spine, shoulders, and proximal limbs. It began with seborrheic dermatitis and alopecia, and progressed to gait abnormalities, stiffness, and an inability to jump. This condition has been described in slightly more cats than dogs, and is speculated be often misclassified as myositis ossificans[110] owing to sometimes intimate association of connective tissue and muscle (**Fig. 38**). Although this is not a malignant condition, its debilitating effects often create quality of life issues, and in humans it is linked to genetic mutations in the bone morphogenetic pathway.[111]

Other

This last section of this review focuses on CT reports not associated with any of the joints, or tumors. Three of these involve trauma to muscular structures, with 1 acute iliopsoas disruption with multiple intramuscular hypoattenuating areas,[112] 2 resulting in fibrotic myopathy of the iliopsoas[16] and tensor fascia lata. All were seen as abnormal enlargement of the muscle with heterogenous increased contrast enhancement, and the tensor fascia lata had additional mild mineralization.[113] Given the diffuse nature of all of these cases, myositis or partial tearing would be the top differentials, rather than a usually more focal neoplastic disease. Often, focal muscular enhancement must be deciphered with prior intramuscular injections taken into account, particularly at larger institutions where other individuals have been managing the patient (**Fig. 39**).

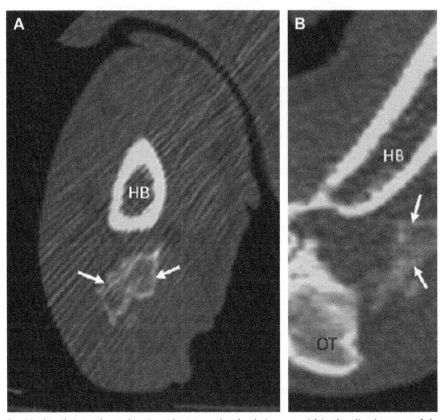

Fig. 38. (*A, B*) A moderately mineral attenuating body is seen within the distal aspect of the triceps musculature, denoted by white arrows, and not affecting the underlying bone. HB, humeral bone; OT, olecranon tuber. (*From* Tambella AM, Palumbo Piccionello A, Dini F, et al. Myositis ossificans circumscripta of the triceps muscle in a Rottweiler dog. Vet Comp Orthop Traumatol 2013;26(2):155; with permission.)

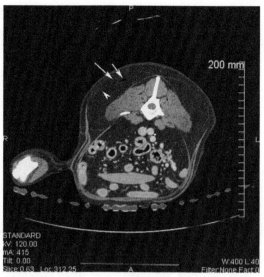

Fig. 39. Small foci of gas attenuation (*white arrows*) and mild contrast enhancement are noted (*arrowhead*) owing to previous subcutaneous injection for preanesthesia. This is a common finding and should not be confused with a wound, clinical steatitis, or possibly spread of a sarcoma, depending on its proximity.

This focal nature also applies to foreign bodies and their associated inflammation, abscess, gas, or regional lymphadenopathy. Grass awns, although regional in the United States and usually within the respiratory tract, can migrate to more distal locations in the paralumbar area, most notably the diaphragmatic crus tract to the third and fourth lumbar vertebrae, but also to the abdomen and pelvic limbs less commonly. In 54 cases described by Vansteenkiste and Lamb,[114] a seed or seed fragment was only seen in 10 cases (19%), but rather lesions seen on CT were the secondary change (52 of 54, or 96%). Depending on your area, grass awns may be a frequent offender migrating foreign body, but may only be on your list of differentials because of that, rather than based on visualization of the seed on CT images.

If a condition is suspected to involve a vascular component or the specific vessels in question need to be identified, angiography can easily make these highly conspicuous. Although this can be slightly challenging technically, it usually requires the use of a power injector to create a tight bolus of contrast and timing boluses to catch arterial and venous phases; however, it can create excellent vascular data that can have surrounding information subtracted through selection of high attenuating objects only for visualization, and can be manipulated in very diagnostic ways, especially on 3D reconstruction. This view is especially useful in the imaging of arteriovenous fistulae, which can be congenital or acquired, and often cause large hemorrhagic masses surrounding them. These fistulae often have nests of tiny capillary beds that can be highly confusing without the presence of contrast. This has been reported in the appendicular skeleton of dogs, cats, and horses,[115–118] but used 3D volume rendering in the forelimb of a cat with nonhealing ulcers of the front digits and acquired aberrant neovascularization[118] (**Fig. 40**).

Last, although diffuse idiopathic skeletal hyperostosis usually bridges at least 4 consecutive vertebral bodies along their ventral surface without associated intervertebral disc disease or osteoarthritis in the associated facet joints, it has been reported in

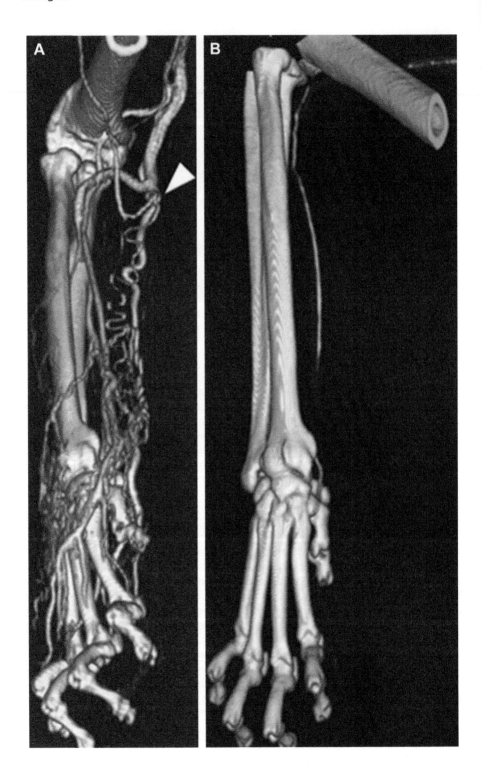

the appendicular skeleton. This was described on CT as multiple lamellar or trabecular bony proliferations at insertion sites of ligaments and tendons, and along long bones resembled variably thick periosteal lifting (**Fig. 41**).[119]

PEARLS, PITFALLS, AND VARIANTS

- Metal is highly attenuating to x-rays, causing the information reaching CT detectors encounters a metallic object to be flawed and inconsistent from different ray projections. This leads to streaking artifacts where the computer cannot resolve the inconsistencies (see **Figs. 1** and **30**). This makes recheck of conditions with orthopedic implants, which are often metallic and sometimes voluminous difficult, although specific computational manipulations of the data can be applied to minimize these artifacts; these manipulations not be available to all CT users.
- Very small differences in attenuation exist between soft tissues, making their conspicuity sometimes low when they are in contact with one another. In terms of Hounsfield units, the 2 ranges often overlap. Soft tissues that are vascularized can often be increased in attenuation with the addition of intravenous iodinated contrast material.
- With processing algorithms designed to enhance edges mathematically, this often make edges more jagged in 3D reconstructions, or enhances the effect of noise on an image, making the image seem to be grainy or striped. This can sometimes be mistaken for fissures in the medial coronoid process (see **Fig. 20**). For that reason, reconstruction in a "smoother" soft tissue algorithm may be more suitable for some applications.
- Remember the gravitational effects on fluid and organ shape owing to the recumbency of the patient. Some surgeons prefer the animal to be imaged as they will be placed on a surgery table to minimize these effects.
- Radiographs only detect a 30% to 50% change in bone mineral density when the lesion is greater than 2 cm in diameter[120] and CT detects 23% more lytic lesions than radiographs in humans with plasma cell tumors.[121] Remember that screening with radiographs has its merits associated with low risk and cost, but also large limitations. CT is more specific for the evaluation of early skeletal lesions.[17,20]
- Make sure to interpret all images with history and clinical relevance in mind; for instance, most chondrodystrophic animals have a degree of curvature and rotational abnormality of the antebrachium, but not all elbows are secondarily subluxated or degenerative, nor cause clinically significant lameness.

WHAT THE REFERRING VETERINARIAN NEEDS TO KNOW

- Being careful with positioning and technique up front will make interpretation of the received images easier and more accurate, especially if you are not the one

---

Fig. 40. (*A, B*) High-pass filter 3-dimensional rendering of a nonselective angiogram in the antebrachii of this cat revealed large anomalous, acquired arteriovenous fistulae, presumed neovascularization from a chronic bleeding wound on the dorsal manus in the right (but the left side of the image, *A*), with comparison normal left antebrachium (image on the right, *B*). The white arrowhead denotes the truncation of the cephalic vein, and suspected origin of anomalous vessels. (*From* Santoro D, Pease A, Linder KE, et al. Post-traumatic peripheral arteriovenous fistula manifesting as digital haemorrhages in a cat: diagnosis with contrast-enhanced 3D CT imaging. Vet Dermatol 2009;20(3):209; with permission.)

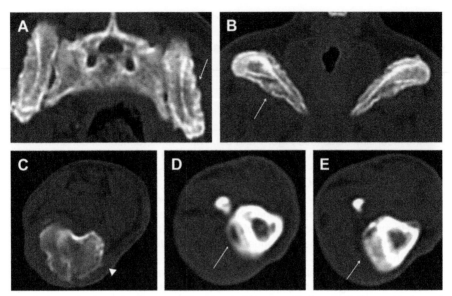

Fig. 41. Note the irregular bony proliferation (*white arrows*) along soft tissue attachments on the ilia (*A*), ischia (*B*), and multiple locations along the distal femur (*arrowhead; C*) and distal tibia (*arrows; D, E*), diagnosed as diffuse idiopathic skeletal hyperostosis (DISH). Vertebral proliferation was also noted, but not bridging as more classic definitions denote. (*From* Oh J, Lee JH, Cho KO, et al. Diffuse idiopathic skeletal hyperostosis with prominent appendicular bone proliferation in a dog. J Vet Med Sci 2015;77(4):495; with permission.)

interpreting. "Just sending the patient through" may give you nondiagnostic images, even in the case of such a forgiving modality as CT. There are of course cases when the condition of the patient precludes good positioning, such as a dyspneic cat. Specific positioning aids and publications have addressed this issue[122] (**Fig. 42**).

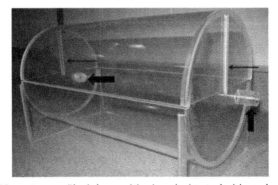

Fig. 42. The VetMousetrap, a Plexiglas positioning device to hold awake cats, yet be user friendly enough to allow for close monitoring, continued therapeutic, and a quick release. The 2 thin arrows denote access for catheters, and the thick arrows are ports for oxygen management. (*From* Oliveira CR, Ranallo FN, Pijanowski GJ, et al. The VetMousetrap: a device for computed tomographic imaging of the thorax of awake cats. Vet Radiol Ultrasound 2011;52(1):44; with permission.)

- Not all formats of digital images are created equal, or compatible with the software you or the individual you are sending the images to has. For that reason, human radiologists created the format DICOM, a format that does not digitally compress images, and is "universal" rather than proprietary for different digital image companies. This format requires special viewing software that is not often included in most computer software packages, but may be obtained free online (eg, Clear Canvas or OsiriX.)
- DICOM format does, however, take a large amount of memory for each image. Depending on the size of the part you are imaging, your slice thickness, and the number of images generated, the size of the entire study may be prohibitive to send electronically or record on portable media for clients.
- Different tissues are more conspicuous with different processing algorithms, and particularly with different window and level settings while viewing images. For instance, subtle contrast enhancement is confused by the noise in a bone processing algorithm, and best constructed with a soft tissue algorithm. Viewing a bone study on a wide lung window width and low level makes all the soft tissues and bones similar shades of gray and obstructing bony changes. Lungs cannot be seen on soft tissue window width and level, because the presence of air makes them all black.
- Cone beam CT has been made recently popular by veterinary vendors. Instead of fan-beam technology, x-rays are emitted from scanner x-rays tubes in a cone shape, creating huge amounts of data at once, that only modern computers are capable of handling. This decreases the cost of the scanner significantly and reduces the amount of radiation needed, but increases scan times, and increases scatter significantly, decreasing the resolution of the images by magnitudes, thus better at larger structures than small ones.

SUMMARY

CT of the musculoskeletal system can provide very detailed information about bony structures with very rapid acquisition, and with the addition of radiopaque contrast information about vascularity of soft tissues, but has specific parameters to interpretation of that information. As CT becomes more commonplace in larger veterinary institutions, there is no doubt the amount of CT data published in veterinary applications will increase, leading to more accurate acquisition methods and recognition of disease entities.

REFERENCES

1. Goldman LW. Principles of CT and CT technology. J Nucl Med Technol 2007; 35(3):115–28 [quiz: 129–30].
2. Benlloch-Gonzalez M, Grapperon-Mathis M, Bouvy B. Computed tomography assisted determination of optimal insertion points and bone corridors for transverse implant placement in the feline tarsus and metatarsus. Vet Comp Orthop Traumatol 2014;27(6):441–6.
3. Petazzoni M, Nicetto T. Rapid prototyping to design a customized locking plate for pancarpal arthrodesis in a giant breed dog. Vet Comp Orthop Traumatol 2014;27(1):85–9.
4. Stadler K, Hartman S, Matheson J, et al. Computed tomographic imaging of dogs with primary laryngeal or tracheal airway obstruction. Vet Radiol Ultrasound 2011;52(4):377–84.

5. Stadler K, O'Brien R. Computed tomography of nonanesthetized cats with upper airway obstruction. Vet Radiol Ultrasound 2013;54(3):231–6.

6. Strohm PC, Uhl M, Hauschild O, et al. What is the value of the whole body spiral CT in the primary radiological imaging of severely injured children? Z Orthop Unfall 2008;146(1):38–43 [in German].

7. Oblak ML, Boston SE, Woods JP, et al. Comparison of concurrent imaging modalities for staging of dogs with appendicular primary bone tumours. Vet Comp Oncol 2015;13(1):28–39.

8. Wang SI, Mathews KG, Robertson ID, et al. The effects of patient positioning and slice selection on canine acetabular angle assessment with computed tomography. Vet Radiol Ultrasound 2005;46(1):39–43.

9. Barnes JE. Characteristics and control of contrast in CT. Radiographics 1992; 12(4):825–37.

10. Cogar SM, Cook CR, Curry SL, et al. Prospective evaluation of techniques for differentiating shoulder pathology as a source of forelimb lameness in medium and large breed dogs. Vet Surg 2008;37(2):132–41.

11. Agnello KA, Puchalski SM, Wisner ER, et al. Effect of positioning, scan plane, and arthrography on visibility of periarticular canine shoulder soft tissue structures on magnetic resonance images. Vet Radiol Ultrasound 2008;49(6):529–39.

12. Newton CD, Nunamaker DM. Textbook of small animal orthopaedics. Philadelphia: Lippincott; 1985. p. 1140.

13. Lande R, Reese SL, Cuddy LC, et al. Prevalence of computed tomographic subchondral bone lesions in the scapulohumeral joint of 32 immature dogs with thoracic limb lameness. Vet Radiol Ultrasound 2014;55(1):23–8.

14. Kunkel KA, Rochat MC. A review of lameness attributable to the shoulder in the dog: part one. J Am Anim Hosp Assoc 2008;44(4):156–62.

15. Rochat MC. Emerging causes of canine lameness. Vet Clin North Am Small Anim Pract 2005;35(5):1233–9, vii.

16. da Silva YL, Costa RZ, Pinho KE, et al. Effects of iodinated contrast agent, xylocaine and gadolinium concentration on the signal emitted in magnetic resonance arthrography: a samples study. Radiol Bras 2015;48(2):69–73.

17. Kunkel KA, Rochat MC. A review of lameness attributable to the shoulder in the dog: part two. J Am Anim Hosp Assoc 2008;44(4):163–70.

18. Marcellin-Little DJ, DeYoung DJ, Ferris KK, et al. Incomplete ossification of the humeral condyle in spaniels. Vet Surg 1994;23(6):475–87.

19. Moores AP, Agthe P, Schaafsma IA. Prevalence of incomplete ossification of the humeral condyle and other abnormalities of the elbow in English Springer Spaniels. Vet Comp Orthop Traumatol 2012;25(3):211–6.

20. Butterworth SJ, Innes JF. Incomplete humeral condylar fractures in the dog. J Small Anim Pract 2001;42(8):394–8.

21. Rovesti GL, Flückiger M, Margini A, et al. Fragmented coronoid process and incomplete ossification of the humeral condyle in a Rottweiler. Vet Surg 1998; 27(4):354–7.

22. Robin D, Marcellin-Little DJ. Incomplete ossification of the humeral condyle in two Labrador retrievers. J Small Anim Pract 2001;42(5):231–4.

23. Carrera I, Hammond GJ, Sullivan M. Computed tomographic features of incomplete ossification of the canine humeral condyle. Vet Surg 2008;37(3):226–31.

24. Tromblee TC, Jones JC, Bahr AM, et al. Effect of computed tomography display window and image plane on diagnostic certainty for characteristics of dysplastic elbow joints in dogs. Am J Vet Res 2007;68(8):858–71.

25. Kunst CM, Pease AP, Nelson NC, et al. Computed tomographic identification of dysplasia and progression of osteoarthritis in dog elbows previously assigned OFA grades 0 and 1. Vet Radiol Ultrasound 2014;55(5):511–20.
26. Lappalainen AK, Mölsä S, Liman A, et al. Evaluation of accuracy of the Finnish elbow dysplasia screening protocol in Labrador retrievers. J Small Anim Pract 2013;54(4):195–200.
27. LaFond E, Breur GJ, Austin CC. Breed susceptibility for developmental orthopedic diseases in dogs. J Am Anim Hosp Assoc 2002;38(5):467–77.
28. Frazho JK, Graham J, Peck JN, et al. Radiographic evaluation of the anconeal process in skeletally immature dogs. Vet Surg 2010;39(7):829–32.
29. Gasch EG, Labruyere JJ, Bardet JF. Computed tomography of ununited anconeal process in the dog. Vet Comp Orthop Traumatol 2012;25(6):498–505.
30. Coppieters E, Gielen I, Verhoeven G, et al. Erosion of the medial compartment of the canine elbow: occurrence, diagnosis and currently available treatment options. Vet Comp Orthop Traumatol 2015;28(1):9–18.
31. Vermote KA, Bergenhuyzen AL, Gielen I, et al. Elbow lameness in dogs of six years and older: arthroscopic and imaging findings of medial coronoid disease in 51 dogs. Vet Comp Orthop Traumatol 2010;23(1):43–50.
32. Hornof WJ, Wind AP, Wallack ST, et al. Canine elbow dysplasia. The early radiographic detection of fragmentation of the coronoid process. Vet Clin North Am Small Anim Pract 2000;30(2):257–66, v.
33. Meyer-Lindenberg A, Fehr M, Nolte I. Co-existence of ununited anconeal process and fragmented medial coronoid process of the ulna in the dog. J Small Anim Pract 2006;47(2):61–5.
34. Quinn R, Preston C. Arthroscopic assessment of osteochondrosis of the medial humeral condyle treated with debridement and sliding humeral osteotomy. Vet Surg 2014;43(7):814–8.
35. Grondalen J, Grondalen T. Arthrosis in the elbow joint of young rapidly growing dogs. V. A pathoanatomical investigation. Nord Vet Med 1981;33(1):1–16.
36. Gendler A, Keuler NS, Schaefer SL. Computed tomographic arthrography of the normal canine elbow. Vet Radiol Ultrasound 2015;56(2):144–52.
37. Waldt S, Bruegel M, Ganter K, et al. Comparison of multislice CT arthrography and MR arthrography for the detection of articular cartilage lesions of the elbow. Eur Radiol 2005;15(4):784–91.
38. Groth AM, Benigni L, Moores AP, et al. Spectrum of computed tomographic findings in 58 canine elbows with fragmentation of the medial coronoid process. J Small Anim Pract 2009;50(1):15–22.
39. Lappalainen AK, Mölsä S, Liman A, et al. Radiographic and computed tomography findings in Belgian shepherd dogs with mild elbow dysplasia. Vet Radiol Ultrasound 2009;50(4):364–9.
40. Reichle JK, Park RD, Bahr AM. Computed tomographic findings of dogs with cubital joint lameness. Vet Radiol Ultrasound 2000;41(2):125–30.
41. Krotscheck U, Böttcher PB, Thompson MS, et al. Cubital subchondral joint space width and CT osteoabsorptiometry in dogs with and without fragmented medial coronoid process. Vet Surg 2014;43(3):330–8.
42. Phillips A, Burton NJ, Warren-Smith CM, et al. Topographic bone density of the radius and ulna in Greyhounds and Labrador Retrievers with and without medial coronoid process disease. Vet Surg 2015;44(2):180–90.
43. Dickomeit MJ, Böttcher P, Hecht S, et al. Topographic and age-dependent distribution of subchondral bone density in the elbow joints of clinically normal dogs. Am J Vet Res 2011;72(4):491–9.

44. House MR, Marino DJ, Lesser ML. Effect of limb position on elbow congruity with CT evaluation. Vet Surg 2009;38(2):154–60.

45. Burton NJ, Warren-Smith CM, Roper DP, et al. CT assessment of the influence of dynamic loading on physiological incongruency of the canine elbow. J Small Anim Pract 2013;54(6):291–8.

46. Skinner OT, Warren-Smith CM, Burton NJ, et al. Computed tomographic evaluation of elbow congruity during arthroscopy in a canine cadaveric model. Vet Comp Orthop Traumatol 2015;28(1):19–24.

47. Eljack H, Werner H, Bottcher P. Sensitivity and specificity of 3D models of the radioulnar joint cup in combination with a sphere fitted to the ulnar trochlear notch for estimation of radioulnar incongruence in vitro. Vet Surg 2013;42(4): 365–70.

48. Holsworth IG, Wisner ER, Scherrer WE, et al. Accuracy of computerized tomographic evaluation of canine radio-ulnar incongruence in vitro. Vet Surg 2005; 34(2):108–13.

49. Worth AJ, Bridges JP, Jones G. Reduction in the incidence of elbow dysplasia in four breeds of dog as measured by the New Zealand Veterinary Association scoring scheme. N Z Vet J 2010;58(4):190–5.

50. Kramer A, Holsworth IG, Wisner ER, et al. Computed tomographic evaluation of canine radioulnar incongruence in vivo. Vet Surg 2006;35(1):24–9.

51. Gemmill TJ, Hammond G, Mellor D, et al. Use of reconstructed computed tomography for the assessment of joint spaces in the canine elbow. J Small Anim Pract 2006;47(2):66–74.

52. Gemmill TJ, Mellor DJ, Clements DN, et al. Evaluation of elbow incongruency using reconstructed CT in dogs suffering fragmented coronoid process. J Small Anim Pract 2005;46(7):327–33.

53. Wikibooks. Online OsiriX Documentation/Making OsiriX run faster. Available at: https://en.wikibooks.org/wiki/Online_OsiriX_Documentation/Making_OsiriX_run_faster. Accessed September 18, 2015.

54. Crosse KR, Worth AJ. Computer-assisted surgical correction of an antebrachial deformity in a dog. Vet Comp Orthop Traumatol 2010;23(5):354–61.

55. Dismukes DI, Fox DB, Tomlinson JL, et al. Use of radiographic measures and three-dimensional computed tomography imaging in surgical correction of an antebrachial deformity in a dog. J Am Vet Med Assoc 2008;232(1):68–73.

56. de Bakker E, Gielen I, van Caelenberg A, et al. Computed tomography of canine elbow joints affected by primary and concomitant flexor enthesopathy. Vet Radiol Ultrasound 2014;55(1):45–55.

57. de Bakker E, Samoy Y, Gielen I, et al. Medial humeral epicondylar lesions in the canine elbow. A review of the literature. Vet Comp Orthop Traumatol 2011;24(1): 9–17.

58. de Bakker E, Saunders J, Gielen I, et al. Radiographic findings of the medial humeral epicondyle in 200 canine elbow joints. Vet Comp Orthop Traumatol 2012; 25(5):359–65.

59. Evans HE, Miller ME. Miller's anatomy of the dog. 4th edition. St Louis (MO): Elsevier; 2013. p. 850.

60. Jaeger GH, Canapp SOJ. Carpal and tarsal injuries, in clean run. South Hadley (MA): Clean Run Productions; 2008. p. 74–6.

61. Fitzpatrick N. Carpal and Metacarpal injuries in working dogs - Misdiagnosis or Surgical candidate. Proceedings of the European Society of Veterinary Orthopaedics and Traumatology Congress 2008;14:78–82.

62. Ober CP, Jones JC, Larson MM, et al. Computed tomographic and cross-sectional anatomic characterization of myofascial compartments and soft tissue spaces in the manus in cadavers of dogs without forelimb disease. Am J Vet Res 2010;71(2):138–49.

63. Ober CP, Jones JC, Larson MM, et al. Modeling of the spread of infection in the interdigital spaces of the manus in limbs from clinically normal dogs. Am J Vet Res 2010;71(3):268–74.

64. Ober CP, Jones JC, Larson MM, et al. Comparison of ultrasound, computed tomography, and magnetic resonance imaging in detection of acute wooden foreign bodies in the canine manus. Vet Radiol Ultrasound 2008;49(5):411–8.

65. Casteleyn C, den Ouden I, Coopman F, et al. The ligaments of the canine hip joint revisited. Anat Histol Embryol 2015;44(6):433–40.

66. PennHip. PennHIP hip improvement program. Available at: http://info.antechimagingservices.com/pennhip/navigation/general/what-is-PennHIP.html. Accessed September 18, 2015.

67. Farese JP, Todhunter RJ, Lust G, et al. Dorsolateral subluxation of hip joints in dogs measured in a weight-bearing position with radiography and computed tomography. Vet Surg 1998;27(5):393–405.

68. Ginja MM, Ferreira AJ, Jesus SS, et al. Comparison of clinical, radiographic, computed tomographic, and magnetic resonance imaging methods for early prediction of canine hip laxity and dysplasia. Vet Radiol Ultrasound 2009; 50(2):135–43.

69. Andronescu AA, Kelly L, Kearney MT, et al. Associations between early radiographic and computed tomographic measures and canine hip joint osteoarthritis at maturity. Am J Vet Res 2015;76(1):19–27.

70. Lopez MJ, Lewis BP, Swaab ME, et al. Relationships among measurements obtained by use of computed tomography and radiography and scores of cartilage microdamage in hip joints with moderate to severe joint laxity of adult dogs. Am J Vet Res 2008;69(3):362–70.

71. Dueland RT, Adams WM, Patricelli AJ, et al. Canine hip dysplasia treated by juvenile pubic symphysiodesis. Part I: two year results of computed tomography and distraction index. Vet Comp Orthop Traumatol 2010;23(5):306–17.

72. Fujiki M, Misumi K, Sakamoto H. Laxity of canine hip joint in two positions with computed tomography. J Vet Med Sci 2004;66(8):1003–6.

73. Gatineau M, Dupuis J, Beauregard G, et al. Palpation and dorsal acetabular rim radiographic projection for early detection of canine hip dysplasia: a prospective study. Vet Surg 2012;41(1):42–53.

74. Vanden Berg-Foels WS, Schwager SJ, Todhunter RJ, et al. Femoral head shape differences during development may identify hips at risk of degeneration. Ann Biomed Eng 2011;39(12):2955–63.

75. Chalmers HJ, Dykes NL, Lust G, et al. Assessment of bone mineral density of the femoral head in dogs with early osteoarthritis. Am J Vet Res 2006;67(5): 796–800.

76. Vanden Berg-Foels WS, Schwager SJ, Todhunter RJ, et al. Femoral head bone mineral density patterns may identify hips at risk of degeneration. Ann Biomed Eng 2011;39(1):75–84.

77. D'Amico LL, Xie L, Abell LK, et al. Relationships of hip joint volume ratios with degrees of joint laxity and degenerative disease from youth to maturity in a canine population predisposed to hip joint osteoarthritis. Am J Vet Res 2011; 72(3):376–83.

78. Claus AM, Totterman SM, Sychterz CJ, et al. Computed tomography to assess pelvic lysis after total hip replacement. Clin Orthop Relat Res 2004;(422): 167–74.
79. Cook SD, Patron LP, Salkeld SL, et al. Correlation of computed tomography with histology in the assessment of periprosthetic defect healing. Clin Orthop Relat Res 2009;467(12):3213–20.
80. Ragetly CA, Evans R, Mostafa AA, et al. Multivariate analysis of morphometric characteristics to evaluate risk factors for cranial cruciate ligament deficiency in Labrador Retrievers. Vet Surg 2011;40(3):327–33.
81. Mostafa AA, Griffon DJ, Thomas MW, et al. Morphometric characteristics of the pelvic limbs of Labrador Retrievers with and without cranial cruciate ligament deficiency. Am J Vet Res 2009;70(4):498–507.
82. Samii VF, Dyce J, Pozzi A, et al. Computed tomographic arthrography of the stifle for detection of cranial and caudal cruciate ligament and meniscal tears in dogs. Vet Radiol Ultrasound 2009;50(2):144–50.
83. Han S, Cheon H, Cho H, et al. Evaluation of partial cranial cruciate ligament rupture with positive contrast computed tomographic arthrography in dogs. J Vet Sci 2008;9(4):395–400.
84. Paek M, Engiles JB, Mai W. Prevalence, association with stifle conditions, and histopathologic characteristics of tibial tuberosity radiolucencies in dogs. Vet Radiol Ultrasound 2013;54(5):453–8.
85. Towle HA, Griffon DJ, Thomas MW, et al. Pre- and postoperative radiographic and computed tomographic evaluation of dogs with medial patellar luxation. Vet Surg 2005;34(3):265–72.
86. Smith TJ, Baltzer WI, Löhr C, et al. Primary synovial osteochondromatosis of the stifle in an English Mastiff. Vet Comp Orthop Traumatol 2012;25(2):160–6.
87. Fitch RB, Wilson ER, Hathcock JT, et al. Radiographic, computed tomographic and magnetic resonance imaging evaluation of a chronic long digital extensor tendon avulsion in a dog. Vet Radiol Ultrasound 1997;38(3):177–81.
88. Aper R, Kowaleski MP, Apelt D, et al. Computed tomographic determination of tibial torsion in the dog. Vet Radiol Ultrasound 2005;46(3):187–91.
89. Gielen I, Van Ryssen B, Coopman F, et al. Comparison of subchondral lesion size between clinical and non-clinical medial trochlear ridge talar osteochondritis dissecans in dogs. Vet Comp Orthop Traumatol 2007;20(1):8–11.
90. Dingemanse WB, Van Bree HJ, Duchateau L, et al. Comparison of clinical and computed tomographic features between medial and lateral trochlear ridge talar osteochondrosis in dogs. Vet Surg 2013;42(3):340–5.
91. Lacourt M, Gao C, Li A, et al. Relationship between cartilage and subchondral bone lesions in repetitive impact trauma-induced equine osteoarthritis. Osteoarthritis Cartilage 2012;20(6):572–83.
92. Johnson KA, Muir P, Nicoll RG, et al. Asymmetric adaptive modeling of central tarsal bones in racing greyhounds. Bone 2000;27(2):257–63.
93. Bergh MS, Piras A, Samii VF, et al. Fractures in regions of adaptive modeling and remodeling of central tarsal bones in racing Greyhounds. Am J Vet Res 2012;73(3):375–80.
94. Goldman S, Pirotte BJ. Brain tumors. Methods Mol Biol 2011;727:291–315.
95. Vanel M, Blond L, Vanel D. Imaging of primary bone tumors in veterinary medicine: which differences? Eur J Radiol 2013;82(12):2129–39.
96. Alexander JW. Selected skeletal dysplasias: craniomandibular osteopathy, multiple cartilaginous exostoses, and hypertrophic osteodystrophy. Vet Clin North Am Small Anim Pract 1983;13(1):55–70.

97. Ferrell EA, Berry CR, Thrall DE. Interpretation paradigms for the appendicular skeleton. In: Thrall DE, editor. Textbook of veterinary diagnostic radiology. St Louis (MO): Saunders; 2007. p. 222–39.
98. Karnik KS, Samii VF, Weisbrode SE, et al. Accuracy of computed tomography in determining lesion size in canine appendicular osteosarcoma. Vet Radiol Ultrasound 2012;53(3):273–9.
99. McEntee MC, Page RL, Mauldin GN, et al. Results of irradiation of infiltrative lipoma in 13 dogs. Vet Radiol Ultrasound 2000;41(6):554–6.
100. McEntee MC, Thrall DE. Computed tomographic imaging of infiltrative lipoma in 22 dogs. Vet Radiol Ultrasound 2001;42(3):221–5.
101. Vignoli M, Ohlerth S, Rossi F, et al. Computed tomography-guided fine-needle aspiration and tissue-core biopsy of bone lesions in small animals. Vet Radiol Ultrasound 2004;45(2):125–30.
102. Vignoli M, Terragni R, Rossi F, et al. Whole body computed tomographic characteristics of skeletal and cardiac muscular metastatic neoplasia in dogs and cats. Vet Radiol Ultrasound 2013;54(3):223–30.
103. Seely S. Possible reasons for the high resistance of muscle to cancer. Med Hypotheses 1980;6(2):133–7.
104. Martano M, Morello E, Buracco P. Feline injection-site sarcoma: past, present and future perspectives. Vet J 2011;188(2):136–41.
105. McEntee MC, Page RL. Feline vaccine-associated sarcomas. J Vet Intern Med 2001;15(3):176–82.
106. Seguin B. Feline injection site sarcomas. Vet Clin North Am Small Anim Pract 2002;32(4):983–95, viii.
107. Thomas R, Valli VE, Ellis P, et al. Microarray-based cytogenetic profiling reveals recurrent and subtype-associated genomic copy number aberrations in feline sarcomas. Chromosome Res 2009;17(8):987–1000.
108. Travetti O, di Giancamillo M, Stefanello D, et al. Computed tomography characteristics of fibrosarcoma – a histological subtype of feline injection-site sarcoma. J Feline Med Surg 2013;15(6):488–93.
109. Freire M, Meuten D, Lascelles D. Pathology of articular cartilage and synovial membrane from elbow joints with and without degenerative joint disease in domestic cats. Vet Pathol 2014;51(5):968–78.
110. Tambella AM, Palumbo Piccionello A, Dini F, et al. Myositis ossificans circumscripta of the triceps muscle in a Rottweiler dog. Vet Comp Orthop Traumatol 2013;26(2):154–9.
111. Klang A, Kneissl S, Glänzel R, et al. Imaging diagnosis: fibrodysplasia ossificans progressiva in a cat. Vet Radiol Ultrasound 2013;54(5):532–5.
112. Rossmeisl JH Jr, Rohleder JJ, Hancock R, et al. Computed tomographic features of suspected traumatic injury to the iliopsoas and pelvic limb musculature of a dog. Vet Radiol Ultrasound 2004;45(5):388–92.
113. Kalff S, Parry A, Gemmill T. Traumatic fibrotic myopathy of the tensor fascia lata muscle in a Whippet. Vet Comp Orthop Traumatol 2013;26(4):328–31.
114. Vansteenkiste DP, Lee KC, Lamb CR. Computed tomographic findings in 44 dogs and 10 cats with grass seed foreign bodies. J Small Anim Pract 2014; 55(11):579–84.
115. Aiken SW, Jakovljevic S, Lantz GC, et al. Acquired arteriovenous fistula secondary to castration in a dog. J Am Vet Med Assoc 1993;202(6):965–7.
116. Lewis DC, Harari J. Peripheral arteriovenous fistula associated with a subcutaneous hemangiosarcoma/hemangioma in a cat. Feline Pract 1992;20:27–9.

117. Parks AH, Guy BL, Rawlings CA, et al. Lameness in a mare with signs of arteriovenous fistula. J Am Vet Med Assoc 1989;194(3):379–80.

118. Santoro D, Pease A, Linder KE, et al. Post-traumatic peripheral arteriovenous fistula manifesting as digital haemorrhages in a cat: diagnosis with contrast-enhanced 3D CT imaging. Vet Dermatol 2009;20(3):206–13.

119. Oh J, Lee JH, Cho KO, et al. Diffuse idiopathic skeletal hyperostosis with prominent appendicular bone proliferation in a dog. J Vet Med Sci 2015;77(4):493–7.

120. Rybak LD, Rosenthal DI. Radiological imaging for the diagnosis of bone metastases. Q J Nucl Med 2001;45(1):53–64.

121. Wolf MB, Murray F, Kilk K, et al. Sensitivity of whole-body CT and MRI versus projection radiography in the detection of osteolyses in patients with monoclonal plasma cell disease. Eur J Radiol 2014;83(7):1222–30.

122. Oliveira CR, Ranallo FN, Pijanowski GJ, et al. The VetMousetrap: a device for computed tomographic imaging of the thorax of awake cats. Vet Radiol Ultrasound 2011;52(1):41–52.

Musculoskeletal MRI

Jaime E. Sage, DVM, MS[a],*, Patrick Gavin, DVM, PhD[b,c]

KEYWORDS

- Musculoskeletal MRI • Small animal MRI • Shoulder joint MRI • Stifle joint MRI
- Elbow joint MRI • Carpal/Tarsal joint MRI

KEY POINTS

- MRI is unparalleled in the imaging of musculoskeletal disease because it allows for multiplanar images with a large field of view and superior soft tissue resolution.
- MRI is equally well suited to detecting conditions of osseous, articular, and soft tissue origin, making MRI the most comprehensive diagnostic imaging modality.
- For musculoskeletal imaging in particular, fluid-sensitive sequences are used to easily detect conditions related to trauma, infection, inflammation, and neoplasia; these sequences include T2-weighted, proton density with fat saturation, and short tau inversion recovery.
- The MRI features of common disorders affecting the shoulder, elbow, stifle, carpal, and tarsal joints are included in this article.

MRI has the unique ability to detect abnormal fluid content and is, therefore, unparalleled in its role of detection, diagnosis, prognosis, treatment planning, and follow-up of musculoskeletal disease. MRI in companion animals should be considered in the following circumstances:

- A definitive diagnosis cannot be made on radiographs
- A patient is nonresponsive to medical or surgical therapy
- Prognostic information is desired
- Assessing surgical margins and traumatic and/or infectious joint and bone disease
- Ruling out subtle developmental or early aggressive bone lesions

The MRI features of common disorders affecting the shoulder, elbow, stifle, carpal, and tarsal joints are included in this article.

Patients with electronic devices such as pacemakers and newly placed metallic bone implants should not be scanned. Bone implants that have had sufficient time

The authors have nothing to disclose.
[a] MRVets, P.C., 14900 Avery Ranch Boulevard C200, #101, Austin, TX 78717, USA; [b] Department of Veterinary Medicine, Washington State University, Pullman, WA 99164-6610, USA; [c] MRVets, P.C., 109 Raven View Drive, Sagle, ID 83860, USA
* Corresponding author.
E-mail address: Jaime@mrvets.com

Vet Clin Small Anim 46 (2016) 421–451
http://dx.doi.org/10.1016/j.cvsm.2015.12.003
0195-5616/16/$ – see front matter © 2016 Elsevier Inc. All rights reserved.

vetsmall.theclinics.com

to secure to the underlying bone and are out of the field of view and isocenter are often acceptable if a 3.0-T or lower strength magnet is used. Because a patient must be stationary to obtain a diagnostic MRI study, anesthesia or heavy sedation is needed in the conscious patient. Therefore, most contraindications for MRI revolve around the patient's ability to safely undergo anesthesia.

MRI techniques are based on sequences that define normal anatomy and detect abnormal fluid accumulation. Sequences used to define anatomy include T1-weighted, gradient echo (GRE) sequences, and proton density (PD). Fluid sensitive sequences including PD fat saturation and short tau inversion recovery (STIR). T2-weighted images are beneficial in assessing normal anatomy and pathologic change and are essential in eliminating magic angle artifact, especially in the shoulder and stifle joints.

MRI systems of 1.5-T or higher, using quadrature surface coils are recommended in obtaining studies of the joints in companion animals. Although subtle soft tissue signal change and anatomic variations may be undetectable with low-field MRI, most pathologic conditions can be accurately diagnosed when patient positioning and MRI technique are optimized. A quadrature surface coil is used for most musculoskeletal studies because of its ease in patient positioning and increased signal-to-noise ratio over linear coils.

Proper patient positioning is essential in obtaining high-resolution images and distinguishing normal anatomy from pathologic conditions. The patient should be placed in lateral recumbency with the imaged joint in a natural flexed position on the coil. This positioning allows for good contact with the coil and decreased motion from respiration but requires the contralateral joint to be imaged separately.

Musculoskeletal MRI studies are susceptible to common MRI artifacts such as

- Patient motion
- Flow
- Incomplete saturation
- Wraparound
- Shading
- Truncation
- Partial volume averaging
- Radiofrequency interference.

Artifacts of particular concern in musculoskeletal imaging include

- Magnetic susceptibility artifact from implants
- Magic angle artifact

Magic angle artifact is unique to musculoskeletal MRI and can mimic pathologic conditions in tendons and ligaments when they are positioned at an approximately 55° angle to the main magnetic field. At this angle, there is lengthening of the T2 time of the tightly bound protons within the ligament/tendon, and an area of high signal may occur in short TE sequences (T1, GRE, PD and STIR). This artifact does not occur in long TE sequences (T2 weighted); therefore, T2-weighted images should always be included when imaging the joints.

The information in this article draws significantly and expands on topics covered in the orthopedic chapter of *Practical Small Animal MRI*.[1]

SHOULDER JOINT

MRI is becoming an increasingly popular imaging modality for the shoulder joint, as it provides exquisite soft tissue resolution, sensitivity/specificity for bone pathology, assessment of normal joint anatomy, and a large field of view that is useful in ruling out underlying cervical spinal, brachial plexus, or bone disease in a noninvasive manner. Forelimb lameness secondary to shoulder conditions is common, but it is often difficult to obtain a definitive diagnose on physical examination and radiography alone. Ultrasound imaging is beneficial in viewing conditions of the supporting ligaments, tendons, and joint, but is operator dependent, has a small field of view, and is limited in evaluating the medial compartment.

Arthroscopy provides diagnostic and therapeutic intervention but is invasive, is less readily available, and lacks evaluation of extra-articular soft tissues and bone. Computed tomography (CT) is excellent in confirming bone lesions but has poor soft tissue resolution.

MRI of the shoulder joint allows visualization of the joint capsule, articular margin, tendons (supraspinatus, infraspinatus, biciptal, teres minor, subscapularis), scapular and brachial muscles, scapula and humerus, caudal cervical spine, and brachial plexus structures.[2] Developmental, traumatic, infectious and neoplastic disorders of the caudal cervical, axilla, and proximal forelimb are visualized in one imaging procedure.[3]

This article covers the more common afflictions of the shoulder joint including osteochondrosis, supraspinatus tendinopathy, bicipital tenosynovitis, neoplasia, and foreign bodies near the joint.

Determining the underlying cause of forelimb lameness is often challenging and includes a broad differential list involving pathology of the caudal cervical spine, axilla, scapula, humerus, shoulder joint, and extra-articular forelimb soft tissues. Even when the pain and lameness is isolated to the shoulder joint, both intra-articular and extra-articular etiologies remain. Often, arthroscopy is reported as the gold standard with disregard of the multitude of extra-articular disorders.

The ideal MRI protocol for proximal forelimb pain/lameness includes sequences designed to visualize the caudal cervical spine, axillary region, shoulder joint, and scapular and brachial soft tissues while maintaining high spatial resolution. **Fig. 1** shows images of a normal shoulder.

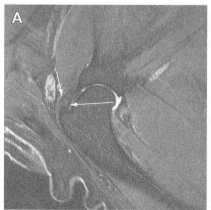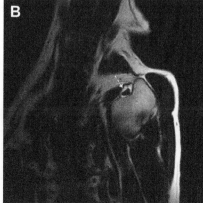

Fig. 1. STIR sagittal (*A*) and T2-weighted transverse (*B*) images of a normal shoulder. A normal degree of T2/STIR signal of the supraspinatus tendon insertion at the fibrocartilaginous junction (*arrows*) is seen and should not be confused with a pathologic condition. The bicipital tendon should be located in the mid aspect of intertubercular groove and should have a nearly round shape (*dashed arrow*).

The patient should be placed in lateral recumbency with the affected limb downward and at an approximately 90° angle (**Fig. 2**). If the contralateral limb is to be imaged, the patient needs to be rolled and repositioned in appropriate lateral recumbency.

Standard imaging sequences should include a T1-weighted sequence to define anatomic abnormalities and fluid-sensitive sequences such as STIR, PD with fat saturation, and T2 with fat saturation sequences, which are fundamental in the diagnosis of conditions. A T2-weighted sagittal sequence is needed to eliminate erroneous interpretation caused by magic angle. Although many combinations of sequences are acceptable, the most reliable sequences, especially when a radiologist is not available to guide the study, is to include a T2 sagittal sequence of the cervical and cranial thoracic spine and a STIR dorsal sequence of the axilla through the brachial plexus bilaterally, in addition to focused sequences of the shoulder joint. T1-weighted sagittal, T2-weighted sagittal, STIR or fat-suppressed PD or T2-weighted sagittal, transverse, and dorsal imaging (to the bicipital tendon) are adequate for imaging the shoulder joint.[4]

Osteochondrosis

Shoulder osteochondrosis is a common developmental disorder most frequently seen in young, athletic, large- to giant-breed dogs. Articular margin abnormalities can be easily missed on radiographs because of the curved surface of the humeral head but are readily seen on MRI. The humeral epiphysis is of high signal on T1, T2, and PD images, and a change in the contour and signal of the articular defect is easily seen.[5] Cartilaginous flaps and active inflammation of the underlying bone, if present, are seen as a high signal on the STIR or T2 fat-saturated sequence (**Fig. 3**). Chronic osteochondrosis lesions are occasionally seen in middle to older-aged patients and are typically of low signal on all sequences, indicative of sclerotic bone without associated inflammation (**Fig. 4**). Most chronic osteochondrosis lesions lacking high signal on fluid-sensitive sequences are considered incidental, and alternate causes for the lameness are often found.

Supraspinatus Trauma

Supraspinatus tendinopathy is the most common traumatic disease process of the shoulder joint. Bicipital tenosynovitis was once thought to be the most common cause of acquired shoulder disease and, although it still occurs independently, most cases of

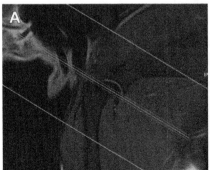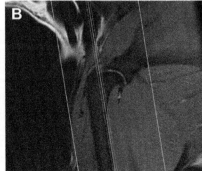

Fig. 2. PD fat-saturated sagittal images of the shoulder joint with proper slice orientation for planning transverse (*A*) and coronal (*B*) images, respectively.

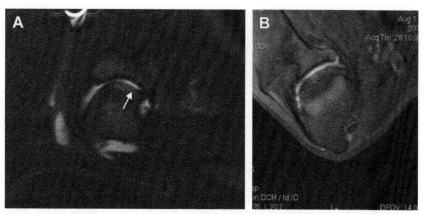

Fig. 3. Sagittal STIR (*A*) and PD fat-saturated transverse (*B*) images of the shoulder joint. There is marked flattening of the caudal humeral head articular margin and underlying hyperintensity of the subchondral bone (*arrow*).

chronic cranial shoulder pain are caused by repetitive strain injury of the supraspinatus tendon. Repetitive trauma of the supraspinatus insertion along the medial aspect of the greater tubercle results in a collagenous mass that is hyperintense on T2/STIR and fat-suppressed proton density sequences.

This mass effect compresses and causes medial displacement of the underlying bicipital tendon within the intertubercular groove[6] (**Fig. 5**). With chronicity, there is fatty replacement at the myotendinous junction of the supraspinatus tendon evidenced by high T1/T2, low STIR signal on MRI studies. On arthroscopy, impingement of the

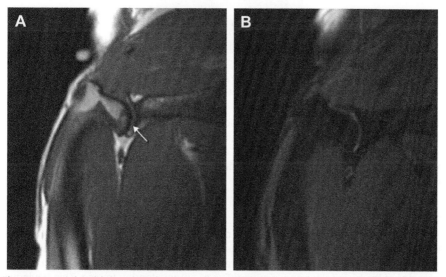

Fig. 4. T1-weighted (*A*) and PD fat-saturated sagittal (*B*) images of a nonactive osteochondrosis lesion (*arrow*) in a 6-year-old dog without underlying subchondral inflammation, significant joint effusion, or degenerative changes. This patient's clinical signs were attributable to multiple chronic foreign body abscesses.

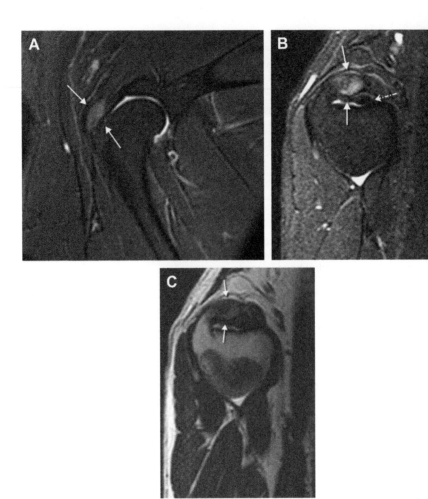

Fig. 5. STIR sagittal (*A*), STIR transverse (*B*), and T2-weighted transverse (*C*) images show enlargement and hyperintensity of the supraspinatus tendon (*solid arrows*) with compression and medial displacement of the bicipital tendon (*dashed arrow*).

bicipital tendon by the supraspinatus tendon may be underinterpreted because of joint distention during the procedure.[7] On MRI, an extracapsular primary cause of the lameness can be identified, which may, in turn, alter treatment protocol. MRI has, therefore, helped to reshape therapeutic management and outcomes in patients with chronic shoulder lameness.

Bicipital Tenosynovitis

Primary bicipital tendon trauma is a less common cause of shoulder conditions than supraspinatus tendinopathy but does occur. The distinction between primary and secondary bicipital tendinopathy can be therapeutically significant. A decrease in overall diameter of the bicipital tendon is suggestive of chronic tendon fraying. This fraying is often associated with T2 and STIR or fat-suppressed hyperintensity of the tendon, consistent with core tendon damage (**Figs. 6** and **7**). With severe thinning of the bicipital tendon, impending tendon rupture is of concern.

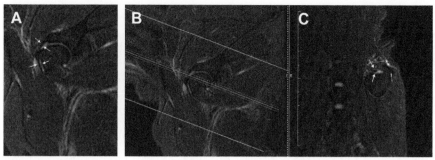

Fig. 6. STIR sagittal (*A, B*) and transverse (*C*) images with severe thinning of the bicipital tendon proximal and distal to the intertubercular groove (*arrows*).

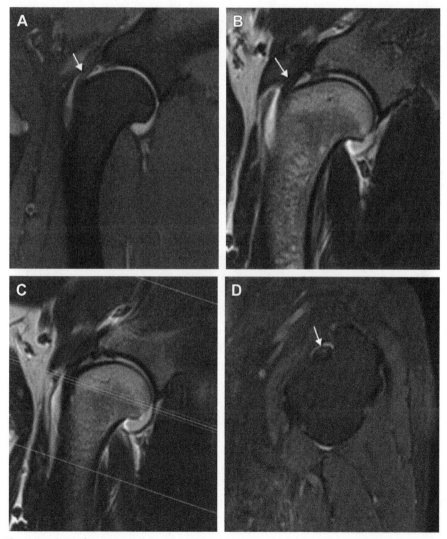

Fig. 7. High PD fat-saturated (*A, D*) and T2 (*B, C*) signal of the bicipital tendon within the intertubercular groove (*arrow*). Confirmation of high PD or STIR within the tendon is necessary to rule out a magic angle artifact.

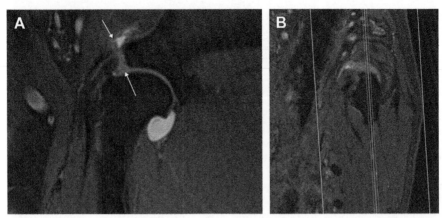

Fig. 8. PD fat-saturated sagittal (*A*) and transverse (*B*) images of an origin avulsion of the bicipital tendon (*arrows*) with marked hyperintensity and enlargement of the tendon within the intertubercular groove. Joint distension is also present and is commonly seen in patients with bicipital tendon tears/rupture.

When the bicipital tendon is enlarged, it is likely that a partial tear has occurred, and marked joint effusion is typical (**Fig. 8**). Chronic, repetitive trauma and acute trauma causes inflammation of the synovial membrane and joint capsule (synovitis and capsulitis). Synovitis is seen as a thickened, occasionally irregular synovial lining with decreased T2 signal and with avid contrast enhancement. The bicipital tendon sheath is a continuation of the joint; therefore, similar changes can be seen affecting the tendon sheath lining (**Fig. 9**).

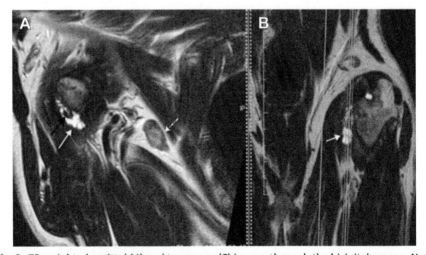

Fig. 9. T2-weighted sagittal (*A*) and transverse (*B*) images through the bicipital groove. Note the tendon sheath distension and irregular, low T2 signal synovial membrane thickening (*arrow*), consistent with bicipital tenosynovitis. The low signal structure within the bicipital tendon sheath represents an osteochondroma (*black arrow*). An enlarged axillary lymph node (*dashed arrow*) is also seen. This patient also has a proximal humeral primary bone tumor.

Infectious

Infectious etiologies affecting the shoulder are uncommon, and frequently involve extra-articular puncture foreign bodies. One of the primary advantages of MRI over ultrasound scan and arthroscopy is the ability to detect conditions over a large field of view. A study of the shoulder joint with concern for a foreign body should include a portion of the neck, caudal cervical and thoracic spine, brachial plexus, shoulder joint, and scapular and brachial soft tissues and osseous structures.

The fluid-sensitive sequences with fat saturation are essential in detecting pockets of fluid accumulation that surround foreign bodies. High STIR signal fluid accumulation surrounding a low T1/T2/STIR structure is often pathognomonic for a foreign body.[8] Detection and pursuance of the course and termination site of a draining tract is often easily accomplished with the STIR sequence (**Fig. 10**). Unlike CT examination, contrast is rarely needed.

The multiplanar features of MRI are well suited for foreign body localization, assessment of joint and osseous involvement, and lymphadenopathy. Sagittal and dorsal STIR sequences have the largest field of view and allow for quick identification and localization of the lesion. Although transverse fat-suppressed images are most valuable in further localizing the lesion and evaluating involvement of underlying structures, T1-weighted images aid in assessing for subtle bony remodeling caused by osteomyelitis and provide a comparison if contrast is given.

Neoplasia

Perhaps the most consequential use of MRI is the ability to rule out aggressive disease as an underlying cause of lameness that would not otherwise be detected. CT is sensitive to the detection of early lysis, but many neoplasms, particularly those of joint origin, have only soft tissue involvement initially. Additionally, the earliest form of

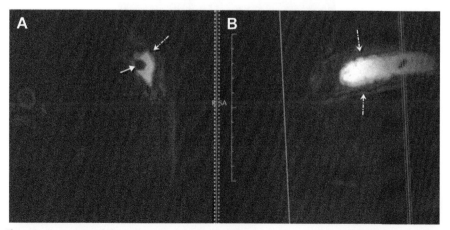

Fig. 10. Transverse (*A*) and sagittal STIR (*B*) images of the scapula highlighting a large, hyperintense fluid pocket (*dashed arrows*) containing a low signal foreign body (*arrow*). This particular foreign body was a chronic porcupine quill.

bone tumor infiltration occurs at a cellular level with increased water content that is detectable on fat-saturated fluid-sensitive MRI sequences.

Tumors affecting the shoulder joint and the surrounding structures include primary bone tumors such as osteosarcoma and soft tissue sarcomas including, but not limited to, malignant histiocytosis, synovial cell sarcoma, fibrosarcoma, and peripheral nerve sheath tumors.

Early bone edema and infiltration from primary bone tumors are best visualized on STIR of fat-suppressed T2 or PD sequences, whereas early cortical lysis and proliferation are best assessed on T1-weighted images (**Fig. 11**). Adjacent soft tissue signal change identified on MRI is often undetectable on radiographs and CT examination.

Primary soft tissue tumors may also be undetectable on radiographs and CT examination if underlying bone change is early or absent (**Fig. 12**).

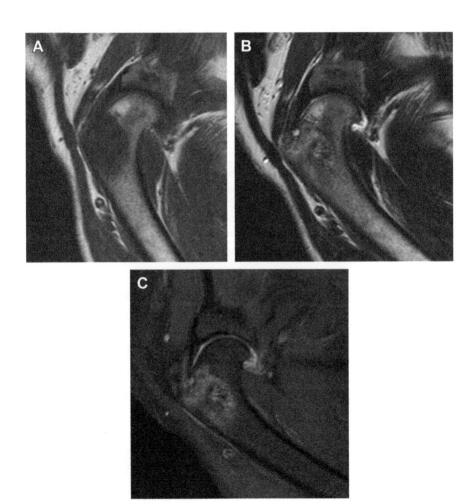

Fig. 11. T1-weighted (*A*), T2-weighted (*B*), and STIR sagittal (*C*) images of a primary bone tumor of the proximal humerus. This lesion is seen on all 3 sequences but is most readily detected on the STIR sequence.

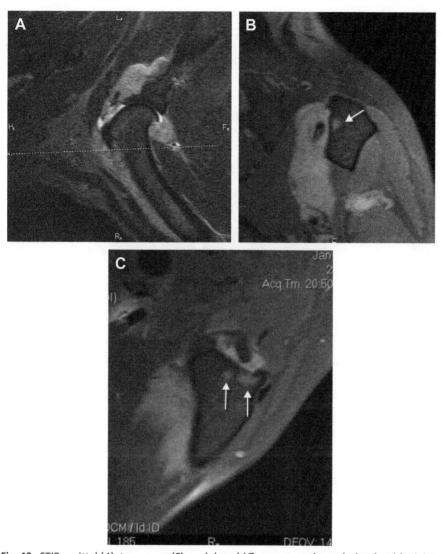

Fig. 12. STIR sagittal (*A*), transverse (*B*), and dorsal (*C*) sequences through the shoulder joint. Severe joint capsule, bicipital tendon sheath, and extra-articular soft tissue thickening and hyperintensity are seen, along with 2 small areas of bone infiltration (*arrows*). Radiographs were normal in this patient with suspected trauma. Histiocytic sarcoma was confirmed on histopathology. MRI is extremely valuable in detecting soft tissue neoplasia with early bone involvement.

ELBOW JOINT

The elbow joint is less frequently imaged with MRI compared with the shoulder joint partially because of an increased incidence of lameness caused by shoulder conditions and partially because of more common causes of elbow pain being more accurately diagnosed on radiographs and CT examination when compared with conditions of the shoulder and stifle joints. However, extra-articular soft tissues elbow injuries do occur and often need to be ruled out even in patients with presumed elbow dysplasia.

MRI is accurate in diagnosing fragmented medial coronoid process of the ulna, elbow incongruity, osteoarthrosis and acute and chronic tendon injuries of the biceps brachii, triceps tendon, and deep digital flexor tendon at the level of the elbow joint. **Fig. 13** shows images of a normal elbow.[9]

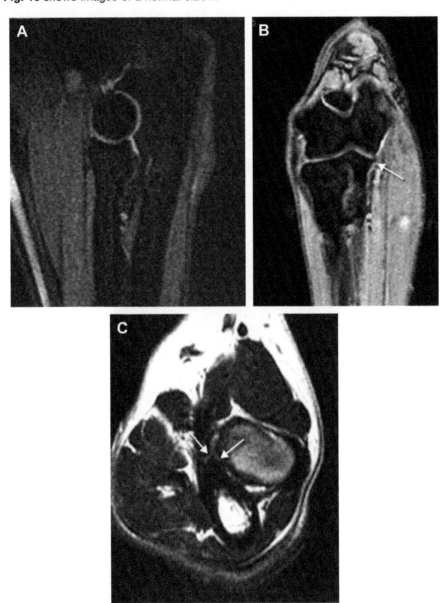

Fig. 13. STIR sagittal (*A*), T1-weighted GRE dorsal (*B*), and T2-weighted transverse (*C*) images of a normal elbow joint. The medial coronoid process is readily identified on the dorsal and transverse images (*arrows*). Joint congruity is best assessed on sagittal fluid-sensitive sequences.[9]

The patient should be scanned in lateral recumbency with the affected limb down. The elbow should be in a natural, flexed position, and transverse and dorsal plane images should be planned parallel to the radius and ulna (**Fig. 14**). If a bilateral study is deemed necessary, each elbow joint should be independently imaged to obtain optimal resolution and positioning.

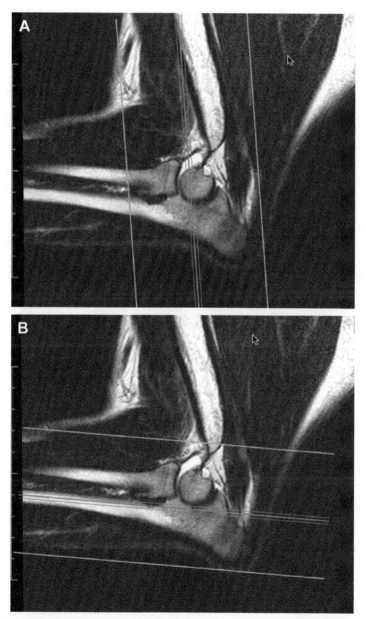

Fig. 14. T2-weighted images of the elbow joint with proper slice orientation for planning transverse (A) and coronal (B) images, respectively.

Dysplasia

Although CT examination is often used to confirm and diagnose elbow dysplasia, especially when underlying medial coronoid fragmentation is present, MRI can also accurately diagnose elbow dysplasia and can depict accompanying subchondral bone change and soft tissue abnormalities.[10] Elbow joint incongruity, either as an underlying component of medial coronoid pathology or perhaps as an unrelated form of elbow dysplasia, is easily seen on multiplanar MRI studies.[11] The fragment associated with the medial coronoid process is best seen on fat-suppressed T2 or PD or STIR images, as the synovial fluid extends into the fissure (**Fig. 15**).

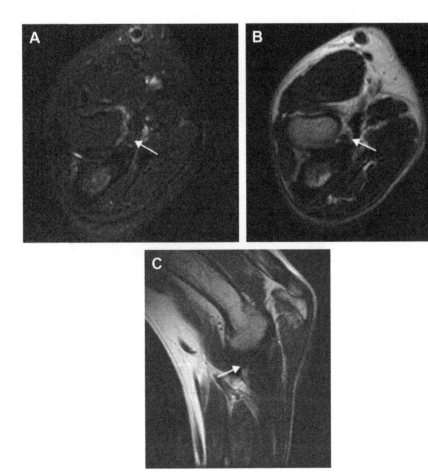

Fig. 15. Transverse STIR (A), transverse T2-weighted (B), and sagittal T2-weighted (C) images of a fragmented medial coronoid process (arrows). High T2/STIR synovial fluid dissects along the fragment.

Joint Osteoarthrosis and Trauma

Osteoarthrosis of the elbow joint is a common occurrence and is readily diagnosed on radiographs. The most important function of MRI of elbow osteoarthrosis is ruling out concurrent neoplastic or trauma injuries.

Joint effusion is appreciated on T2-weighted sequences, periarticular osteophytes are seen on T1-weighted images, and contrast enhancement of the synovial lining is seen on postcontrast T1-weighted images.

Trauma to the insertion of the triceps tendon on the olecranon elicits a marked inflammatory response that is easily appreciated on MRI. Marked, ill-defined T2/STIR hyperintensity proximal to the olecranon and loss of integrity and undulation (with cases of tendon avulsion) of the tendon in the T1 images are seen (**Figs. 16** and **17**). Methemoglobin, if present, will have increased signal on T1 images before contrast.

Trauma to the distal biceps tendon may occur and is seen as contrast enhancing, high T2/STIR signal of the muscle belly (see **Fig. 17**). Rupture of the biceps tendon at its insertion is uncommon.

Injury to the deep digital flexor tendon at its origin on the medial humeral epicondyle can also be seen. High T2/STIR signal is seen surrounding the tendon

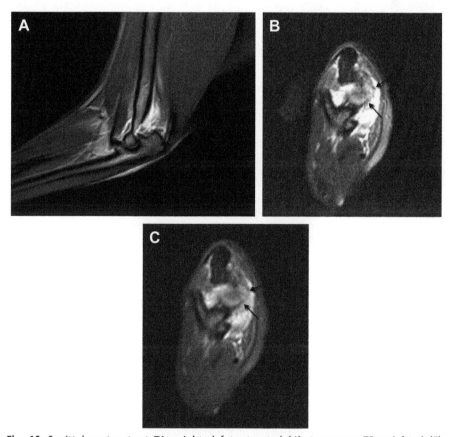

Fig. 16. Sagittal postcontrast T1-weighted fat-saturated (*A*), transverse T2-weighted (*B*), and transverse PD fat-saturated (*C*) images of the elbow joint in a cat with a chronic avulsion of the triceps insertion. There is a low T2 signal/PD fat-saturated signal mass (*arrows*) representing the ruptured distal portion of the tendon and resulting in a collagenous mass with marked surrounding contrast-enhancing, high T2/PD fat-saturated signal inflammation.

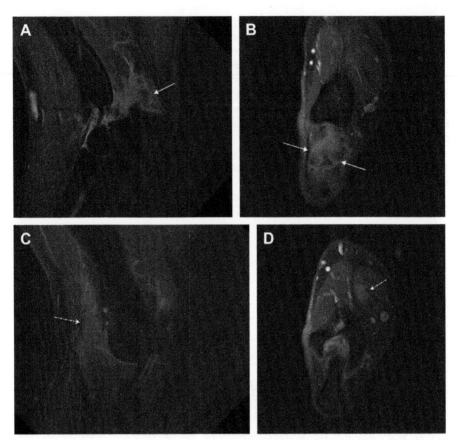

Fig. 17. Sagittal (*A*) and transverse (*B*) postcontrast T1-weighted fat-saturated images of a dog with a chronic triceps tendon avulsion at the insertion. The arrow denotes the thickened avulsion portion of tendon with surrounding inflammation. This patient also has an injury to the distal bicipital muscle belly (*C, D*) (*dashed arrows*).

and is most conspicuous on fat-saturated sequences when the adjacent subcutaneous fat is nulled (**Fig. 18**). Tendon enlargement occurs as the body attempts to repair damaged collagen fibers with new collagen of abnormal structure and composition.

Neoplasia

Neoplastic disease processes of the elbow are uncommon and are typically associated with soft tissue tumors such as synovial cell sarcoma. MRI can easily detect neoplastic lesions affecting the elbow joint and is especially valuable compared with radiographs and CT when bone involvement is not yet present.

Marked joint distension is seen on T2 sequences. Marked synovial membrane irregular thickening with decreased T2 signal and avid contrast enhancement is seen. Early bone involvement is best detected on fat-suppressed T2 sequences (**Fig. 19**).

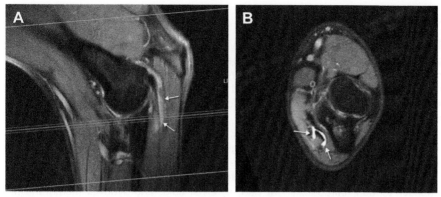

Fig. 18. Parasagittal (*A*) and transverse (*B*) PD fat-saturated images of the elbow joint at the origin of the deep digital flexor on humeral epicondyle. Peritendinous effusion is readily seen on fat-saturated sequences (*arrows*). These sequences are needed to visualize an injury at this location because of adjacent high T2 signal fat.

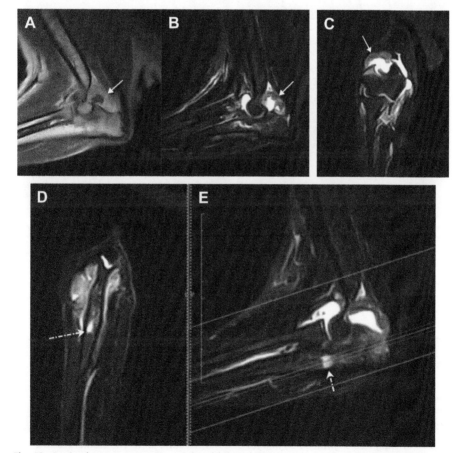

Fig. 19. Sagittal postcontrast T1-weighted (*A*) and STIR images (*B–E*) of synovial cell sarcoma involving the elbow joint. Note the contrast-enhancing, low STIR signal of the thickened, irregular synovial membrane (*arrow*), marked joint effusion, and STIR hyperintensity of the proximal ulna indicating bone infiltration (*dashed arrow*).

STIFLE JOINT

The knee joint is the most commonly imaged human joint, but the veterinary community has been slow to embrace this imaging modality in the equivalent stifle joint as standard of practice before surgical procedures. This lack of acceptance is partially because of the added cost, lack of comfort/experience with MR stifle diagnosis, and the ability to perform diagnostic arthroscopy at the time of surgery.

As with the shoulder joint, arthroscopy has limited visibility and is unable to assess the extra-articular structures and damage below the articular surface, such as intrameniscal damage and subchondral bone damage.

The menisci, cranial and caudal cruciate ligaments, collateral ligaments, long digital extensor tendon, infrapatellar fat pad, synovial fluid, and synovial membrane are clearly identified (**Fig. 20**).[12] The articular cartilage can be visualized in larger patients.

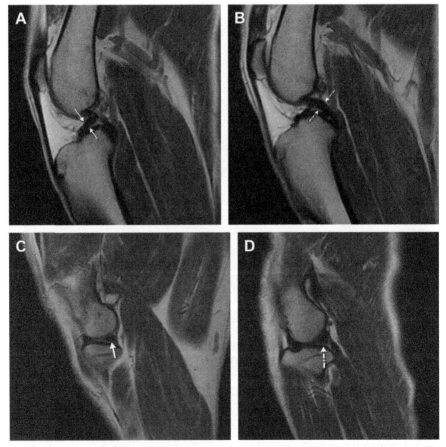

Fig. 20. T1-weighted sagittal (*A–D*) images of a normal stifle joint. The cranial cruciate ligament (*thin, solid arrows*) is a short, low-signal structure that is well visualized. The caudal cruciate ligament (*thin, dashed arrows*) is longer, thicker, and typically more easily seen than the cranial cruciate ligament. The medial menisci (*thick, solid arrow*) and lateral menisci (*thick, dashed arrow*) are low-signal, bowtie-shaped structures.

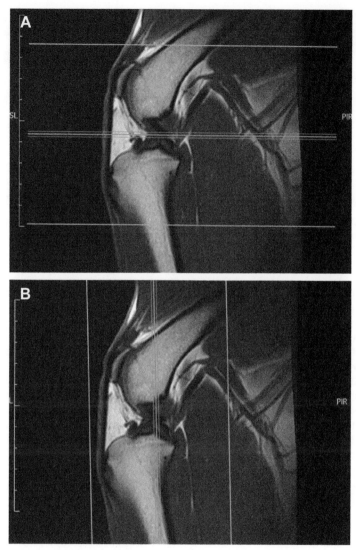

Fig. 21. T1-weighted sagittal images of the stifle joint with proper slice orientation for planning transverse (A) and coronal (B) images, respectively.

The stifle joint of interest should be positioned downward on the surface coil at a 90° angle. Transverse and sagittal images should be planned perpendicular and parallel to the patellar tendon (**Fig. 21**). T1-weighted sagittal, T2-weighted sagittal, STIR or fat-saturated T2-weighted or PD sagittal and transverse, and PD or T1-weighted dorsal images are recommended.

Partial Cranial Cruciate Ligament Tear

Most patients presenting for stifle MR studies are suspected to have partial cranial cruciate ligament ruptures and do not have an obvious drawer sign. These patients typically have a stable joint on manipulation, unilateral hind limb lameness, presumed

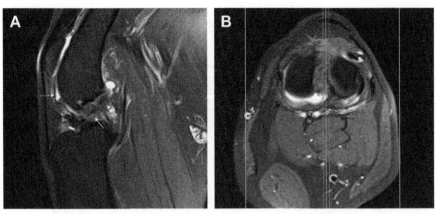

Fig. 22. PD fat-saturated sagittal (*A*) and transverse (*B*) images of the stifle. The cranial cruciate ligament is hyperintense and indistinct (*arrows*), and there is mild joint effusion (*dashed arrow*).

stifle joint effusion on physical examination, and presumed joint effusion and mild arthritic change on radiographs.

These partial tears are diagnosed based on disruption of the normal linear collagen fibers that extend the entire length from the origin to insertion. Damage to these collagen fibers results in inflammation, causing separation of these fibers, especially at their origin and insertion.

On MRI, hyperintensity and loss of the normal low signal of the ligament is readily seen on fluid-sensitive sequences (**Fig. 22**) in addition to subchondral hyperintensity at the origin and insertion of the ligament (**Fig. 23**).[13,14] Because of the normal fan shape of the cranial cruciate ligament at its origin and volume averaging with adjacent synovial fluid, a higher signal intensity is often seen at the origin, and care should be taken to prevent overinterpretation.

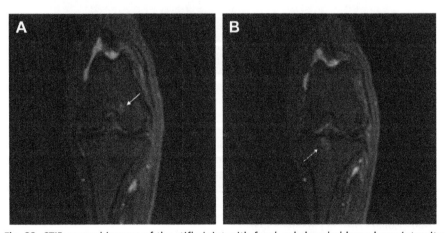

Fig. 23. STIR coronal images of the stifle joint with focal, subchondral bone hyperintensity along the lateral aspect of the intercondylar fossa (*A*) (*solid arrow*) and just medial of midline on the tibial plateau (*B*) (*dashed arrow*), corresponding to the origin and insertion of the cranial cruciate ligament.

The caudal cruciate ligament is shorter and thicker than the cranial cruciate ligament and has uniformly dark appearance on all sequences. Caudal cruciate ligament tears are uncommon in the veterinary patient, although stretching of this ligament is occasionally seen with cranial cruciate ligament injuries.

Traumatic muscle tears, collateral ligament damage, disruption of the long digital extensor tendon, caudal cruciate ligament damage, simple osteoarthritis, patellar cartilaginous damage, and neoplastic disease of the joint and adjacent bone are additional conditions that are seen in patients suspected of having partial cranial cruciate tears.

Menisci

Meniscal damage is estimated to occur in approximately 40% to 60% of patients with cruciate ligament injuries.[15,16] Recognition of meniscal damage is clinically important, as ongoing lameness may occur if these lesions are not addressed during surgical repair of cruciate injuries. Damage to the medial and lateral menisci is often seen as synovial fluid dissecting within intrameniscal tears (**Fig. 24**). Meniscal degeneration and displacement, often associated with a bucket-handle tear, can also be identified (**Fig. 25**). Meniscal signal and anatomic change should ideally be confirmed on more than one plane to prevent overinterpretation owing to volume averaging.

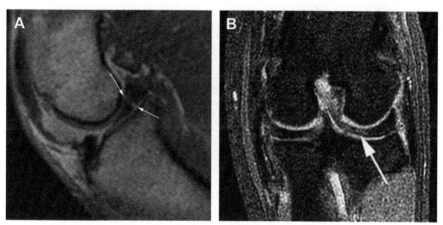

Fig. 24. T2-weighted sagittal (*A*) and coronal (*B*) images of the stifle joint. A distinct hyperintensity of the caudal horn of the lateral meniscus is seen, representing a radial tear (*arrows*).

Neoplasia

In addition to synovial cell sarcoma, adjacent primary bone tumors are common, and early aggressive bone disease needs to be distinguished from intra-articular ligamentous injuries causing stifle pain and lameness. Often, multiple stifle disease processes are present, and the detection of an early neoplastic disease is essential in eliminating unnecessary surgical intervention for less significant traumatic disorders.

Primary neoplastic bone disease is readily seen on fluid-sensitive fat-saturated sequences as severe high signal with possible cortical bone disruption and extension of the disease into the adjacent soft tissues[17] (**Fig. 26**).

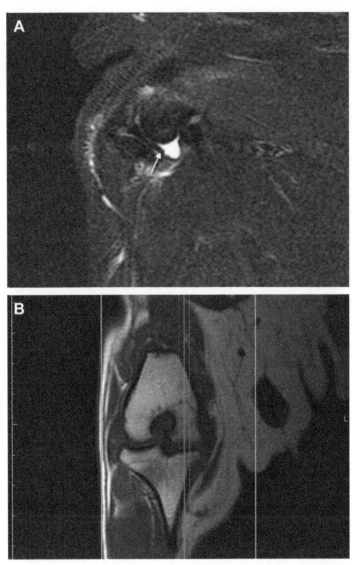

Fig. 25. Sagittal STIR (*A*) and dorsal T1-weighted (*B*) images of the medial meniscus. Notice the thin, flat shape of the caudal horn that may be caused by severe degeneration or a bucket-handle tear (*arrow*). This dog was lame, but the cranial cruciate ligament and remainder of the intra-articular structures were normal with the exception of joint distension.

Synovial cell sarcoma in the stifle joint has a similar appearance on MRI to that of other joints. Marked joint distension is seen on T2 sequences.[18] Marked synovial membrane irregular thickening with decreased T2 signal and avid contrast enhancement is seen. Early bone involvement is best detected on fat-suppressed T2 sequences.

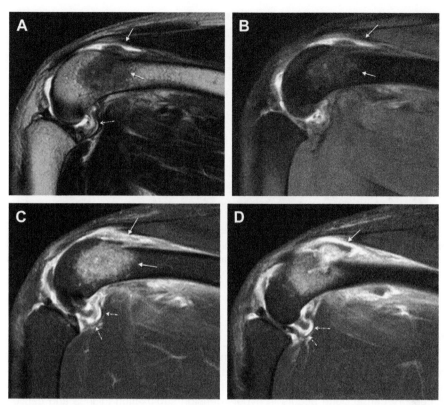

Fig. 26. Sagittal T2 fat-saturated (*A*), STIR (*B*), and postcontrast T1-weighted (*C, D*) images of the stifle joint. There is an aggressive primary bone tumor centered on the metaphyseal region of the distal femur that has broken through the cranial cortex (*arrows*). This patient has stifle synovitis with a thickened, contrast-enhancing synovial membrane (*dashed arrows*) and a probable cranial cruciate ligament rupture.

CARPUS

MRI is less commonly used in small joints such as the carpus and tarsus, but as access to high-field MRI increases in the veterinary community and improvements are made in surface coils, more traumatic, neoplastic and chronic foreign body MRI studies are being performed. **Fig. 27** depicts images of a normal carpus.[19]

The patient should be imaged in lateral recumbency with the affected limb downward on the surface coil. For carpal studies, the limb should be in a straight, neutral, non–weight-bearing position similar to positioning for a lateral carpal radiograph. Transverse and dorsal sequences are planned relative to the carpal bones (**Fig. 28**).

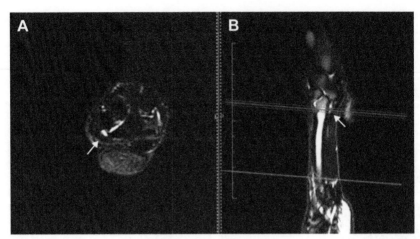

Fig. 27. Transverse STIR (*A*) and sagittal T2-weighted (*B*) images of a normal carpus. The arrow is pointing to the normal, low signal ligament of the accessory carpal bone, which is commonly damaged during hyperextension injuries.

Trauma

Hyperextension carpal injuries are common in athletic and working dogs. The extent of soft tissue trauma sustained in these injuries is grossly underappreciated by other imaging modalities. Additionally, rupture of the ligament of the accessory carpal bone occurs in hyperextension subluxation injuries and can be identified on MRI examination. High STIR or fat-suppressed T2 or PD images will

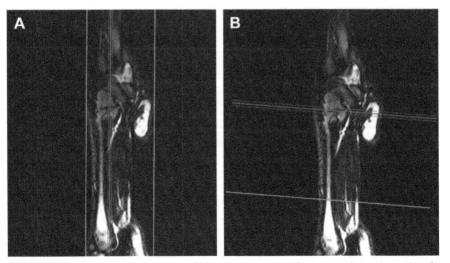

Fig. 28. T2-weighted sagittal images of the carpal joint with proper slice orientation for planning coronal (*A*) and transverse (*B*) images, respectively.

reveal joint effusion and peritendonous fluid accumulation. Lack of visualization of a distinct, continuous low-signal ligament of the accessory carpal bone is diagnostic for rupture of this ligament, as this ligament should be well visualized on sagittal and transverse T1-weighted and T2-weighted images (**Fig. 29**).

Infectious

Fluid-sensitive sequences are well suited for identifying foreign bodies, which are often seen in the foot area, because of a pocket of fluid that accumulates circumferential to the low-signal foreign body (**Fig. 30**).[8] T1-weighted sequences are primarily helpful with anatomic disturbances such as secondary osteomyelitis.

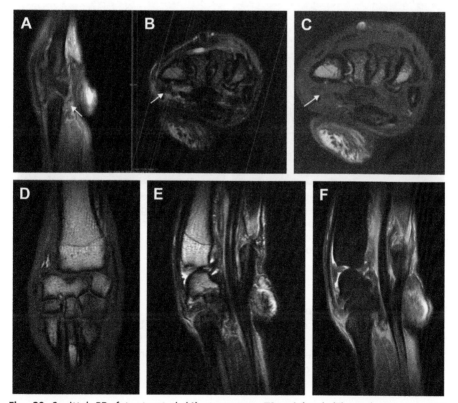

Fig. 29. Sagittal PD fat-saturated (*A*), transverse T2-weighted (*B*), and transverse (*C*) T1-weighted images through the site of the ligament of the accessory carpal bone in a working dog with a hyperextension injury. Note the discontinuity of the ligament of the accessory carpal bone (*arrows*). On the second row of images, dorsal T1-weighted (*D*), sagittal T2-weighted (*E*), and sagittal PD fat-saturated (*F*) images highlight soft tissue edema and peritendinous effusion.

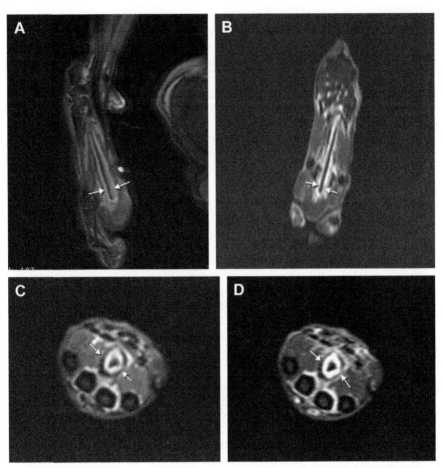

Fig. 30. Sagittal PD fat-saturated (*A*), coronal postcontrast T1-weighted (*B*), PD fat-saturated transverse (*C*), and transverse postcontrast T1-weighted (*D*) images (*left to right, top to bottom*) of a high signal fluid pocket surrounding a low signal, linear foreign body (*arrows*) in the palmar metacarpal region. Contrast is often unnecessary, as fluid-sensitive sequences show the extent of the pathology.

TARSUS

The patient should be imaged in lateral recumbency with the affected limb downward on the surface coil. For tarsal studies, the limb should be in a neutral, non–weight-bearing flexed position similar to positioning for a lateral tarsal radiograph. **Fig. 31** shows images of a normal tarsus.[20] Transverse and dorsal sequences are planned relative to the calcaneal bone (**Fig. 32**).

Osteochondrosis

Tarsal osteochondrosis is historically diagnosed on radiographs and occasionally with the aid of CT studies, but clinicians are beginning to acknowledge the soft tissue component of the disease that has previously been overlooked. In cases of osteochondrosis, extra-articular soft tissue inflammation can cause

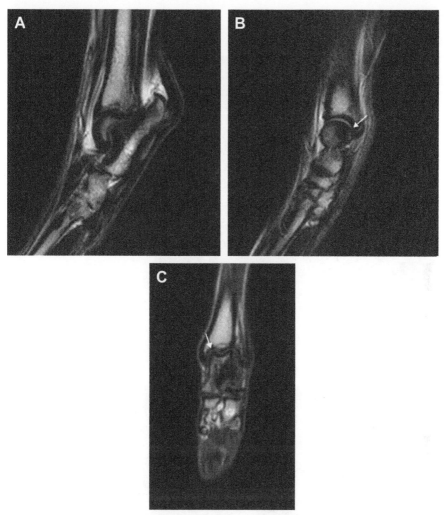

Fig. 31. Dorsal T1-weighted (C) and sagittal T2-weighted (A, B) images of a normal tarsus. The medial trochlear ridge of the talus bone is clearly seen on parasagittal (B) and dorsal (C) images (*arrows*).

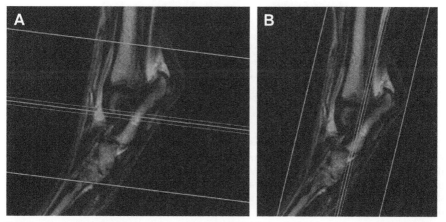

Fig. 32. T2-weighted sagittal images of the tarsus with proper slice orientation for planning transverse (A) and coronal (B) images, respectively.

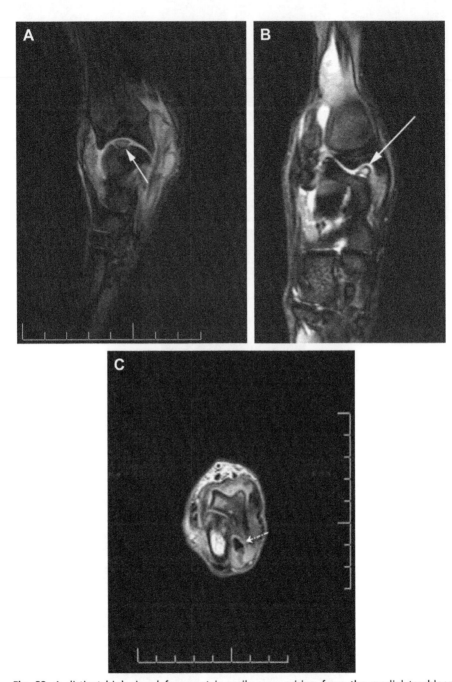

Fig. 33. A distinct high-signal fragment is easily seen arising from the medial trochlear ridge of the talus bone (*A, B*) (*arrow*). Medial joint incongruity is also noted. Impingement of the deep digital flexor tendon (*C*) (*dashed arrow*) with alteration of the normally round shape of the tendon can also occur secondary to joint inflammation from underlying osteochondrosis.

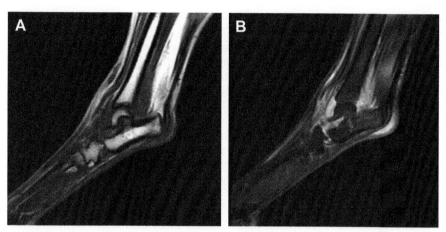

Fig. 34. Sagittal pre- (*A*) and postcontrast (*B*) T1-weighted images of the tarsus in a patient with tarsal trauma. Joint and peritendinous effusion are seen.

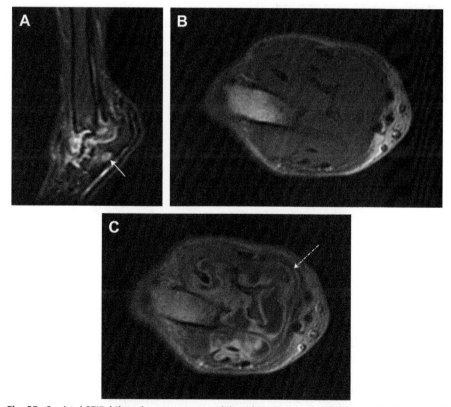

Fig. 35. Sagittal STIR (*A*) and transverse pre- (*B*) and postcontrast (*C*) T1-weighted images of synovial cell sarcoma involving the tarsus. Note the severely thickened, irregular and contrast-enhancing synovial membrane (*dashed arrow*) and the focal calcaneal bone involvement (*arrow*).

impingement of the deep digital flexor tendon along the medial aspect of the calcaneal bone.

MR studies allow clear visualization of the osteochondrosis lesion, incongruity of the joint, and the secondary periarticular inflammatory proliferative soft tissue change that can result in impingement of the deep digital flexor in the region of the sustentaculum tali (**Fig. 33**). These soft tissues changes, secondary to tarsal osteochondrosis, contribute to the patient's lameness.

Trauma

Like the carpus, tarsal trauma is common and often involves the intra-articular, extra-articular, ligamentous, and tendinous soft tissues. Although subluxation injuries and fractures can be evaluated radiographically and with CT examination, the soft tissues are best evaluated with MRI (**Fig. 34**).

Neoplasia

Neoplasia affecting the tarsus and adjacent structures are readily seen on MR studies, as are foreign bodies (**Fig. 35**).

SUMMARY

MRI is particularly valuable in defining normal anatomy and ruling out pathologic conditions and is, therefore, the most comprehensive diagnostic imaging modality of osseous, articular, and soft tissue disease. MRI has changed and will continue to change our understanding of musculoskeletal disease processes and thereby alter treatment options and improve prognosis.

REFERENCES

1. Gavin P, Bagley R. Practical small animal MRI. Ames (IA): Wiley-Blackwell; 2009. p. 233–72. Chapter 3.
2. Schaefer S, Forrest L. Magnetic resonance imaging of the canine shoulder: an anatomic study. Vet Surg 2006;35(8):721–8.
3. Van Bree H, Dingemanse W, Gielen I. MRI and arthroscopy for evaluation of shoulder joint pathology. In: 20th Annual scientific meeting of the European college of veterinary surgeons (ECVS 2011). Ghent (Belgium): Ghent University; July 8, 2011.
4. Agnello K, Puchalski S, Wisner E, et al. Effect of positioning, scan plane, and arthrography on visibility of periarticular canine shoulder soft tissue structures on magnetic resonance images. Vet Radiol Ultrasound 2008;49(6):529–39.
5. Wall C, Cook C, Cook J. Diagnostic sensitivity of radiography, ultrasonography, and magnetic resonance imaging for detecting shoulder osteochondrosis/osteochondritis dissecans in dogs. Vet Radiol Ultrasound 2014;56(1):3–11.
6. Fransson B, Gavin P, Lahmers K. Supraspinatus tendinosis associated with biceps brachii tendon displacement in a dog. J Am Vet Med Assoc 2005;227(9): 1429–33.
7. Murphy S, Ballegeer E, Forrest L, et al. Magnetic resonance imaging findings in dogs with confirmed shoulder pathology. Vet Surg 2008;37(7):631–8.
8. Young B, Klopp L, Albrecht M, et al. Imaging diagnosis: magnetic resonance imaging of a cervical wooden foreign body in a dog. Vet Radiol Ultrasound 2004; 45(6):538–41.

9. Snaps F, Saunders J, Park R, et al. Comparison of spin echo, gradient echo and fat saturation magnetic resonance imaging sequences for imaging the canine elbow. Vet Radiol Ultrasound 1998;39(6):518–23.

10. Snaps F, Ballingand M, Saunders J, et al. Comparison of radiography, magnetic resonance imaging, and surgical findings in dogs with elbow dysplasia. Am J Vet Res 1997;58(12):1367–70.

11. Magnetic resonance arthrography of the cubital joint in dogs affected with fragmented medial coronoid processes. Am J Vet Res 1999;60(2):190–3.

12. Baird D, Hathcock J, Rumph P, et al. Low-field magnetic resonance imaging of the canine stifle joint: normal anatomy. Vet Radiol Ultrasound 1998;39(2):87–97.

13. Banfield CM, Morrison W. Magnetic resonance arthrography of the canine stifle joint technique and applications in eleven military dogs. Vet Radiol Ultrasound 2000;41(3):200–13.

14. Widmer W, Buckwalter K, Braunstein E, et al. Radiographic and magnetic resonance imaging of the stifle joint in experimental osteoarthritis in dogs. Vet Radiol Ultrasound 1994;35(5):371–84.

15. Casale S, McCarthy R. Complications associated with lateral fabellotibial suture surgery for cranial cruciate ligament injury in dogs: 363 cases (1997–2005). J Am Vet Med Assoc 2009;234(2):229–35.

16. Ralphs S, Whitney W. Arthroscopic evaluation of menisci in dogs with cranial cruciate ligament injuries: 100 cases (1999-2000). J Am Vet Med Assoc 2002;221(11):1601–4.

17. Davis GJ, Kapatkin A, Craig L, et al. Comparison of radiography, computed tomography, and magnetic resonance imaging for evaluation of appendicular osteosarcoma in dogs. J Am Vet Med Assoc 2002;220(8):1171–6.

18. Evans P, Gassel A, Huber M. Veterinary medicine today. J Am Vet Med Assoc 2004;224(4):511–2.

19. Nordberg C, Johnson K. Magnetic resonance imaging of normal canine carpal ligaments. Vet Radiol Ultrasound 1999;40(2):128–36.

20. Deruddere K, Milne M, Wilson K, et al. Magnetic resonance imaging, computed tomography, and gross anatomy of the canine tarsus. Vet Surg 2014;43(8):912–9.

Ultrasound Imaging of the Hepatobiliary System and Pancreas

Martha Moon Larson, DVM, MS

KEYWORDS

- Liver • Gallbladder • Bile duct • Pancreas • Obstruction • Neoplasia • Mucocele
- Pancreatitis

KEY POINTS

- The normal and abnormal appearance of the liver is variable and subjective. Interpretation should take into consideration all aspects of the case, using cytology/histopathology for the final diagnosis when appropriate.
- Ultrasound assessment of the biliary system is extremely useful for the diagnosis of obstruction and inflammation.
- The canine pancreas is not a well-visualized organ. Anatomy and adjacent landmarks should be used to find the pancreatic area to search for pancreatic disease.
- The ultrasound appearance of pancreatitis, pancreatic abscess, pancreatic neoplasia, and pseudocyst can all appear similar.

 Video content accompanies this article at http://www.vetsmall.theclinics.com

INTRODUCTION

Ultrasonography is a valuable noninvasive imaging modality for the evaluation of hepatic and biliary disease. Indications for hepatic ultrasound include hepatomegaly, cranial abdominal masses, icterus, ascites, detection of portosystemic shunts, and search for metastases. Ultrasound is commonly used to guide needle placement for fine-needle aspiration and true-cut biopsy.

Normal Ultrasound Appearance of the Liver

The liver is a coarse, moderately echogenic organ located between the diaphragm cranially and stomach and right kidney caudally (**Fig. 1**A, B). The hepatic echogenicity is similar to the cranial pole of the right kidney (can be slightly more or less echogenic)

The author has nothing to disclose.
Department of Small Animal Clinical Sciences, Virginia-Maryland College of Veterinary Medicine, Duckpond Drive, Blacksburg, VA 24061, USA
E-mail address: moonm@vt.edu

Vet Clin Small Anim 46 (2016) 453–480
http://dx.doi.org/10.1016/j.cvsm.2015.12.004   **vetsmall.theclinics.com**

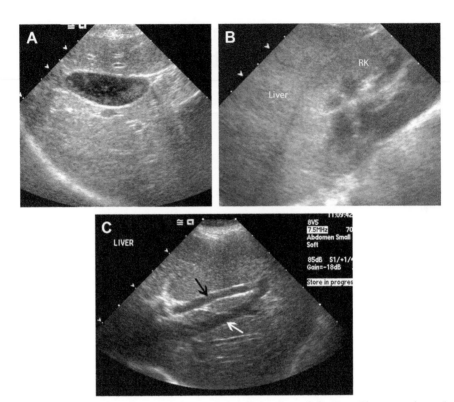

Fig. 1. (*A*) Longitudinal image of the normal right portion of the liver. The parenchyma is coarsely echogenic and broken up only by vessels and gallbladder. (*B*) Cranial pole of the right kidney (RK) is noted in the renal fossa of the caudate liver lobe. The echogenicities of the right renal cortex and liver parenchyma are very similar. (*C*) Transverse image of the left liver. The left portal vein (*black arrow*) extends toward the hepatic periphery. The left hepatic vein (*white arrow*) is located more dorsally.

and hypoechoic to the spleen. Normal cats can deposit large amounts of fat in the renal cortex, which can result in an apparent hypoechoic liver.[1] Alternatively, obese cats can have a moderately hyperechoic liver without pathologic hepatic lipidosis.[2–4] Because assessment of echogenicity is highly subjective, mild changes should be considered with caution, and correlated with serum chemistries, signalment, and clinical signs.

Hepatic size is also a subjective assessment. With microhepatia, the gallbladder may appear large relative to hepatic volume, and cranial displacement of the stomach limits the imaging window. An enlarged liver may extend well beyond the rib cage, often with rounded margins. Hepatic and portal veins course through the hepatic parenchyma; portal veins are characterized by their more echogenic margins, with color Doppler flow toward the hepatic periphery (potentially toward the transducer). Hepatic veins (less echogenic margins) extend toward the hilus and caudal vena cava (usually away from the transducer) (**Fig. 1C**). The caudal vena cava travels through the dorsal aspect of liver, with the portal vein located immediately ventral. At the hepatic hilus, the portal vein branches into a larger left and smaller right branch.

Normal Ultrasound Appearance of the Gallbladder and Bile Duct

The gallbladder is a round/ovoid structure, located ventrally and to the right of midline. A duplicate or septated gallbladder is occasionally seen as a normal variation in cats and is caused by an abnormality in embryonic development (**Fig. 2**).[5] Normal gallbladder wall thickness in cats is less than 1 mm, with slightly greater thickness (1–2 mm) noted in normal dogs.[6,7] Gallbladder volume can be measured using the ellipsoid formula (length × width × height × 0.52).[8,9] Normal gallbladder volume in dogs is less than or equal to 1 mL/kg body weight. In cats, approximate normal gallbladder volume is 2.4 mL (no association between body weight and volume).[8,9] The gall bladder is normally filled with anechoic bile but frequently contains sludge (mobile, dependent, echogenic, nonshadowing sediment) (**Fig. 3**). The significance of biliary sludge is uncertain and is present within the lumen in normal dogs.[10] However, a more recent report indicates that the presence of sludge may indicate dysmotility of the gallbladder and cholestasis.[11]

In normal dogs, the common bile duct is not consistently visualized; if seen, it should be less than 3 mm in diameter.[8,12] In the cat, the common bile duct is identified immediately ventral to the portal vein as an anechoic tubular structure surrounded by hyperechoic fat and can be followed to the duodenal papilla (**Fig. 4**). Normal diameter in the cat is 4 mm or less.[13] Intrahepatic bile ducts are not visible unless pathologically dilated.

Ultrasound Appearance of the Abnormal Liver

Diffuse disease

The ultrasound appearance of diffuse hepatic disease is characterized by changes in size, shape, and echogenicity. However, as noted earlier, assessment of these characteristics is inherently subjective. Caution must be used in the diagnosis of diffuse liver disease based solely on the ultrasonographic appearance.[14] As a result, ultrasonography is less valuable for recognizing or differentiating diffuse liver disease, and a biopsy is almost always necessary for diagnosis.

When visible, a hyperechoic liver parenchyma results in an abnormal echogenicity of liver compared with adjacent organs (hyperechoic to renal cortex, isoechoic or

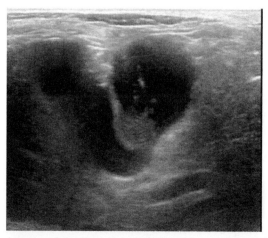

Fig. 2. Longitudinal image of the liver of a normal cat. Two ovoid anechoic structures are noted representing a bilobed gallbladder.

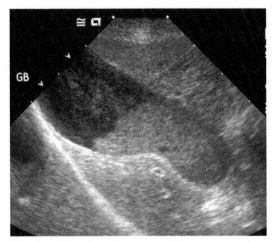

Fig. 3. Longitudinal image of the right liver and gallbladder. A moderate amount of echogenic, nonshadowing biliary sludge is located in the dependent portion of the gallbladder lumen.

hyperechoic to spleen), loss of visualization of the prominent periportal echoes, and increased attenuation of sound as it passes through the hyperechoic liver (**Fig. 5**). A lower frequency than expected may be needed for adequate organ penetration.

Hyperechoic hepatic parenchyma
- Vacuolar hepatopathy
  - Hepatic lipidosis
  - Steroid hepatopathy
- Chronic hepatitis
  - Cholangiohepatitis
  - Cirrhosis
- Neoplasia (variable)
  - Mast cell tumor
  - Lymphosarcoma

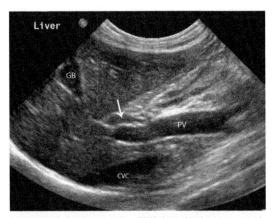

Fig. 4. Longitudinal image of the liver and gallbladder (GB) in a normal cat. The portal vein (PV) lies ventral to the caudal vena cava (CVC). The bile duct (*arrow*) is a linear anechoic structure identified immediately dorsal to the portal vein.

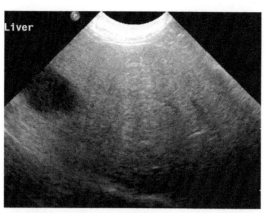

Fig. 5. Longitudinal image of the liver and gallbladder in a dog with a hyperechoic liver secondary to steroid hepatopathy. The normally prominent portal markings are not visible, and the deeper portions of the liver are attenuated. The liver has a very dense, uniform parenchymal texture, similar to the spleen.

Hepatic lipidosis is the most common hepatic disease in the cat. The liver is typically hyperechoic to adjacent falciform fat and enlarged. As noted earlier, in some obese cats, the liver is hyperechoic to falciform fat, without disease present. The calculated accuracy of ultrasound in the diagnosis of hepatic lipidosis was only approximately 70% in one study.[14] Steroid hepatopathy secondary to hyperadrenocorticism or iatrogenic corticosteroid administration may cause a hyperechoic liver, either uniformly hyperechoic or hyperechoic parenchyma with poorly defined hypoechoic nodules.

Chronic hepatitis or cirrhosis commonly results in hyperechogenicity secondary to fibrosis.[15] The liver size may be normal to small with irregular margins secondary to hypoechoic regenerative nodules. Ascites may be present. Hepatic parenchyma in cats with cholangitis/cholangiohepatitis complex (CCHC) may be normal, hyperechoic, hypoechoic, or heterogeneous, either enlarged or normal size.[8,16,17] Biliary abnormalities typically accompany this disease (see section on Ultrasound Appearance of Biliary Disease).

Some diffuse hepatic diseases result in a mottled liver and hyperechoic background with poorly defined hypoechoic nodules (**Fig. 6**).[14]

- Chronic hepatitis
- Vacuolar hepatopathy
- Nodular hyperplasia
- Fibrosis
- Toxic hepatopathy
- Storage diseases
- Combination of more than one disease

Decreased hepatic echogenicity
Decreased hepatic echogenicity is suspected when portal vein markings have increased prominence and the liver is hypoechoic to the right renal cortex (**Fig. 7**). Diseases resulting in hypoechoic hepatic parenchyma are less common.[15]

- Acute suppurative hepatitis
- Lymphosarcoma

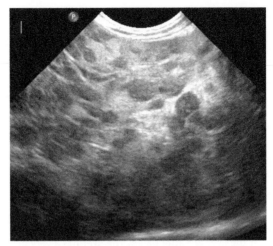

Fig. 6. Longitudinal image of the liver in a dog with diabetes mellitus. The liver is mottled, with a hyperechoic background and diffuse hypoechoic nodules. Vacuolar hepatopathy was diagnosed on fine-needle aspiration.

- Leukemia
- Amyloidosis

Focal disease

Hepatic nodules or masses may be isoechoic, hyperechoic, hypoechoic, mixed echogenicity, cavitated, gas containing, or cystic. Target lesions (nodules with hypoechoic rim and hyperechoic center) are more often associated with malignant disease (**Fig. 8**).[18]

Focal disease:
- Nodular hyperplasia
- Primary or metastatic neoplasia
- Abscess

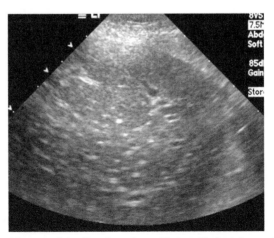

Fig. 7. Longitudinal image of the liver in a dog with hepatic lymphoma. The liver is hypoechoic, with very prominent portal vein markings.

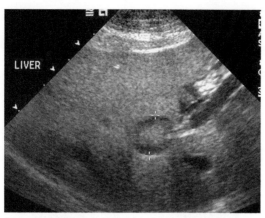

Fig. 8. Longitudinal image of the liver in a cat with pancreatic carcinoma. A target lesion (nodule with hypoechoic rim and hyperechoic center) representing a metastatic nodule is present (*between calipers*).

- Hematoma
- Cyst
- Cystadenoma
- Hepatocutaneous syndrome (superficial necrolytic dermatitis)

Nodular hyperplasia can be of any echogenicity and, although more often a focal nodule, can be quite large and even cavitated.[19,20] Nodular hyperplasia is a differential for every focal hepatic disease. Metastatic neoplasia is the most common form of hepatic neoplasia in the dog and typically originates from the pancreas, spleen, and gastrointestinal (GI) tract.[21] Metastatic lesions may be hyperechoic, hypoechoic, or mixed echogenicity and cannot be reliably differentiated from primary hepatic neoplasia (see **Fig. 8**).[22–24] Primary tumors can be solitary masses, multifocal, or diffuse coalescing nodular disease (**Fig. 9**).[21–24] Hepatocellular carcinoma is the most common primary malignant tumor in the canine liver; other differentials include cholangiocarcinoma, lymphosarcoma, hemangiosarcoma, leiomyosarcoma, and fibrosarcoma. Mast cell tumor may appear normal despite diffuse infiltration; diffuse nodular disease may also be present.[25] Cystadenoma, a benign cystic focal or multifocal hepatic tumor, is the most common form of hepatic neoplasia in cats (**Fig. 10**).[26,27] Cholangiocarcinoma is the most frequent malignant form. There are no individual distinguishing features that allow an ultrasound diagnosis of a specific form of neoplasia. Cytology and histopathology are necessary for a definitive diagnosis.[28]

Abscesses and hematomas have a variable appearance depending on age.[29–31] Abscesses may be hypoechoic nodules or thick-walled cavitated masses containing fluid or gas (resulting in echogenic interfaces with acoustic shadowing and reverberation artifact) (**Fig. 11**, Video 1). Hematomas can appear similar to abscesses, although usually do not contain gas. Hepatic cysts are relatively common and usually considered incidental findings (although may be associated with polycystic kidney disease). They are characterized by thin, well-defined walls and anechoic contents with acoustic enhancement. Hepatocutaneous syndrome (superficial necrolytic dermatitis) has been reported in both dogs and cats and results in variably sized hypoechoic nodules surrounded by hyperechoic hepatic parenchyma. This formation creates a

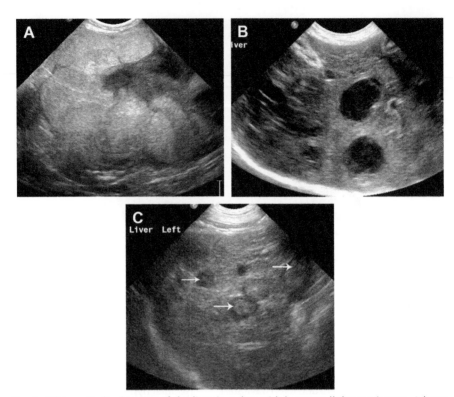

Fig. 9. (*A*) Longitudinal image of the liver in a dog with hepatocellular carcinoma. A large, irregularly marginated hyperechoic mass occupies most of the liver lobe. (*B*) Longitudinal image of the liver in a dog with hepatic hemangiosarcoma. Multiple cavitated masses are present. (*C*) Longitudinal image of the left liver in a dog with diffuse mast cell tumor. Multiple hypoechoic nodules (some with target appearance) are noted (*arrows*).

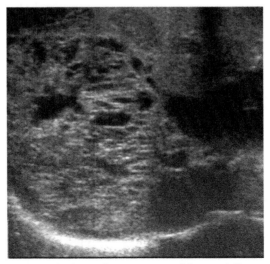

Fig. 10. Large cystic mass in the liver of a cat presented for renal disease. The cystadenoma was an incidental finding on abdominal ultrasound examination.

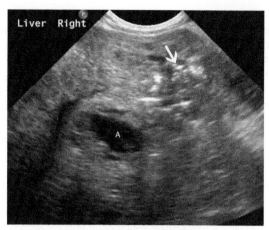

Fig. 11. Longitudinal image of the right liver in a dog with hepatic abscess. A thick-walled cavitated abscess (A) is noted adjacent to an additional area of abscess containing gas with multiple hyperechoic foci (*arrow*).

honeycomb appearance and is seen in conjunction with characteristic dermal lesions **(Fig. 12)**.[32,33]

Ultrasound Appearance of Biliary Disease

Ultrasound is extremely useful in the diagnosis of diseases of the biliary system and can be used to detect structural abnormalities of the gallbladder, abnormal contents (choleliths, choledocoliths, abnormal accumulation of sludge), inflammation, obstruction, and neoplasia.

Gallbladder wall thickening is a nonspecific abnormality and may be secondary to primary gallbladder disease or systemic disease with secondary gallbladder effects.[8,12,34,35] Wall thickening may have a layered appearance, with a central hypoechoic layer surrounded by more echoic layers creating an onionskin appearance, or be diffusely irregular and hyperechoic.

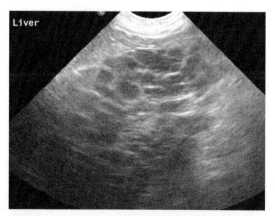

Fig. 12. Transverse image of a dog with hepatocutaneous syndrome. Hypoechoic nodules are distributed throughout the hepatic parenchyma creating a honeycomb appearance.

- Inflammatory disease
  - Cholangitis, cholecystitis, adjacent inflammation (hepatitis, pancreatitis)
- Cystic mucinous hyperplasia
- Systemic disease
  - Right-sided congestive heart failure
  - Hypoproteinemia
  - Portal hypertension
  - Anaphylaxis

Cholangiohepatitis and cholecystitis are primary inflammatory diseases of the gallbladder that may result in hyperechoic, irregular wall thickening (**Fig. 13**). Echogenic foci with reverberation artifact representing gas in the gallbladder wall are present with emphysematous cholecystitis. Adjacent inflammation, such as hepatitis and pancreatitis, can also cause gallbladder wall thickening. Systemic diseases, including right-sided congestive heart failure, hypoproteinemia, portal hypertension, and anaphylaxis, can cause gallbladder wall edema and thickening (**Fig. 14A**). Cystic mucinous hyperplasia is characterized by a hyperplastic gallbladder epithelium with cystic accumulations of mucus and papillary projections into the gallbladder lumen and appears as sessile or polypoid masses along a variably thickened gallbladder wall (**Fig. 14B**).[8,36] The clinical significance of cystic mucinous hyperplasia is unknown but may be a predisposing factor in the development of gallbladder mucocele; cystic mucinous hyperplasia has been documented as an incidental finding at necropsy.[37] Focal wall thickening may be seen with neoplasia (adenomas, adenocarcinoma), cystic mucinous hyperplasia, and cholecystitis. Occasionally small volumes of anechoic peritoneal effusion surround the gallbladder, mimicking wall thickening.

Biliary sludge is a common finding in asymptomatic dogs with a prevalence of 53% (see **Fig. 3**).[10] Biliary sludge has been found in 35% to 48% of dogs irrespective of health status.[38,39] A recent study reported that dogs with biliary sludge have decreased gallbladder emptying when compared with dogs without biliary sludge.[11] It is hypothesized that biliary stasis and biliary sludge lead to further inspissation of bile and accumulation of mucus forming a gallbladder mucocele.[8,40,41]

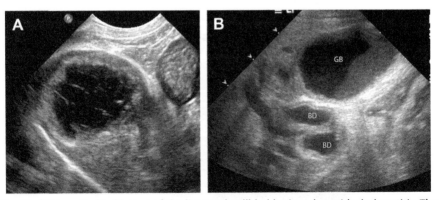

Fig. 13. (*A*) Longitudinal image of the liver and gallbladder in a dog with cholecystitis. The gallbladder wall is thickened and irregular. (*B*) Transverse image of the liver and gallbladder in a cat with cholangitis/cholangiohepatitis. The gallbladder (GB) wall is thickened (>1 mm) and irregular. Sludge is noted in the gallbladder lumen. The bile duct (BD) is tortuous, thickened, and dilated.

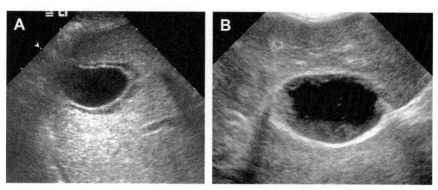

Fig. 14. (*A*) Longitudinal image of the gallbladder in a dog with hypoproteinemia and ascites. The gallbladder wall is thickened, with a double-layered appearance. (*B*) Transverse image of the gallbladder in a dog with cystic mucinous hyperplasia. The gallbladder wall is irregularly thickened and is likely an incidental finding in this older dog.

Choleliths (stones within the gallbladder) and choledocholiths (stones within the bile duct and peripheral ducts) are occasionally seen in both dogs and cats. Choleliths are most often incidental findings, although they have the potential to result in biliary obstruction or may arise secondary to inflammation and biliary stasis. Cholangiohepatitis is often associated with feline cholelithiasis and may be a predisposing factor in the pathogenesis.[42] Choleliths appear hyperechoic, often with acoustic shadowing, and are usually mobile. Stones within the bile ducts are less common and may be present more often in cats in association with CCHC (**Fig. 15**). Choledocholiths are a relatively common cause of extrahepatic biliary obstruction in cats, usually located in the distal bile duct, close to or into the duodenal papilla.[43]

Gallbladder mucoceles are an accumulation of gelatinous to semisolid mucus and inspissated bile distending the gallbladder lumen and are currently the most clinically significant gallbladder disease in dogs.[41,44–47] Mucoceles are diagnosed when the gall bladder is distended by excessive amounts of echogenic, centralized, non-mobile sludge. Echogenic striations extend to the periphery (**Fig. 16**). Bile duct dilation may

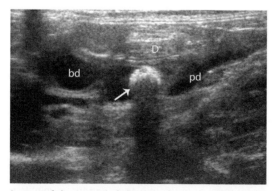

Fig. 15. Transverse image of the cranial abdomen of a cat presenting for icterus and vomiting. An obstructing echogenic choledocholith (*arrow*) with distal shadowing is identified in the lumen of the dilated bile duct (bd) at the level of the duodenal papilla. The pancreatic duct (pd) is also obstructed and dilated. D, duodenum.

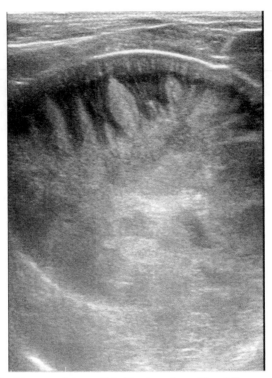

Fig. 16. Longitudinal image of the gallbladder in a dog with a biliary mucocele. A centralized echogenic accumulation of non-dependent biliary sludge, with peripheral echogenic striations is present. The gallbladder wall is thickened.

occur because of obstruction from inspissated bile. Gallbladder distension may result in pressure necrosis of the wall and subsequent rupture. Signs of gallbladder rupture include discontinuity of the gallbladder wall, focal free fluid, and adjacent hyperechoic mesentery (**Fig. 17**). Rupture may be present without ultrasound changes.[41,44,48] Because of fewer mucus-secreting glands in the feline gallbladder, biliary mucoceles in cats are considered less common.[43,49]

CCHC is the second most common form of hepatic disease in cats and the most common inflammatory disease.[8,50] In many cases, no ultrasound abnormalities are present. However, when present, ultrasound findings include thickened gallbladder wall (often with a palisade type mucosal irregularity), biliary sludge (within gallbladder or bile duct), choleliths or choledocholiths, and thickened, tortuous, and sometimes dilated bile duct (see **Figs. 13**B and **15**; **Fig. 18**A).[8,16,17,42,51,52]

Gallbladder dysmotility (biliary dyskinesia) has recently been reported in dogs and has been associated with gallbladder mucoceles, cholelithiasis, biliary sludge, hyperadrenocorticism, hypothyroidism, and dyslipidemias.[8,11,45] Gallbladder motility studies can be performed using various protocols that assess gallbladder emptying. After a 12-hour fast, gallbladder volume is measured (gallbladder length × height × width × 0.52). One and 2 hours after a meal or prokinetic agent (erythromycin) is administered, gallbladder volume is reassessed. Gallbladder volume should be less than 1 mL/kg or have a greater than 25% reduction in gallbladder volume (ejection fraction). If gallbladder volume or ejection fraction is abnormal, gallbladder dysmotility is assumed.[8,9]

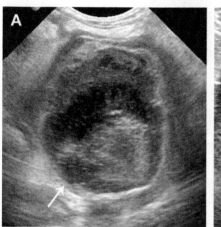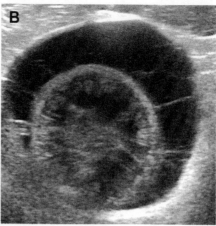

Fig. 17. (*A*) Longitudinal image of the gallbladder in a dog with a mucocele and gallbladder wall rupture. Centralized nondependent biliary sludge is noted. The gallbladder wall is thickened but is poorly visualized in the craniodorsal aspect (*arrow*). Hyperechoic fat is noted surrounding the gallbladder consistent with adjacent inflammation and focal peritonitis. (*B*) Longitudinal image of the gallbladder in a dog presented for elevated liver enzymes. A characteristic gallbladder mucocele is surrounded by well-defined and contained anechoic fluid. A ruptured gallbladder that was completely sealed off by omentum was noted at surgery.

Extrahepatic biliary obstruction results in a retrograde dilation of the biliary system.[53] With complete obstruction, the gall bladder and cystic duct distend within 24 hours, with progressive dilation of the common bile duct within 48 hours. It should be noted that gallbladder distension may be minimal in the face of chronic cholecystitis or hepatic inflammation.[8] Progressive dilation of the common bile duct and hepatic ducts occur during the next 3 to 4 days, with dilation of lobar and interlobar ducts seen by 7 days (see **Figs. 13**B and **18**; **Fig. 19**, Video 2). Multiple tortuous, irregularly branching anechoic tracks (without Doppler signal) are noted. The most common causes of obstruction in the dog include pancreatitis, neoplasia in the adjacent pancreas, duodenum, bile duct, or liver, and sludge associated with biliary mucocele. In the cat, tumors and inflammation of the common bile duct, pancreas, and duodenum, along with choledocholithiasis, are more commonly noted.[43] In a study of 30 cats with extrahepatic biliary obstruction, 97% had a bile duct diameter greater than 5 mm, with the degree of dilation mostly influenced by the duration of obstruction.[43] Gallbladder dilation was noted in only 43% and, thus, is not a reliable indication of obstruction.[43] Sludge accumulation within the bile duct associated with cholangiohepatitis and causing extrahepatic biliary obstruction is not easily differentiated from a neoplastic mass in the bile duct (see **Fig. 19**). It is important to note that incomplete or early obstruction may not cause visible biliary dilation. In addition, bile duct dilation may be persistent, even after resolution of the obstruction.

Contrast-Enhanced Ultrasound Evaluation of the Liver

Contrast-enhanced ultrasound (using microbubble contrast agents) has been used for the improved detection and evaluation of focal liver nodules and the differentiation of benign from malignant disease.[54–57] Both blood pool agents that stay within the intravascular space (such as SonoVue [sulphur hexafluoride microbubbles] and Definity [perflutren lipid microsphere]) and other agents that have a true parenchymal phase

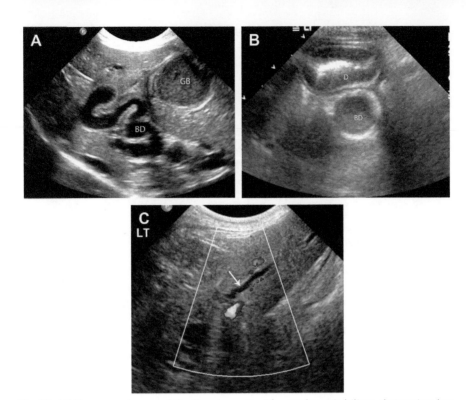

Fig. 18. (*A*) Transverse image of the liver in a cat with extrahepatic biliary obstruction (secondary to sludge accumulation). The bile duct (BD) is dilated (>4 mm), thickened, and tortuous. Much sludge is noted in the gallbladder (GB). (*B*) Transverse right lateral intercostal image of the proximal duodenum (D) of a dog presenting for vomiting and icterus. The BD is markedly dilated (1 cm) as it approaches the duodenum. A focal pancreatic carcinoma obstructed the duodenal papilla resulting in extrahepatic biliary obstruction. (*C*) Dilated intrahepatic bile ducts develop with prolonged complete biliary obstruction. A dilated intrahepatic duct (*arrow*) is confirmed by the absence of a color Doppler signal.

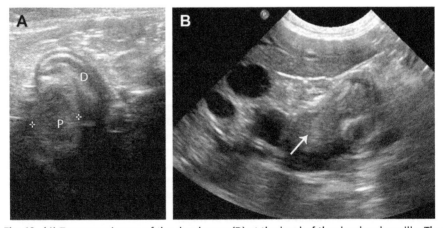

Fig. 19. (*A*) Transverse image of the duodenum (D) at the level of the duodenal papilla. The terminal portion of the bile duct (*marked by calipers*) is distended with an echogenic plug (P) of inspissated bile resulting in obstruction. (*B*) Longitudinal image of a dilated, tortuous bile duct in a cat with biliary obstruction. A large plug of echogenic material is noted in the terminal portion of the bile duct (*arrow*). This material was diagnosed as a biliary carcinoma at surgery. Inspissated bile and neoplastic masses are not easily differentiated on ultrasound.

due to phagocytosis of the contrast agent by the reticuloendothelial system (such as Sonozoid [perflubutane]) have been described for this use. Malignant nodules are typically hypoechoic to surrounding, uniformly enhanced liver parenchyma during peak enhancement (portal phase or parenchymal phase). Benign nodules are typically iso-echoic to surrounding enhanced parenchyma. In one study, these findings correlated with malignancy with a sensitivity of 93.8%, specificity of 100%, and a positive predictive value of 100%.[54] However, some benign tumors can demonstrate contrast findings of malignancy; a definitive diagnosis still requires a biopsy with cytopathologic or histopathologic evaluation.

Elastography

Elastography uses ultrasound to evaluate the elasticity of tissues (relative compressibility) and has been used in the identification of neoplastic and fibrotic lesions in humans.[58–60] Stiffness of tissue is inversely proportional to elasticity (or deformation). Elasticity can be measured by comparing compressibility of adjacent tissues in the ultrasound window using a superimposed color map that represents relative stiffness (strain imaging). Alternatively, stiffness can be more quantitatively assessed using measurement of a shear wave velocity within the tissue of interest (shear wave elastography). There are several limitations to shear wave elastography in veterinary practice, including variables introduced by depth of tissue, patient weight, and sex. In addition, patient motion is a significant limitation and results in unreliable shear wave velocity measurements. Additional studies of elastography in veterinary patients will provide a better assessment of feasibility.

PANCREAS

Ultrasound imaging of the canine and feline pancreas is an important noninvasive tool in the diagnosis of pancreatic disease. The ultrasound appearance of the pancreas is less conspicuous than other abdominal organs, such as the kidney or spleen. The pancreas can be visualized in many dogs and most cats, but the anatomic landmarks are essential in defining the pancreatic area.

Anatomy

In both dogs and cats, the pancreas is divided into the right and left limbs, joined at the body. In the dog, the right limb is the easiest to identify, located dorsomedial to the descending duodenum, ventral to the right kidney, and medial to the ascending colon. In dogs with a deep chested conformation, a right lateral intercostal window is extremely helpful (**Fig. 20**A, B, F). The duodenum and adjacent right pancreatic limb can be located in the dorsal aspect of the 10th to 12th intercostal space and followed caudally, either in transverse or longitudinal planes. The anatomy of the feline right pancreatic limb is similar; although the pancreas is much more conspicuous in the cat than the dog, the right limb is typically less well visualized than the left (**Fig. 21**A). The pancreatic body (both canine and feline) lies immediately caudal and dorsal to the pyloroduodenal junction, ventral to the portal vein, and medial to the proximal duodenum (**Fig. 20**C). The left limb in the dog lies dorsal and caudal to the body of the stomach, cranial to the transverse colon. It follows the course of the splenic vein as it travels from the splenic hilus medially to the portal vein at the level of the pancreatic body (**Fig. 20**D, E). The canine left limb is more difficult to consistently visualize because of shadowing and reverberation artifact from gas in the stomach and transverse colon. It is much easier to visualize in the cat and is consistently

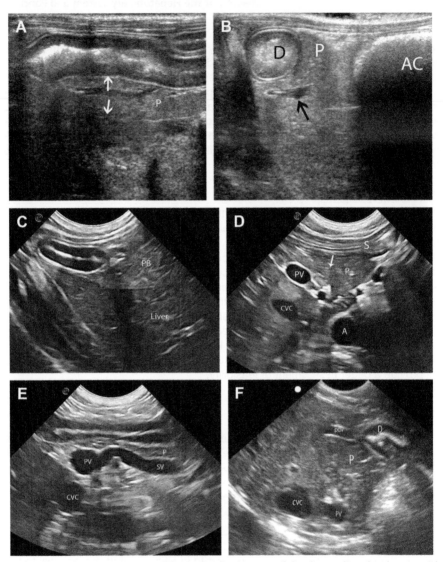

Fig. 20. Normal canine pancreas. (*A*) Longitudinal image of the descending duodenum with the right pancreatic limb (P) noted dorsally between arrows. The pancreaticoduodenal vein is an anechoic vessel coursing through the right pancreatic limb. (*B*) Transverse image of the descending duodenum (D) with the right pancreatic limb (P) located medially. The ascending colon (AC) is noted medial to the pancreas. Arrow denotes pancreaticoduodenal vein. (*C*) Longitudinal image of the proximal aspect of the descending duodenum just after it leaves the pylorus. The pancreatic body (PB) is located medially. (*D*) Longitudinal image of the left pancreatic limb (transducer is oriented transverse to the patient). The stomach (S) is just ventral to the left pancreas (P), with the portal vein (PV) noted just dorsal. The caudal vena cava (CVC) and aorta (A) are located dorsal and to the left of the portal vein. The white arrow indicates the pancreatic duct. (*E*) Same ultrasound window but located slightly more caudal. The splenic vein (SV) is identified coursing toward the right, into the portal vein (PV). The left pancreas (P) is located just ventral to the splenic vein. The caudal vena cava (CVC) is located dorsal to the portal vein. (*F*) Right lateral intercostal window illustrating the pancreas (P) located medial to the duodenum (D). The pancreaticoduodenal vein (pdv) is noted within the pancreatic parenchyma. The caudal vena cava (CVC) and portal vein (PV) are located to the left and dorsal.

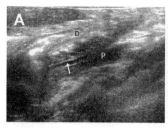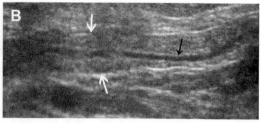

Fig. 21. Normal feline pancreas. (*A*) Longitudinal image of the right limb of the pancreas (P) located just dorsal to the descending duodenum (D). The white arrow notes pancreatic duct. (*B*) Longitudinal image of the left limb of the pancreas (*white arrows*). The pancreatic duct is noted by the black arrow. The transducer is oriented transverse to the patient.

identified caudal to the gastric body, extending toward the spleen and left kidney (**Fig. 21**B).

Normal Appearance

The pancreas is isoechoic or slightly hypoechoic to surrounding mesentery and liver and, in the dog, may have indistinct margins (see **Fig. 20**). The pancreatic parenchyma often has a uniform, homogeneous appearance; but a heterogeneous appearance, with hyperechoic foci, is also common in normal dogs.[61–63] The pancreaticoduodenal vein extends through the right limb, coursing caudally in an undulating fashion, parallel to the descending duodenum. This position creates a helpful landmark to identify the right pancreatic area in the dog but is less conspicuous in the cat. The pancreatic duct can be visualized as an anechoic tubular structure with highly echogenic walls (see **Fig. 21**). The duct is very prominent in the feline pancreas but is not as easily seen in the dog. The reported normal thickness of the canine pancreas depends on the study and may be up to 3 cm in thickness. One large study reported the upper limit of normal thickness as 1.6 cm (3.5 mm–16.0 mm) or about 1.0 cm in medium-sized dogs (15–30 kg).[62] The mean diameter of the pancreatic duct is reported to be 0.8 mm in medium-sized dogs, with a range of 0.1 to 1.2 mm in all dogs.[62] Normal ranges for the feline pancreatic body and left limb width are 0.3 to 1.0 cm, with a mean of approximately 5.0 mm. The right limb is smaller, at 0.3 to 0.6 cm. The pancreatic duct diameter ranges from 0.7 to 2.5 mm, with a mean of about 1.0 mm.[64,65] There is a slight increase in pancreatic duct diameter with increasing age.[65,66]

Ultrasound Appearance of Pancreatic Disease

The diagnosis of pancreatic disease is based on a combination of imaging and clinicopathological findings. The ultrasound appearance of various pancreatic diseases overlaps; in some cases no changes are visible despite histologic pancreatic disease. Histopathology of the pancreas is considered the gold standard, but is not feasible in most patients. Multiple pancreatic samples are required for a reliable diagnosis because of potentially very localized disease. Serum-specific canine pancreatic lipase (cPL) and feline pancreatic lipase (fPL) are generally considered the most specific noninvasive tests for pancreatitis in the dog and cat.[67]

Acute Pancreatitis: Canine

Inflammation, edema, necrosis, and hemorrhage associated with acute pancreatitis result in an enlarged, irregularly marginated, hypoechoic pancreas in the dog (**Fig. 22**, Video 3). The affected areas may be diffuse or very focal. Peripancreatic

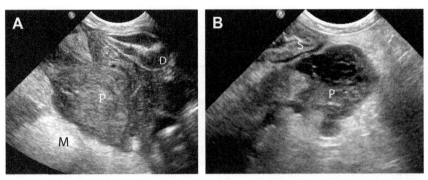

Fig. 22. Canine pancreatitis. (*A*) Acute pancreatitis in the right limb of a dog. The pancreas (P) is enlarged, hypoechoic, with irregular margins. The adjacent mesentery (M) is hyperechoic, consistent for focal steatitis. D, duodenum. (*B*) Acute pancreatitis in the left limb of a dog. The pancreas (P) is enlarged and hypoechoic, and surrounded by hyperechoic mesentery. S, stomach.

steatitis and fat necrosis results in surrounding hyperechoic mesentery with or without fluid accumulation. The descending duodenum may be thickened with poor definition of wall layers, fluid-filled and nonmotile, or corrugated secondary to duodenitis. Focal peritoneal effusion may be present. Pancreatitis is a common cause of extrahepatic biliary obstruction; fibrosis, edema, and inflammation of the bile duct can occur as it extends through the inflamed pancreatic parenchyma.

Chronic Pancreatitis: Canine

Chronic pancreatitis seems to be relatively common in the dog, with postmortem studies indicating an incidence as high as 34% and 65%.[68,69] Chronic pancreatitis can be subclinical or result in chronic, intermittent GI signs. The role of ultrasound in the diagnosis of chronic pancreatitis is unknown. In many cases of histologically proven chronic pancreatitis, there are no ultrasound changes. A small, irregular, mixed echogenic pancreas, nodular echotexture, hyperechoic foci (possibly due to mineralization, fat, or fibrosis) or diffuse hyperechogenicity may suggest chronic disease (**Fig. 23**).[61,63,68–71] A hyperechoic pancreas due to normal aging changes in humans does not seem to happen in dogs. In one study, only 7% (5 of 74) of normal dogs had a hyperechoic pancreatic parenchyma; there was no association between pancreatic echogenicity, age, or body condition score.[61] In another study, chronic pancreatitis was induced in dogs by pancreatic duct ligation. After 12 weeks, the mean pancreatic echogenicity increased significantly because of fibrous tissue and fat replacement of atrophied exocrine pancreatic tissue.[72] There seems to be a correlation between pancreatic hyperechogenicity and hyperadrenocorticism.[61] A hyperechoic pancreas was noted in 40% (37 of 92) dogs with hyperadrenocorticism. This finding may be due to subclinical pancreatitis (elevated cPL has been noted in dogs with hyperadrenocorticism with no signs of pancreatitis[73]), benign fat deposition, or possibly mineralization.

Feline Pancreatitis

Feline pancreatitis may result in an enlarged (thickened), hypoechoic, hyperechoic, or mixed echogenic pancreas with irregular or scalloped margins (**Fig. 24**). The surrounding mesentery may become hyperechoic because of focal steatitis, with fluid accumulation secondary to focal peritonitis.[53,74–78] Ultrasound imaging of the feline pancreas

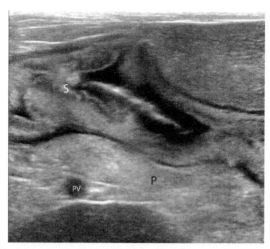

Fig. 23. Longitudinal image of the left pancreatic limb (transverse to the patient). The pancreas (P) is uniformly hyperechoic, which can be seen with chronic pancreatitis. PV, portal vein; S, stomach.

lacks the specificity to differentiate chronic and acute forms of the disease; in many cases, feline chronic pancreatitis has no ultrasound changes at all or the changes are so subtle that they cannot be identified.[76,77,79] Agreement between ultrasonography and lipase assays in cats with suspicion of pancreatitis is only slight to fair,[76] which may be due to false-positive ultrasound results in cats with previous pancreatitis and persistent ultrasound changes but normal lipase assays.[76] Silent chronic pancreatitis without enzyme release but with sufficient ultrasonographic change could also cause a false-positive result.[76] Finally, there may be insufficient changes in acoustic impedance between normal and abnormal pancreas to allow an ultrasound diagnosis of pancreatitis.[76]

Pancreatitis in cats is frequently accompanied by diseases in other organs, including hepatic lipidosis, inflammatory liver disease, bile duct obstruction, inflammatory bowel disease, and diabetes mellitus.[80,81] Pancreatitis (based on serum markers

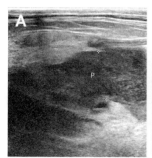
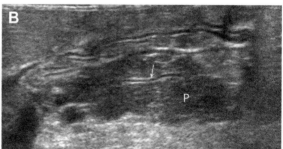

Fig. 24. Feline pancreatitis. (*A*) The left pancreatic limb (P) is markedly thickened, hypoechoic, and irregular. Surrounding mesentery is hyperechoic. This cat had acute onset of clinical signs; ultrasound changes are consistent with acute, severe pancreatitis. (*B*) The left pancreatic limb (P) is thickened and hypoechoic, with irregular margins. These changes are consistent with feline pancreatitis but do not appear as severe or acute as the cat in (*A*). Pancreatic duct is noted by the arrow.

and ultrasound changes) seems to be common in cats at the time of diagnosis of diabetes, and an additional cohort of diabetic cats might develop pancreatitis during the next 6 months.[81] The pancreatitis in these cats was subclinical. It is important to do a complete ultrasound examination in any cat suspected of having pancreatitis.

Pancreatic Edema

Hypoechoic/anechoic fissures running through the pancreatic parenchyma, outlining and separating individual pancreatic lobules, are seen with pancreatic edema (**Fig. 25**). Edema often occurs with pancreatitis but can also occur secondary to nonpancreatic disease, such as hypoalbuminemia and portal hypertension.[82]

Focal Pancreatic Disease

Pancreatic pseudocyst

Pancreatic pseudocysts are focal collections of pancreatic enzymes, blood, and products of tissue digestion contained within a nonepithelialized fibrous sac and are a potential sequela to pancreatitis in both dogs and cats.[63,83,84] Pseudocysts appear generally hypoechoic or anechoic, may have acoustic enhancement, usually contain echogenic debris, and may be surrounded by a thick wall (**Fig. 26A**). It is difficult to differentiate a pancreatic pseudocyst from a pancreatic abscess or neoplastic mass on ultrasound examination alone.

Pancreatic abscess

Abscesses are collections of purulent material and necrotic tissue within the pancreas or extending into adjacent tissues. Pancreatic abscesses develop from secondary infection of necrotic pancreatic tissue and are a serious and often fatal complication of acute pancreatitis. Abscesses may appear as ill-defined mass lesions within the pancreas, containing both hypoechoic and hyperechoic areas (**Fig. 26B**).[63,85–87] Echogenic foci with distal shadowing indicating gas may be present within the lumen. A thick or poorly defined wall may surround the abscess.

Pancreatic nodular hyperplasia

Nodular hyperplasia of the pancreas seems to be common in older cats and dogs and is likely not clinically significant.[88] Hypoechoic small nodules (3–10 mm in cats) distributed diffusely within normal pancreatic parenchyma may be seen as an incidental finding on ultrasound examination (**Fig. 27**).[63,89] However, nodular hyperplasia cannot be reliably differentiated from malignant pancreatic neoplasia. A biopsy is needed for a definitive diagnosis.

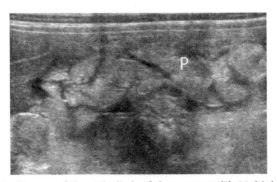

Fig. 25. Longitudinal image of the right limb of the pancreas (P). Multiple anechoic fissure extend through the parenchyma consistent with edema.

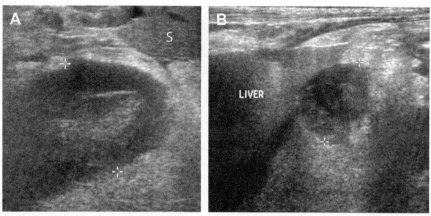

Fig. 26. (*A*) Transverse image of the cranial abdomen in a dog with previously diagnosed pancreatitis. A large, mixed echogenic mass (*between calipers*) has formed in the area of the left pancreatic limb. Pseudocyst was diagnosed on fine-needle aspiration. S, spleen. (*B*) Focal hypoechoic mass (*between calipers*) present in the body of the pancreas. Abscess was diagnosed at necropsy. Note that pseudocyst, abscess, focal pancreatitis, and neoplasia are all differentials for this appearance.

Pancreatic neoplasia

Pancreatic endocrine tumors (insulinomas are most common) are suspected in some animals with hypoglycemia. These tumors are generally small (usually <2.5 cm), focal, hypoechoic solitary or multiple nodules, which may be located in any part of the pancreas (**Fig. 28**A).[63,90] Because they are easily missed, a negative ultrasound

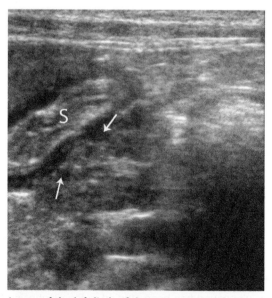

Fig. 27. Transverse image of the left limb of the pancreas in an asymptomatic cat. Multiple small hypoechoic nodules are noted in the pancreatic parenchyma (*arrows*). Cystic adenomatous hyperplasia was diagnosed on fine-needle aspiration and was likely an incidental finding. S, stomach.

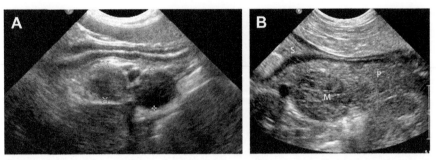

Fig. 28. (A) Longitudinal image of the right pancreatic limb in a dog with hypoglycemia. Two hypoechoic nodules (*between calipers*) are noted dorsal to the descending duodenum. Insulinoma was diagnosed on histopathology after surgical removal. (B) Longitudinal image of the left limb of the pancreas (transverse to the patient) in a dog presented for vomiting. A focal hypoechoic mass (M) is identified in the left pancreas (P), located just caudal to the body of the stomach (S). Pancreatic carcinoma was diagnosed on fine-needle aspiration.

examination should not rule out insulinomas. Metastatic lesions in adjacent lymph nodes or liver may be more reliably imaged.

Pancreatic exocrine tumors (carcinomas are most common) are a differential for any mass lesion within the pancreas. They may obstruct the common bile duct or extend into adjacent stomach or duodenum. Ultrasound examination cannot reliably differentiate neoplasia from pancreatitis, pseudocyst, abscess, or nodular hyperplasia. A focal mass is the most common ultrasound appearance for malignant neoplasia (**Fig. 28**B).[63,89] The only ultrasound feature unique to malignant pancreatic neoplasia versus nodular hyperplasia in cats is the presence of a single mass greater than 2.0 cm in at least one dimension.[89] In this study, feline pancreatic neoplasias tended to have a single, larger mass lesion, whereas nodular hyperplasia tended to have multiple, smaller nodules. Metastatic spread of pancreatic neoplasia to the mesentery (carcinomatosis) can occur, resulting in a nodular-appearing omentum and peritoneal effusion.

NEWER ULTRASOUND IMAGING TECHNIQUES
Endosonography

Endoscopic ultrasound (EUS) (ultrasound transducer placed on the tip of an endoscope) has been used to more carefully evaluate both the canine and feline pancreas.[91,92] With this technique, the transducer tip is just a few millimeters from the pancreas (imaged through the duodenal or gastric wall), allowing the use of high frequencies. Lack of intervening gas is also an advantage with this technique. Cats with pancreatitis were imaged using EUS. Although there was no difference in the diagnosis of pancreatitis between EUS and abdominal ultrasound, pancreatic margins and parenchymal detail were better visualized on EUS. EUS has been used to guide fine-needle aspiration of the pancreas in dogs. Disadvantages of EUS include specialized equipment, general anesthesia, and the expertise and experience needed for this procedure.

Contrast-Enhanced Ultrasound

Contrast-enhanced ultrasound has been studied in the diagnosis of pancreatic disease in the dog and cat.[93-97] Contrast enhancement of the pancreas correlates with perfusion and can be used to evaluate areas of inflammation (more intensely enhancing) and necrosis (nonenhancement). In dogs with acute pancreatitis, mean pixel and peak intensity of the pancreatic parenchyma were significantly higher than normal dogs after contrast administration.[93] All dogs with pancreatitis had a decrease in pixel intensity 10 to 15 days after the initial examination.

SUPPLEMENTARY DATA

Supplementary data related to this article can be found at http://dx.doi.org/10.1016/j. cvsm.2015.12.004.

REFERENCES

1. Yeager AE, Anderson WI. Study of association between histologic features and echogenicity of architecturally normal cat kidneys. Am J Vet Res 1989;50:860–3.
2. Ibrahim WH, Bailey N, Sunvold GD, et al. Effects of carnitine and taurine on fatty acid metabolism and lipid accumulation in the liver of cats during weight gain and weight loss. Am J Vet Res 2003;64:1265–77.
3. Nicoll RG, O'Brien RT, Jackson MW. Qualitative ultrasonography of the liver in obese cats. Vet Radiol Ultrasound 1998;39:47–50.
4. Drost WT, Henry GA, Meinkoth JH, et al. Quantification of hepatic and renal cortical echogenicity in clinically normal cats. Am J Vet Res 2000;61:1016.
5. Moentk J, Biller DS. Bilobed gallbladder in a cat: ultrasonographic appearance. Vet Radiol Ultrasound 1993;34:354.
6. Hittmair KM, Vielgrader HD, Loupal G. Ultrasonographic evaluation of gallbladder wall thickness in cats. Vet Radiol Ultrasound 2001;42:149.
7. Spalding KA. Gallbladder wall thickness. Vet Radiol Ultrasound 1993;34:270–3.
8. Center SA. Diseases of the gallbladder and biliary tree. Vet Clin North Am Small Anim Pract 2009;39:543–98.
9. Ramstedt K, Center SA, Randolph J, et al. Changes in gallbladder volume in healthy dogs after food was withheld for 12 hours followed by ingestion of a meal or a meal containing erythromycin. Am J Vet Res 2008;69:647–51.
10. Bromel C, Barthez P, Leveille R, et al. Prevalence of gallbladder sludge in dogs as assess by ultrasonography. Vet Radiol Ultrasound 1998;39:206–10.
11. Tsukagoshi T, Ohno K, Tsukamoto A, et al. Decreased gallbladder emptying in dogs with biliary sludge or gallbladder mucocele. Vet Radiol Ultrasound 2012;53:84–91.
12. d'Anjou M-A. Liver. In: Penninck D, d'Anjou M-A, editors. Atlas of small animal ultrasonography. Ames (IA): Wiley-Blackwell; 2008. p. 243.
13. Leveille R, Biller DS, Shiroma JT. Sonographic evaluation of the common bile duct in cats. J Vet Intern Med 1996;10:296–9.
14. Feeney DA, Anderson KL, Ziegler LE. Statistical relevance of ultrasonographic criteria in the assessment of diffuse liver disease in dogs and cats. Am J Vet Res 2008;69:212–21.
15. Biller DS, Kantrowitz B, Miyabayashi T. Ultrasonography of diffuse liver disease. A review. J Vet Intern Med 1992;6:71–6.
16. Newell SM, Selcer BA, Girard E, et al. Correlation between ultrasonographic findings and specific hepatic diseases in cats: 72 cases (1985-1997). J Am Vet Med Assoc 1998;213:94.
17. Marolf AJ, Leach L, Gibbons DS, et al. Ultrasonographic findings of feline cholangitis. J Am Anim Hosp Assoc 2012;48:36–42.
18. Cuccovillo A, Lamb CR. Cellular features of sonographic target lesions of the liver and spleen in 21 dogs and a cat. Vet Radiol Ultrasound 2002;43:275–8.

19. Stowater JL, Lamb CR, Schelling SH. Ultrasonographic features of canine hepatic nodular hyperplasia. Vet Radiol Ultrasound 1990;31:268–72.

20. Lamb CR. Ultrasonography of the liver and biliary tract. Probl Vet Med 1991;3: 555–73.

21. Liptak J. Hepatobiliary tumors. In: Withrow SJ, MacEwen EG, editors. Small animal clinical oncology. Philadelphia: WB Saunders; 2007. p. 484–92.

22. Nyman HT, Kristensen AT, Flagstad A, et al. A review of the sonographic assessment of tumor metastases in liver and superficial lymph nodes. Vet Radiol Ultrasound 2004;45:438–48.

23. Whiteley MB, Feeney DA, Whiteley LO, et al. Ultrasonographic appearance of primary and metastatic canine hepatic tumors. A review of 48 cases. J Ultrasound Med 1989;8:621–30.

24. Murakami T, Feeney DA, Bahr K. Analysis of clinical and ultrasonographic data by use of logistic regression models for prediction of malignant versus benign causes of ultrasonographically detected focal liver lesions in dogs. Am J Vet Res 2012;73:821–9.

25. Sato AF, Solano M. Ultrasonographic findings in abdominal mast cell disease: a retrospective study of 19 patients. Vet Radiol Ultrasound 2004;45:51–7.

26. Liptak JM, Dernell WS, Withrow SJ. Liver tumors in cats and dogs. Compend Cont Educ Small Anim Pract 2004;26:50–7.

27. Nyland TG, Koblick PD, Tellyer SE. Ultrasonographic evaluation of biliary cystadenomas in cats. Vet Radiol Ultrasound 1999;40:300.

28. Warren-Smith CMR, Andrew S, Mantis P, et al. Lack of associations between ultrasonographic appearance of parenchymal lesions of the canine liver and histological diagnosis. J Small Anim Pract 2012;53:168–73.

29. Schwarz LA, Penninck DG, Leveille-Webster C. Hepatic abscesses in 13 dogs: a review of the ultrasonographic findings, clinical data and therapeutic options. Vet Radiol Ultrasound 1998;39:357–65.

30. Sergeeff JS, Armstrong PJ, Bunch SE. Hepatic abscesses in cats: 14 cases (1985-2002). J Vet Intern Med 2004;18:295–300.

31. vanSonnenberg E, Simeone JF, Mueller PR, et al. Sonographic appearance of hematoma in the liver, spleen, and kidney: a clinical, pathologic, and animal study. Radiology 1983;147:507–10.

32. Jacobson LS, Kirberger RM, Nesbit JW. Hepatic ultrasonography and pathological findings in dogs with hepatocutaneous syndrome: new concepts. J Vet Intern Med 1995;9:399–404.

33. Nyland TG, Barthez PY, Ortega TM, et al. Hepatic ultrasonographic and pathologic findings in dogs with canine superficial necrolytic dermatitis. Vet Radiol Ultrasound 1996;37:200–4.

34. Quantz JE, Miles MS, Reed AL, et al. Elevation of alanine transaminase and gallbladder wall abnormalities as biomarkers of anaphylaxis in canine hypersensitivity patients. J Vet Emerg Crit Care (San Antonio) 2009;19:536–44.

35. Rivers BJ, Walter PA, Johnston GR, et al. Acalculous cholecystitis in four canine cases: ultrasonographic findings and use of ultrasonographic-guided, percutaneous cholecystocentesis in diagnosis. J Am Anim Hosp Assoc 1997;33:207–14.

36. Neer TA. Review of disorders of the gallbladder and extrahepatic biliary tract in the dog and cat. J Vet Intern Med 1992;6:186–92.

37. Kovatch R, Hildebrandt P, Marcus L. Cystic mucinous hyperplasia of the mucosa of the gall bladder in the dog. Pathol Vet 1965;2:574–84.

38. Secchi P, Poppl AG, Ilha A, et al. Prevalence, risk factors, and biochemical markers in dogs with ultrasound-diagnosed biliary sludge. Res Vet Sci 2012; 93:1185–9.

39. Bandyopadhyay S, Varshney J, Hoque M, et al. Prevalence of cholecystic disease in dogs: an ultrasonographic evaluation. Asian J Anim Vet Adv 2007;2: 234–8.

40. Mehler S, Bennet R. Canine extrahepatic biliary tract disease and surgery. Compendium 2006;28:302–14.

41. Besso J, Wrigley R, Gliatto J, et al. Ultrasonographic appearance and clinical findings in 14 dogs with gallbladder mucocele. Vet Radiol Ultrasound 2000;41: 261–71.

42. Eich CS, Ludwig LL. The surgical treatment of cholelithiasis in cats: a study of nine cases. J Am Anim Hosp Assoc 2002;38:290.

43. Gaillot HA, Penninck DG, Webster CR, et al. Ultrasonographic features of extra-hepatic biliary obstruction in 30 cats. Vet Radiol Ultrasound 2007;48:439–47.

44. Pike F, Berg J, King N, et al. Gallbladder mucocele in dogs: 30 cases (2000-2002). J Am Vet Med Assoc 2004;224:1615–22.

45. Aguirre AL, Center SA, Randolph JF, et al. Gallbladder disease in Shetland sheepdogs: 38 cases (1995-2005). J Am Vet Med Assoc 2007;231:79–88.

46. Uno T, Okamoto K, Onaka T, et al. Correlation between ultrasonographic imaging of the gallbladder and gallbladder content in eleven cholecystectomised dogs and their prognoses. J Vet Med Sci 2009;71:1295–300.

47. Choi J, Kim A, Keh S, et al. Comparison between ultrasonographic and clinical findings in 43 dogs with gallbladder mucoceles. Vet Radiol Ultrasound 2014; 55:202–7.

48. Worley D, Hottinger H, Lawrence H. Surgical management of gallbladder muco-celes in dogs: 22 cases (1999-2003). J Am Vet Med Assoc 2004;225:1418–22.

49. Bennett SL, Milne M, Slocombe RF, et al. Gallbladder mucocoele and concurrent hepatic lipidosis in a cat. Aust Vet J 2007;85:397–400.

50. Zawie DA, Garvey MS. Feline hepatic disease. Vet Clin North Am Small Anim Pract 1984;14:1201–30.

51. Callahan JE, Haddad JL, Brown DC, et al. Feline cholangitis: a necropsy study of 44 cats (1986-2008). J Feline Med Surg 2011;13:570–6.

52. Brain PH, Barrs VR, Martin P, et al. Feline cholecystitis and acute neutrophilic cholangitis: clinical findings, bacterial isolates and response to treatment in six cases. J Feline Med Surg 2006;8:91–103.

53. Nyland TG, Gillett NA. Sonographic evaluation of experimental bile duct ligation in the dog. Vet Radiol 1982;23:252–60.

54. Nakamura K, Takagi S, Sasaki N, et al. Contrast-enhanced ultrasonography for characterization of canine focal liver lesions. Vet Radiol Ultrasound 2010;51: 79–85.

55. Kanemoto H, Ohno K, Nakashima K, et al. Characterization of canine focal liver lesion with contrast-enhanced ultrasound using a novel contrast agent–Sonazoid. Vet Radiol Ultrasound 2009;50:188–94.

56. Vančić M, Long F, Seiler G. Contrast harmonic ultrasonography of splenic masses and associated liver nodules in dogs. J Am Vet Med Assoc 2009;234:88–94.

57. O'Brien RT. Improved detection of metastatic hepatic hemangiosarcoma nodules with contrast ultrasound in three dogs. Vet Radiol Ultrasound 2007;48:146–8.

58. White J, Gay J, Farnsworth R, et al. Ultrasound elastography of the liver, spleen, and kidneys in clinically normal cats. Vet Radiol Ultrasound 2014;55:428–34.

59. Holdsworth A, Bradley K, Birch S, et al. Elastography of the normal canine liver, spleen and kidneys. Vet Radiol Ultrasound 2014;55:620–7.
60. Jeon S, Lee G, Lee S, et al. Ultrasonographic elastography of the liver, spleen, kidneys, and prostate in clinically normal beagle dogs. Vet Radiol Ultrasound 2015;56:425–31.
61. Granger LA, Hilferty M, Francis T, et al. Variability in the ultrasonographic appearance of the pancreas in healthy dogs compared to dogs with hyperadrenocorticism. Vet Radiol Ultrasound 2015;56(5):540–8.
62. Penninck DG, Zeyen U, Taeymans ON, et al. Ultrasonographic measurement of the pancreas and pancreatic duct in clinically normal dogs. Am J Vet Res 2013;74:433–7.
63. Hecht S, Henry G. Sonographic evaluation of the normal and abnormal pancreas. Clin Tech Small Anim Pract 2007;22:115–21.
64. Etue SM, Penninck DG, Labato MA, et al. Ultrasonography of the normal feline pancreas and associated anatomical landmarks: a prospective study of 20 cats. Vet Radiol Ultrasound 2001;42:330–6.
65. Hecht S, Penninck DG, Mahoney O, et al. Relationship of pancreatic duct dilation to age and clinical findings in cats. Vet Radiol Ultrasound 2006;47:287–94.
66. Larson MM, Panciera DL, Ward DL, et al. Age-related changes in the ultrasound appearance of the normal feline pancreas. Vet Radiol Ultrasound 2005;46: 238–42.
67. Oppliger S, Hartnack S, Riond B, et al. Agreement of the serum Spec fPL™ and 1,2-O-dilauryl-rac-glycero-3-glutaric acid-(6′-methylresorufin) ester lipase assay for the determination of serum lipase in cats with suspicion of pancreatitis. J Vet Intern Med 2013;27:1077–82.
68. Watson PJ, Roulois AJA, Scase T, et al. Prevalence and breed distribution of chronic pancreatitis at post-mortem examination in first-opinion dogs. J Small Anim Pract 2007;48:609–18.
69. Newman S, Steiner J, Woosley K, et al. Localization of pancreatic inflammation and necrosis in dogs. J Vet Intern Med 2004;18:488–93.
70. Watson PJ, Archer J, Roulois AJ, et al. Observational study of 14 cases of chronic pancreatitis in dogs. Vet Rec 2010;167:968–76.
71. Bostrom MB, Xenoulis PG, Newman SJ, et al. Chronic pancreatitis in dogs: a retrospective study of clinical, clinicopathological, and histopathological findings in 61 cases. Vet J 2013;195:73–7.
72. Morita Y, Takiguchi M, Yasuda J, et al. Endoscopic ultrasonographic findings of the pancreas after pancreatic duct ligation in the dog. Vet Radiol Ultrasound 1998;39:557–62.
73. Mawby DI, Whittemore JC, Fecteau KA. Canine pancreatic-specific lipase concentrations in clinically healthy dogs and dogs with naturally occurring hyperadrenocorticism. J Vet Intern Med 2014;28:1244–50.
74. Saunders HM, VanWinkle TJ, Drobatz K, et al. Ultrasonographic findings in cats with clinical, gross pathologic, and histologic evidence of acute pancreatitic necrosis: 20 cases (1994-2001). J Am Vet Med Assoc 2002;221:1724–30.
75. Williams JM, Panciera DL, Larson MM, et al. Ultrasonographic findings of the pancreas in cats with elevated serum pancreatic lipase immunoreactivity. J Vet Intern Med 2013;27:913–8.
76. Oppliger S, Hartnack S, Reusch CE, et al. Agreement of serum feline pancreas-specific lipase and colorimetric lipase assays with pancreatic ultrasonographic findings in cats with suspicion of pancreatitis: 161 cases (2008-2012). J Am Vet Med Assoc 2014;244:1060–5.

77. Ferreri JA, Hardam E, Kimmel SE, et al. Clinical differentiation of acute necrotizing from chronic nonsuppurative pancreatitis in cats: 63 cases (1996-2001). J Am Vet Med Assoc 2003;223:469–74.

78. Armstrong PJ, Williams DA. Pancreatitis in cats. Top Companion Anim Med 2012; 27:140–7.

79. Bazelle J, Watson P. Pancreatitis in cats: is it acute, is it chronic, is it significant? J Feline Med Surg 2014;16:395–406.

80. Simpson KW. Pancreatitis and triaditis in cats: causes and treatment. J Small Anim Pract 2015;56:40–9.

81. Zini E, Hafner M, Kook P, et al. Longitudinal evaluation of serum pancreatic enzymes and ultrasonographic findings in diabetic cats without clinically relevant pancreatitis at diagnosis. J Vet Intern Med 2015;29:589–96.

82. Lamb CR. Pancreatic edema in dogs with hypoalbuminemia or portal hypertension. J Vet Intern Med 1999;13:498–500.

83. VanEnkevort BA, O'Brien RT, Young KM. Pancreatic pseudocysts in 4 dogs and 2 cats: ultrasonographic and clinicopathologic findings. J Vet Intern Med 1999;13: 309–13.

84. Jerram RM, Warman CG, Davies ESS, et al. Successful treatment of a pancreatic pseudocyst by omentalisation in a dog. N Z Vet J 2004;52:197–201.

85. Anderson JR, Cornell KK, Parnell NK, et al. Pancreatic abscess in 36 dogs: a retrospective analysis of prognostic indicators. J Am Anim Hosp Assoc 2008; 44:171–9.

86. Lee M, Kang J, Chang D, et al. Pancreatic abscess in a cat with diabetes mellitus. J Am Anim Hosp Assoc 2015;51:180–4.

87. Johnson MD, Mann FA. Treatment for pancreatic abscesses via omentalization with abdominal closure versus open periteoneal drainage in dogs: 15 cases (1994-2004). J Am Vet Med Assoc 2006;228:397–402.

88. Newman SJ, Steiner JM, Woosley K, et al. Correlation of age and incidence of pancreatic exocrine nodular hyperplasia in the dog. Vet Pathol 2005;42:510–3.

89. Hecht S, Penninck DG, Keating JH. Imaging findings in pancreatic neoplasia and nodular hyperplasia in 19 cats. Vet Radiol Ultrasound 2007;48:45–50.

90. Bryson ER, Snead ECR, McMillan C, et al. Insulinoma in a dog with pre-existing insulin-dependent diabetes mellitus. J Am Anim Hosp Assoc 2007;4:65–9.

91. Kook PH, Baloi P, Ruetten M, et al. Feasibility and safety of endoscopic ultrasound-guided fine needle aspiration of the pancreas in dogs. J Vet Intern Med 2012;26:513–7.

92. Schweighauser A, Gaschen F, Gaschen L, et al. Evaluation of endosonography as a new diagnostic tool for feline pancreatitis. J Feline Med Surg 2009;11: 492–8.

93. Rademacher N, Schur D, Gaschen F, et al. Contrast-enhanced ultrasonography of the pancreas in healthy dogs and in dogs with acute pancreatitis. Vet Radiol Ultrasound 2016;57:58–64. [Epub ahead of print].

94. Rademacher N, Ohlerth S, Scharf G, et al. Contrast-enhanced power and color Doppler ultrasonography of the pancreas in healthy and diseased cats. J Vet Intern Med 2008;22:1310–6.

95. Leinonen MR, Raekallio MR, Vainio OM, et al. Quantitative contrast-enhanced ultrasonographic analysis of perfusion in the kidneys, liver, pancreas, small intestine, and mesenteric lymph nodes in healthy cats. Am J Vet Res 2010;71: 1305–11.

96. Vanderperren K, Haers H, Van der Vekens E, et al. Description of the use of contrast-enhanced ultrasonography in four dogs with pancreatic tumours. J Small Anim Pract 2014;55:164-9.

97. Lim SY, Nakamura K, Morishita K, et al. Qualitative and quantitative contrast-enhanced ultrasonographic assessment of cerulean-induced acute pancreatitis in dogs. J Vet Intern Med 2014;28:496-503.

Computed Tomography and MRI of the Hepatobiliary System and Pancreas

Angela J. Marolf, DVM

KEYWORDS

- Computed tomography ● MRI ● Liver ● Biliary system ● Pancreas

KEY POINTS

- CT and MRI are useful in the evaluation of liver, biliary tract, and pancreatic disorders.
- The use of intravenous contrast provides additional information that can aid in distinguishing different disease processes.
- The lack of superimposition of adjacent stomach and bowel gas and decreased operator dependence of these imaging modalities leads to more accurate assessments of the cranial abdomen.

INTRODUCTION

Abdominal radiography and ultrasound have been performed in dogs and cats for evaluation of liver, biliary, and pancreatic abnormalities for many years in veterinary medicine. Abdominal ultrasound in particular has been used for diagnosis of biliary, pancreatic, and parenchymal liver diseases. Advantages to abdominal ultrasound include ability to perform the study on awake or sedated patients, use of nonionizing sound waves, and the ability of ultrasound to distinguish fluid and soft tissue changes. Disadvantages to sonographically evaluating the hepatobiliary system and pancreas include incomplete assessment of the organs because of overlying stomach and bowel gas that interferes with the ultrasound wave propagation and patient discomfort or poor compliance during the study. Additionally, ultrasound is highly operator dependent, and thorough evaluation of these organs is limited by experience level of the sonographer.

Disclosure statement: The author has nothing to disclose.
Department of Environmental and Radiological Health Sciences, College of Veterinary Medicine and Biomedical Sciences, Colorado State University, 300 West Drake Road, Fort Collins, CO 80523-1620, USA
E-mail address: angela.marolf@colostate.edu

Vet Clin Small Anim 46 (2016) 481–497
http://dx.doi.org/10.1016/j.cvsm.2015.12.006
0195-5616/16/$ – see front matter

MRI and computed tomography (CT) of the abdomen have been performed in people for years to assess the hepatobiliary system and pancreas. These two imaging modalities are considered the preferred method to diagnose many conditions including pancreatitis, pancreatic neoplasia, biliary tract abnormalities, and various liver disorders including inflammation and neoplasia.[1–7]

With the increased availability of CT and MRI scanners in veterinary hospitals, these imaging modalities are more readily available for use in dogs and cats for diagnosis of abdominal diseases. The ability to image veterinary patients without superimposition of other organs or bowel gas and perform a complete assessment of the biliary tree, liver, and pancreas offer distinct advantages over current imaging methods. With the advent and increased availability of multislice CT scanners, the speed at which CT studies are performed has increased and the ability to sedate animals for some studies is possible. CT and MRI use intravenous contrast to better evaluate the blood flow to organs and adjacent tissues. CT imaging uses iodinated contrast agents, and MRI uses gadolinium contrast agents.

MRI gives excellent contrast resolution of the soft tissues and provides multiple anatomic planes to visualize organs in the abdomen. The term "intensity" is used to describe tissue characteristics and appearance on various sequences. Tissues that are very bright are hyperintense, dark tissues are hypointense, and tissues of a similar intensity are isointense.

Standard imaging sequences obtained in MRI include T1- and T2-weighted sequences, which demonstrate the molecular differences in various tissues and can detect abnormalities caused by differences in tissue appearance in the sequences. Fluids are typically hypointense on T1-weighted images and hyperintense on T2-weighted images. An additional technique often used in MRI abdominal imaging is called "fat saturation." This technique makes fat appear hypointense on T1- and T2-weighted images and can highlight inflammation and edema in tissues. Disadvantages to MRI are the need for general anesthesia, added expense, and decreased availability compared with ultrasound.

CT imaging provides excellent contrast resolution of soft tissues and bones. Multiple planes are reconstructed with CT imaging allowing for visualization of all anatomic structures in the abdomen. With the ability to perform multiplanar reconstructions (a commercially available software imaging tool), the liver, biliary tract, and pancreas are evaluated in dorsal and sagittal imaging planes in unlimited angles for thorough assessment.

CT terminology uses the term "attenuation" to describe tissue characteristics. Tissues that are bright are hyperattenuating, dark tissues are hypoattenuating, and similar tissues are isoattenuating to each other. Fluids are typically hypoattenuating. Disadvantages to CT imaging include ionizing radiation, added expense, and decreased availability compared with ultrasound.

This article familiarizes the reader with current uses of MRI and CT for the liver, biliary system, and pancreas in dogs and cats.

MRI AND COMPUTED TOMOGRAPHY OF THE NORMAL HEPATOBILIARY SYSTEM AND PANCREAS

The normal appearance of the liver on MRI is uniform hypointensity relative to the spleen on T1- and T2-weighted sequences with homogeneous contrast enhancement. The gallbladder and common bile duct are homogenously hyperintense on T2-weighted images and hypointense on T1-weighted images because of bile being stored within the gallbladder and coursing through the common bile duct (**Fig. 1**).

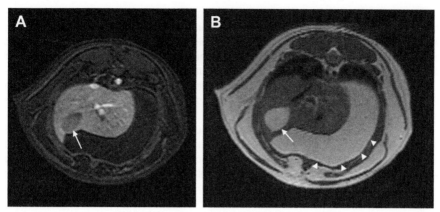

Fig. 1. (*A*) Transverse postcontrast T1-weighted image of the normal liver. Note the hypointense fluid within the gallbladder (*arrow*). Contrast is present in the aorta, caudal vena cava, and hepatic veins. (*B*) Transverse T2-weighted image of the normal liver. Note the hyperintense fluid within the gallbladder (*arrow*). A large amount of hyperintense falciform fat is ventral to the liver (*arrowheads*).

Additionally, the margins of the liver and subjective size should be evaluated. Normal liver margins are smooth.

The pancreas is typically uniformly hyperintense relative to the liver on T1-weighted images and isointense to hypointense on T2 fat-saturated images.[8,9] The pancreas should be a thin, flat organ, so changes in shape and size are also evaluated. The entire pancreas can be assessed on the dorsal and sagittal plane of different sequences, because the right limb follows the duodenum, the body is near the splenic vein as it courses to the portal vein, and the left limb is near the spleen (**Fig. 2**). The pancreatic duct is not well visualized in normal cats because of its small size.[8]

On CT imaging the normal liver is isoattenuating to the spleen with a hypoattenuating gallbladder because of storage of bile. The liver parenchyma uniformly contrast enhances. The common bile duct may not be seen because of its small

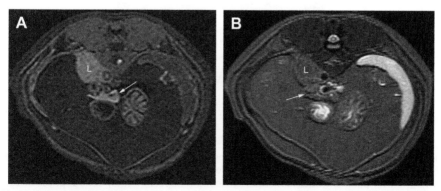

Fig. 2. (*A*) Transverse precontrast T1-weighted image of the normal pancreas (*arrow*). The portion of visible liver is labeled "L." (*B*) Transverse fat-saturated T2-weighted image of the normal pancreas (*arrow*). The visible portion of liver is labeled "L." Compare the appearance of the falciform fat in the image with **Fig. 1**B.

size and lack of enhancement. However, the gallbladder wall thickness and intraluminal biliary contents can be evaluated. The bile should be hypoattenuating with no evidence of contents, such as debris or calculi. To specifically evaluate the hepatic arteries and portal veins, CT angiography must be performed, which is a timed bolus of intravenous contrast followed by multiple specifically timed scans to capture the arterial, venous, and delayed phases of contrast passage through the organ.[10,11] When all three phases are captured, this is termed a three-phase angiogram (**Fig. 3**).

The pancreas is isoattenuating to hypoattenuating to the spleen and liver and uniformly contrast enhances[10] (**Fig. 4**). Again, size and shape of the pancreas and appearance of the surrounding mesentery should be evaluated. With the ability to perform multiplanar reconstructions, the liver, biliary tract, and pancreas are evaluated in multiple imaging planes (**Fig. 5**).

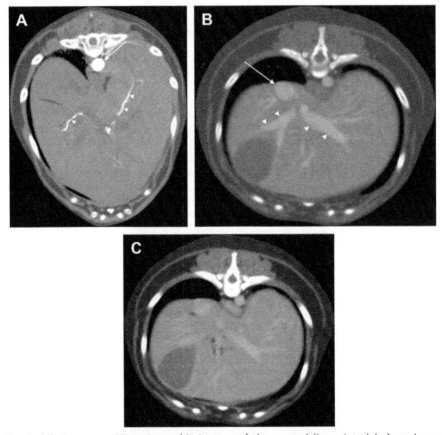

Fig. 3. (A) Transverse CT angiographic images of the normal liver. Arterial-phase image shows thin, linear contrast enhancement of the hepatic arteries (*arrowheads*) and aorta (*arrow*). The liver parenchyma is fairly homogeneous in appearance. (B) Venous-phase image shows contrast enhancement of the hepatic veins (*arrowheads*) and caudal vena cava (*arrow*). Note the hypoattenuating bile in the gallbladder. (C) Delayed-phase image. There is still contrast filling the hepatic veins and caudal vena cava but is less than in the venous phase. There is mild diffuse increased attenuation of the liver parenchyma.

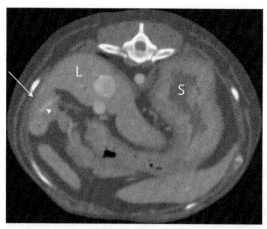

Fig. 4. Transverse CT image of the normal right pancreatic limb (*arrow*) in venous phase of the angiographic study. Note the pancreaticoduodenal vein coursing through the pancreas (*arrowhead*). The visible liver is labeled "L" and the stomach is labeled "S."

ABNORMAL CONDITIONS OF THE HEPATOBILIARY SYSTEM AND PANCREAS
Neoplasia of the Liver and Biliary Tract

Primary liver neoplasia is uncommon in dogs and cats; liver metastasis from other organ neoplasia is more common.[12] Ultrasound is often performed for initial imaging of the liver; however, there is overlap in the appearance of different neoplastic and inflammatory processes.[13,14] Further characterization of liver masses, staging, and surgical planning are reasons to perform cross-sectional imaging with either CT or MRI for suspected liver masses based on abdominal ultrasound or radiographs. Establishing imaging characteristics of primary liver tumors, such as adenocarcinoma, carcinoma, hemangiosarcoma, and biliary carcinomas compared with benign conditions, such as nodular hyperplasia or adenomas, can assist in making diagnoses noninvasively. Also, evaluation of the liver for metastasis and the appearance of these lesions are important. In people, CT and MRI are preferred for diagnosis and staging of liver tumors.[15]

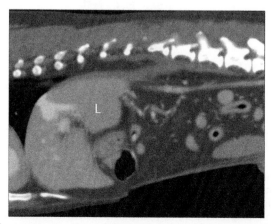

Fig. 5. Sagittal plane reconstruction of the normal liver (L) in venous phase of the angiographic study.

Size, shape, and margination of masses and nodules should be noted; however, these characteristics cannot definitely differentiate tumor types. Several studies in dogs have looked at the CT characteristics of liver masses.[16–18] Two of these studies used CT angiographic methods to evaluate the arterial, venous, and delayed phases to assess tumor type.[16,18] Both studies evaluated hepatocellular carcinomas and nodular hyperplasia. The hepatocellular carcinomas had different enhancement patterns compared with a benign lesion including hypoattenuation in the later phases and heterogeneous, marginal, or central arterial contrast enhancement (**Fig. 6**A–D).

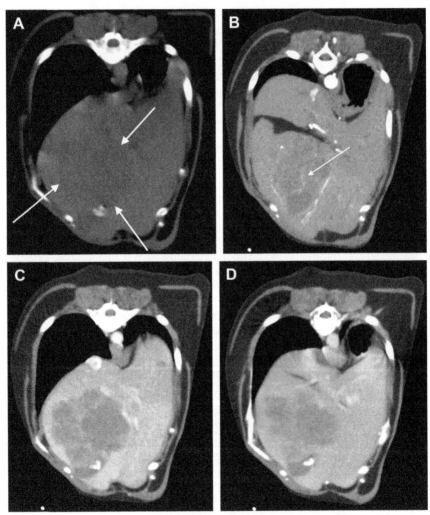

Fig. 6. (A) Transverse CT precontrast image of the liver with a confirmed hepatocellular carcinoma. Note the ill-defined hypoattenuating region in the right ventral liver (*arrows*). (B) Arterial phase. Note the heterogeneous contrast enhancement internally within the poorly defined mass (*arrow*). (C). Venous phase. Note that the mass is becoming more hypoattenuating as the surrounding liver parenchyma shows increased enhancement. (D) Delayed phase. The liver mass shows further hypoattenuation consistent with hepatocellular adenocarcinoma CT characteristics.

Nodular hyperplasia had a diffuse enhancement pattern in the arterial phase and was isoattenuating in the delayed phase. Liver metastatic lesions were also reviewed in one of the studies and were found to be hypoattenuating in both arterial and delayed phases[18] (**Fig. 7**). These differences can potentially be used to distinguish liver masses and metastases noninvasively and assist in therapeutic planning.

MRI of the liver and liver masses has also been performed in dogs and cats. MRI of hepatic lesions using standard gadolinium contrast has shown good sensitivity and specificity for differentiating malignant from benign lesions.[19] Malignant lesions tended to be more heterogeneous and have different enhancement patterns than the surrounding normal liver or benign lesions.[19]

Newer contrast agents that target the hepatobiliary system have been evaluated in dogs.[20–22] These contrast agents are administered intravenously, have a vascular phase, and then concentrate in normal hepatocytes during the later hepatobiliary phase.[23] This allows for normal liver to enhance, whereas lesions that lack normal hepatocytes do not enhance and are hypointense. Using these liver-specific contrast agents, malignant liver masses are characterized by hypointensity in the hepatobiliary phase enabling tumor characterization noninvasively.[21,22] With the use of newer contrast agents, the conspicuity of liver metastasis has been shown to increase compared with other imaging methods.[22] This would allow for better staging of patients with primary tumors diagnosed elsewhere in the body.

Hepatic Lipidosis

Hepatic lipidosis is the most common liver disorder in cats.[24] Ultrasound is commonly performed to evaluate the liver, but there can be overlap in the sonographic

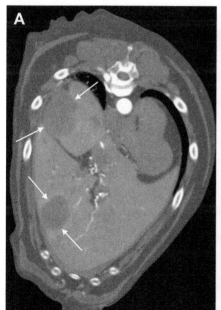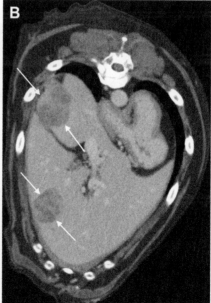

Fig. 7. (*A*) Transverse CT images of the liver with metastasis from a known adrenal adenocarcinoma. Arterial phase. Note the hypoattenuating nodules in the liver (*arrows*). (*B*) Delayed phase. Note the hypoattenuating nodules in the liver (*arrows*). These lesions have consistent CT features of metastasis.

appearance of different disease processes. CT evaluation of the liver in cats has been evaluated to determine normal fat content within the liver and in livers with hepatic lipidosis.[25,26] Mixed results have been shown, and currently CT is not being used for diagnosis of hepatic lipidosis in cats.

Inflammation of the Liver and Biliary Tract

Inflammation of the liver and biliary tract is more common in cats than in dogs. This is caused by the unique ductal anatomy of cats where the common bile duct and pancreatic duct open onto the major duodenal papilla.[27] This relationship allows for infection or inflammation to spread from one area, such as the intestinal tract, into the pancreas and biliary system. As such, cholangitis is second only to hepatic lipidosis as the most common liver disease in cats.[24] Dogs and cats are affected by hepatitis, including acute and chronic forms. Liver size, margination, and parenchymal changes are used to assess the liver in cases of hepatitis. In chronic hepatitis, the liver may be small, irregularly marginated, and have a heterogeneous parenchyma (**Fig. 8**). With acute forms of hepatitis, the liver may be enlarged or have a more normal appearance. Ultrasound is the most common imaging modality to evaluate parenchymal liver disease. However, because there is much overlap in the sonographic changes that can occur with different disease processes, histology is still recommended for definitive diagnosis.[28,29] MRI and CT imaging is commonly used in people to diagnose inflammatory conditions in the liver and biliary tract.[3–5,30] A unique MRI sequence called MRI cholangiography (MRCP) highlights fluid within the biliary tract and pancreatic ducts to diagnose intrahepatic and extrahepatic biliary tract inflammation or obstruction, fluid-filled structures, or inflammation of the pancreas[3,4,30] (**Fig. 9**). In normal dogs, MRCP has been studied and deemed feasible.[31] MRI has been used to assess

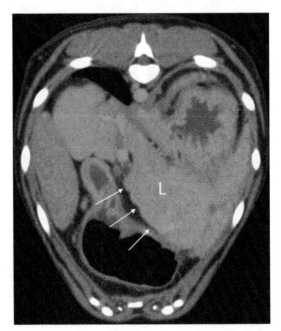

Fig. 8. Transverse CT image of a liver with known chronic hepatitis. Delayed phase. Note the irregular liver margins (*arrows*) and poor enhancement of the liver (L).

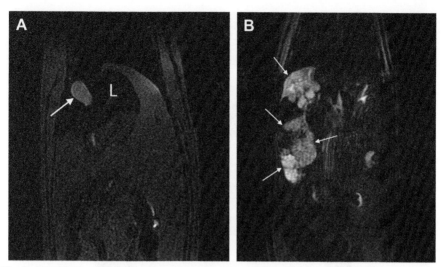

Fig. 9. (*A*) MRCP sequence in dorsal imaging plane of the liver and gallbladder. Note how the liver (L) and other organs are hypointense and the bile within the gallbladder is hyperintense (*arrow*). Fluid is bright on this sequence for easier evaluation of fluid within the biliary tract and pancreatic ducts. (*B*). Same sequence and plane of the liver and cranial abdomen. The lobulated, hyperintense masses within the liver (*arrows*) are biliary cystadenomas. Because these are predominantly fluid-filled masses, they are hyperintense on this sequence.

liver and biliary inflammation in cats.[8,9] The liver parenchymal changes were nonspecific; however, biliary tract changes, such as hyperintense intraluminal gallbladder contents, gallbladder wall enhancement, and increased wall thickness, were indicators of gallbladder and biliary tract inflammation[9] (**Fig. 10**). Calculi in the gallbladder and biliary tract are not common in dogs and cats. However, calculi are diagnosed by CT and MRI (**Fig. 11**). In CT imaging, cholangiographic contrast agents are used

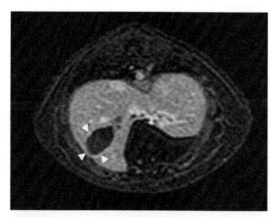

Fig. 10. Transverse MRI postcontrast T1-weighted sequence of the liver and gallbladder. The gallbladder wall is thickened and mildly contrast enhancing (*arrowheads*). The bile is of mixed intensity indicating debris within the bile. These changes are consistent with cholangitis and/or cholecystitis.

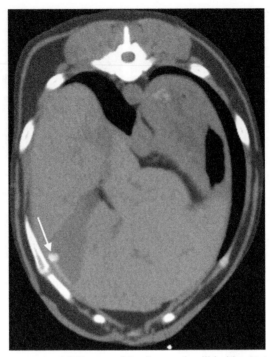

Fig. 11. Transverse precontrast CT image of the liver and gallbladder. Note the hyperattenuating, well-defined cholelith (*arrow*) and hyperattenuating amorphous debris in the dependent portion of the gallbladder.

to highlight the biliary tract.[5,32] CT cholangiography has also been studied in normal dogs and produced high-quality images of the hepatobiliary system.[33] Further studies are needed to determine the usefulness of MRI and CT in diagnosing biliary and liver inflammatory conditions in dogs and cats.

Neoplasia of the Pancreas

Exocrine and endocrine pancreatic neoplasia is rare in dogs and cats. Adenocarcinoma is the most common exocrine tumor and insulinoma is the most common endocrine tumor.[34,35] Diagnosis with ultrasound imaging can be challenging.[36,37] Determining size, location, and metastatic spread of pancreatic tumors is important. In people, CT and MRI are preferred to diagnose and stage pancreatic tumors.[38] In both modalities, differences in the angiographic pattern of enhancement in exocrine or endocrine pancreatic tumors assists in the diagnosis noninvasively.[38,39] CT angiography has been used to diagnose insulinomas in dogs.[40] The angiographic features of canine insulinoma included arterial enhancement, which is a feature of insulinomas in people.[39,40] Pancreatic adenocarcinomas tend to be poorly enhancing in the arterial phase with increased enhancement in the delayed phase[39] (**Fig. 12**). Additional advantages of CT or MRI of pancreatic masses in dogs and cats include evaluation of the liver and adjacent lymph nodes for metastasis.

Inflammation of the Pancreas

Pancreatitis is the most common exocrine pancreatic disease in dogs and cats.[41,42] Regardless of the inciting cause, the result is inflammation of the pancreas, which

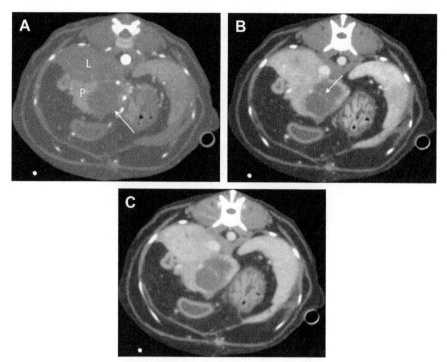

Fig. 12. (*A*) Transverse angiographic CT image of the pancreas with exocrine neoplasia. Arterial phase. Note the hypoattenuating mass (*arrow*) within the pancreas (P). Liver is labeled "L." (*B*) Venous phase. The hypoattenuating mass has mild internal enhancement (*arrow*), whereas the surrounding pancreas is homogeneously enhancing. (*C*) Delayed phase. Mild internal enhancement persists within the mass.

causes subsequent edema and necrosis, which may spread to adjacent tissues.[43,44] Advanced pancreatitis can often be diagnosed with ultrasound, but it can be insensitive because of overlying bowel gas, patient discomfort, or sonographer inexperience. CT and MRI are preferred methods for diagnosing pancreatitis in people.[4,43–47] With CT imaging of the pancreas, size, contrast enhancement, and changes to the surrounding fat and mesentery are used to make a diagnosis.[43,44] With MRI, evaluation of the intensity changes in the pancreas on T1- and T2-weighted sequences, contrast enhancement, pancreatic duct dilation, and surrounding tissues are used to assess the pancreas.[48] In dogs and cats, CT and MRI have been evaluated in diagnosis of inflammation of the pancreas. In a study using sedated CT angiography, dogs with pancreatitis had evidence of pancreatic enlargement, homogeneous to heterogeneous contrast enhancement, and ill-defined margins.[49] Dogs with heterogeneous contrast enhancement may have indicated areas of necrosis with poor blood flow in the pancreas[49,50] (**Fig. 13**). MRI and MRCP have been assessed in cats with pancreatitis.[9] The cats with pancreatitis had changes to their pancreas including T1 hypointense and T2 hyperintense parenchyma (normal pancreas is T1 hyperintense and T2 isointense to hypointense), enlargement, pancreatic duct dilation, and contrast enhancement.[8,9] The intensity changes on T1 and T2 images indicated edema within the pancreas secondary to the inflammation (**Fig. 14**). With CT and MRI, the extrahepatic portion of the common bile duct can be evaluated for evidence of obstruction and dilation secondary to pancreatic inflammation (**Fig. 15**). The surrounding

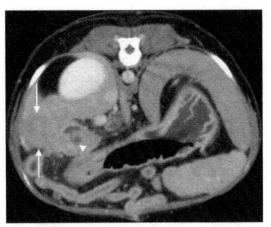

Fig. 13. Transverse angiographic CT delayed-phase image of the pancreas. Note the heterogeneous contrast enhancement of the enlarged pancreas (*arrows*) with ill-defined nonenhancing areas (*arrowhead*). These nonenhancing areas could represent necrosis within the inflamed pancreas.

peripancreatic tissues can show evidence of inflammation and be hyperattenuating on CT and T2 hyperintense on MRI. These usually represent regional steatitis or peritonitis (**Fig. 16**). In a study using CT in dogs with acute abdominal signs, "fat-stranding" or increased attenuation of the mesenteric fat caused by edema was identified in cases with peritonitis and pancreatitis.[51]

Additional Inflammatory Pancreatic Changes

Abscesses, cysts, and pseudocysts are evaluated with CT and MRI. Pseudocysts are considered a sequel to acute pancreatitis and present focal fluid collection that

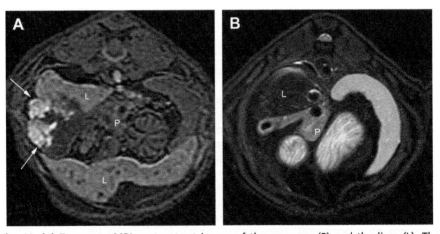

Fig. 14. (*A*) Transverse MRI postcontrast image of the pancreas (P) and the liver (L). The pancreas is hypointense relative to the liver indicating edema and inflammation. There is a biliary cystadenoma present (*arrows*). (*B*) Fat-saturated T2-weighted image of the liver (L) and pancreas (P). The pancreas is hyperintense relative to the liver indicating edema and inflammation.

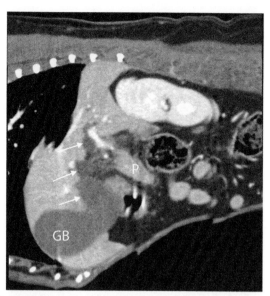

Fig. 15. Sagittal plane CT reconstruction in the delayed phase of the liver and dilated biliary tract. The gallbladder (GB) and dilated common bile duct (*arrows*) are secondary to the inflammation within the pancreas (P).

develops a fibrotic capsule over time.[43] All of these structures have hypoattenuating fluid internally with varying degrees of thickened contrast-enhancing walls on CT imaging. With MRI, fluid-filled structures are typically T2 hyperintense, T1 hypointense with varying degrees of thickened contrast enhancing walls (**Fig. 17**). Fluid-filled

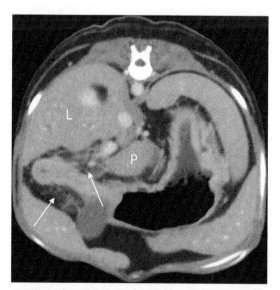

Fig. 16. Transverse angiographic CT image delayed phase of the liver (L) and pancreas (P). Note the peripancreatic linear hyperattenuations (*arrows*) caused by fluid and inflammation secondary to pancreatitis.

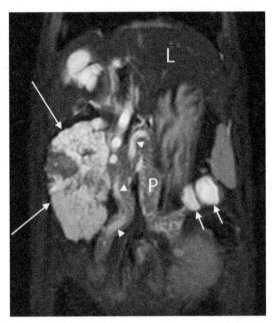

Fig. 17. MRI T2 fat-saturated dorsal plane image of the cranial abdomen. Note the hyperintense pancreas (P) with dilated pancreatic duct (*arrowheads*) and hyperintense cysts within the left pancreatic limb (*short arrows*). Large hyperintense biliary adenomas (*long arrows*) are present within the liver (L).

structures with thicker walls and internal dependent contents can be infected; however, aspirate and analysis of the fluid is necessary for definitive diagnosis.[43] Venous thromboses is diagnosed with CT angiography and MRI and can be sequelae to pancreatitis.[43] This may be caused by intimal injury and inflammatory mediators associated with pancreatitis.[43] In a recent study, 3 of 10 dogs with pancreatitis had venous thrombi identified based on CT evaluation.[49]

SUMMARY

MRI and CT imaging are becoming more common in the diagnosis of hepatobiliary and pancreatic disorders in small animals. With the advent of multislice CT scanners, sedated examinations in veterinary patients are feasible increasing the utility of this imaging modality. CT and MRI provide additional information for dogs and cats with hepatobiliary and pancreatic diseases because of lack of superimposition of structures, operator dependence, and through intravenous contrast administration. This added value provides more information for diagnosis, prognosis, and surgical planning.

REFERENCES

1. Remer EM, Baker ME. Imaging of chronic pancreatitis. Radiol Clin North Am 2002;40(6):1229–42, v.

2. Arvanitakis M, Koustiani G, Gantzarou A, et al. Staging of severity and prognosis of acute pancreatitis by computed tomography and magnetic resonance imaging: a comparative study. Dig Liver Dis 2007;39(5):473–82.

3. Palmucci S, Mauro LA, La Scola S, et al. Magnetic resonance cholangiopancreatography and contrast-enhanced magnetic resonance cholangiopancreatography versus endoscopic ultrasonography in the diagnosis of extrahepatic biliary pathology. Radiol Med 2010;115(5):732–46.

4. Maurea S, Caleo O, Mollica C, et al. Comparative diagnostic evaluation with MR cholangiopancreatography, ultrasonography and CT in patients with pancreatobiliary disease. Radiol Med 2009;114(3):390–402.

5. Saad WE, Ginat D. Computed tomography and magnetic resonance cholangiography. Tech Vasc Interv Radiol 2008;11(2):74–89.

6. Jang HJ, Yu H, Kim TK. Imaging of focal liver lesions. Semin Roentgenol 2009; 44(4):266–82.

7. Ichikawa T, Saito K, Yoshioka N, et al. Detection and characterization of focal liver lesions: a Japanese phase III, multicenter comparison between gadoxetic acid disodium-enhanced magnetic resonance imaging and contrast-enhanced computed tomography predominantly in patients with hepatocellular carcinoma and chronic liver disease. Invest Radiol 2010;45(3):133–41.

8. Marolf AJ, Stewart JA, Dunphy TR, et al. Hepatic and pancreaticobiliary MRI and MR cholangiopancreatography with and without secretin stimulation in normal cats. Vet Radiol Ultrasound 2011;52(4):415–21.

9. Marolf AJ, Kraft SL, Dunphy TR, et al. Magnetic resonance (MR) imaging and MR cholangiopancreatography findings in cats with cholangitis and pancreatitis. J Feline Med Surg 2013;15(4):285–94.

10. Caceres AV, Zwingenberger AL, Hardam E, et al. Helical computed tomographic angiography of the normal canine pancreas. Vet Radiol Ultrasound 2006;47(3): 270–8.

11. Makara M, Chau J, Hall E, et al. Effects of two contrast injection protocols on feline aortic and hepatic enhancement using dynamic computed tomography. Vet Radiol Ultrasound 2015;56(4):367–73.

12. Strombeck DR. Clinicopathologic features of primary and metastatic neoplastic disease of the liver in dogs. J Am Vet Med Assoc 1978;173(3):267–9.

13. Feeney DA, Anderson KL, Ziegler LE, et al. Statistical relevance of ultrasonographic criteria in the assessment of diffuse liver disease in dogs and cats. Am J Vet Res 2008;69(2):212–21.

14. Murakami T, Feeney DA, Bahr KL. Analysis of clinical and ultrasonographic data by use of logistic regression models for prediction of malignant versus benign causes of ultrasonographically detected focal liver lesions in dogs. Am J Vet Res 2012;73(6):821–9.

15. Lu MD, Yu XL, Li AH, et al. Comparison of contrast enhanced ultrasound and contrast enhanced CT or MRI in monitoring percutaneous thermal ablation procedure in patients with hepatocellular carcinoma: a multi-center study in China. Ultrasound Med Biol 2007;33(11):1736–49.

16. Fukushima K, Kanemoto H, Ohno K, et al. CT characteristics of primary hepatic mass lesions in dogs. Vet Radiol Ultrasound 2012;53(3):252–7.

17. Phillips K, Cullen JM, Van Winkle T, et al. CT appearance and vascular characteristics of liver masses in dogs. Proceedings of the American College of Veterinary Radiology, Annual Scientific Meeting. Las Vegas, October 10–13, 2012. p. 103.

18. Kutara K, Seki M, Ishikawa C, et al. Triple-phase helical computed tomography in dogs with hepatic masses. Vet Radiol Ultrasound 2014;55(1):7–15.

19. Clifford CA, Pretorius ES, Weisse C, et al. Magnetic resonance imaging of focal splenic and hepatic lesions in the dog. J Vet Intern Med 2004;18(3):330–8.

20. Marks AL, Hecht S, Stokes JE, et al. Effects of gadoxetate disodium (Eovist((R))) contrast on magnetic resonance imaging characteristics of the liver in clinically healthy dogs. Vet Radiol Ultrasound 2014;55(3):286–91.

21. Yonetomi D, Kadosawa T, Miyoshi K, et al. Contrast agent Gd-EOB-DTPA (EOB.-Primovist(R)) for low-field magnetic resonance imaging of canine focal liver lesions. Vet Radiol Ultrasound 2012;53(4):371–80.

22. Louvet A, Duconseille AC. Feasibility for detecting liver metastases in dogs using gadobenate dimeglumine-enhanced magnetic resonance imaging. Vet Radiol Ultrasound 2015;56(3):286–95.

23. Reimer P, Schneider G, Schima W. Hepatobiliary contrast agents for contrast-enhanced MRI of the liver: properties, clinical development and applications. Eur Radiol 2004;14(4):559–78.

24. Gagne JM, Weiss DJ, Armstrong PJ. Histopathologic evaluation of feline inflammatory liver disease. Vet Pathol 1996;33(5):521–6.

25. Nakamura M, Chen HM, Momoi Y, et al. Clinical application of computed tomography for the diagnosis of feline hepatic lipidosis. J Vet Med Sci 2005;67(11):1163–5.

26. Lam R, Niessen SJ, Lamb CR. X-ray attenuation of the liver and kidney in cats considered at varying risk of hepatic lipidosis. Vet Radiol Ultrasound 2014;55(2):141–6.

27. Smallwood JE. Atlas of feline anatomy for veterinarians. In: Hudson L, Hamilton W, editors. Digestive system. Philadelphia: Saunders, WB; 1993. p. 166–7.

28. Warren-Smith CM, Andrew S, Mantis P, et al. Lack of associations between ultrasonographic appearance of parenchymal lesions of the canine liver and histological diagnosis. J Small Anim Pract 2012;53(3):168–73.

29. Kemp SD, Panciera DL, Larson MM, et al. A comparison of hepatic sonographic features and histopathologic diagnosis in canine liver disease: 138 cases. J Vet Intern Med 2013;27(4):806–13.

30. Vitellas KM, Keogan MT, Freed KS. Radiologic manifestations of sclerosing cholangitis with emphasis on MR cholangiopancreatography. Radiographics 2000;20:959–75.

31. Heo J, Constable P, Naughton J. Dynamic secretin-enhanced magnetic resonance cholangiopancreatography and pancreatic ultrasonography in normal dogs. Proceedings of the American College of Veterinary Radiology, Annual Scientific Meeting. Las Vegas, October 10–13, 2012. p. 105.

32. Schindera ST, Nelson RC, Paulson EK, et al. Assessment of the optimal temporal window for intravenous CT cholangiography. Eur Radiol 2007;17(10):2531–7.

33. Miller J, Brinkman-Ferguson E, Mackin A, Archer T. Cholangiography using 64 multi-detector computed tomography in normal dogs. Proceedings of the American College of Veterinary Radiology, Annual Scientific Meeting. Savannah, GA, October 8–11, 2013. p. 29.

34. Dennis MM, O'Brien TD, Wayne T, et al. Hyalinizing pancreatic adenocarcinoma in six dogs. Vet Pathol 2008;45(4):475–83.

35. Jubb K. In: Jubb K, Kennedy P, Palmer N, editors. The pancreas in pathology of domestic animals. 4th edition. San Diego (CA): Academic Press; 1993.

36. Lamb CR, Simpson KW, Boswood A, et al. Ultrasonography of pancreatic neoplasia in the dog: a retrospective review of 16 cases. Vet Rec 1995;137(3):65–8.

37. Hecht S, Henry G. Sonographic evaluation of the normal and abnormal pancreas. Clin Tech Small Anim Pract 2007;22(3):115–21.

38. Morgan KA, Adams DB. Solid tumors of the body and tail of the pancreas. Surg Clin North Am 2010;90(2):287–307.
39. Zhong L. Magnetic resonance imaging in the detection of pancreatic neoplasms. J Dig Dis 2007;8(3):128–32.
40. Iseri T, Yamada K, Chijiwa K, et al. Dynamic computed tomography of the pancreas in normal dogs and in a dog with pancreatic insulinoma. Vet Radiol Ultrasound 2007;48(4):328–31.
41. De Cock HE, Forman MA, Farver TB, et al. Prevalence and histopathologic characteristics of pancreatitis in cats. Vet Pathol 2007;44(1):39–49.
42. Newman SJ, Steiner JM, Woosley K, et al. Histologic assessment and grading of the exocrine pancreas in the dog. J Vet Diagn Invest 2006;18(1):115–8.
43. Scaglione M, Casciani E, Pinto A, et al. Imaging assessment of acute pancreatitis: a review. Semin Ultrasound CT MR 2008;29(5):322–40.
44. Kim DH, Pickhardt PJ. Radiologic assessment of acute and chronic pancreatitis. Surg Clin North Am 2007;87(6):1341–58, viii.
45. Cappell MS. Acute pancreatitis: etiology, clinical presentation, diagnosis, and therapy. Med Clin North Am 2008;92(4):889–923, ix–x.
46. Fernandez-Esparrach G, Ginès A, Sánchez M, et al. Comparison of endoscopic ultrasonography and magnetic resonance cholangiopancreatography in the diagnosis of pancreatobiliary diseases: a prospective study. Am J Gastroenterol 2007;102(8):1632–9.
47. Takehara Y, Ichijo K, Tooyama N, et al. Breath-hold MR cholangiopancreatography with a long-echo-train fast spin-echo sequence and a surface coil in chronic pancreatitis. Radiology 1994;192(1):73–8.
48. Balci NC, Bieneman BK, Bilgin M, et al. Magnetic resonance imaging in pancreatitis. Top Magn Reson Imaging 2009;20(1):25–30.
49. Adrian AM, Twedt DC, Kraft SL, et al. Computed tomographic angiography under sedation in the diagnosis of suspected canine pancreatitis: a pilot study. J Vet Intern Med 2015;29(1):97–103.
50. Jaeger JQ, Mattoon JS, Bateman SW, et al. Combined use of ultrasonography and contrast enhanced computed tomography to evaluate acute necrotizing pancreatitis in two dogs. Vet Radiol Ultrasound 2003;44(1):72–9.
51. Shanaman MM, Schwarz T, Gal A, et al. Comparison between survey radiography, B-mode ultrasonography, contrast-enhanced ultrasonography and contrast-enhanced multi-detector computed tomography findings in dogs with acute abdominal signs. Vet Radiol Ultrasound 2013;54(6):591–604.

Computed Tomography Imaging in Oncology

Lisa J. Forrest, VMD

KEYWORDS

- CT • Dog • Cat • Oncology • Radiotherapy • IMRT • IGRT

KEY POINTS

- The availability of CT technology in veterinary medicine has increased its use as a first-line imaging modality to evaluate the thorax for primary and metastatic pulmonary tumors, and mediastinal and thoracic wall tumors.
- Often, simultaneous abdominal CT imaging screens for other tumors or metastasis.
- A presurgical CT evaluation helps to inform surgeons about the extent, and whether complete tumor resection is possible.
- Triple-phase vascular CT imaging can identify vascular invasion of tumors.
- CT imaging plays a crucial role in radiotherapy treatment planning, and many linear accelerators have on-board CT imaging for daily image guidance to ensure accurate treatment delivery.

COMPUTED TOMOGRAPHY FOR CANCER STAGING: THORAX

Thoracic imaging is the first step in cancer staging for dogs and cats with known or suspected tumors. Following our colleagues in human oncology along with validation from veterinary literature, thoracic computed tomography (CT) plays an important role in screening for pulmonary and thoracic primary and secondary malignancies.[1–11]

Equipment and Technique

Helical CT scanners allow rapid image acquisition and provide superior delineation of thoracic masses, metastases, and involved thoracic lymph nodes. Dogs and cats are usually under general anesthesia, placed in sternal recumbency, and imaged precontrast and postcontrast administration. At our institution dogs and cats are induced in CT and immediately positioned in sternal recumbency. Using a plexiglass cylinder for cats and small dogs with light or no sedation has also been reported.[12,13]

The author has nothing to disclose.
Department of Surgical Sciences, University of Wisconsin-Madison School of Veterinary Medicine, 2015 Linden Drive, Madison, WI 53706, USA
E-mail address: lforrest@wisc.edu

Vet Clin Small Anim 46 (2016) 499–513
http://dx.doi.org/10.1016/j.cvsm.2015.12.007
0195-5616/16/$ – see front matter © 2016 Elsevier Inc. All rights reserved.

At our institution the thorax protocol on a GE helical CT scanner (GE Healthcare, Hartland, WI) is 120 kVp, 150 to 250 mA, with 1.25 mm contiguous slices for most patients and 2.5 mm for large dogs. The window/level for mediastinum and precontrast evaluation is W = 400/L = 40 and for lung is W = 1500/L = − 700 (**Table 1**). Patients are manually hyperventilated just before slice acquisition to reduce expired CO_2. This decreases respiratory motion on images. Dorsal and sagittal plane reconstructions are obtained in lung window and mediastinal window postcontrast administration.[4] Other protocols also exist in the literature.[9,14–17]

Pulmonary and Thoracic Masses

Sensitivity of CT for metastasis detection is far superior to radiographs.[1,2,5,6,8,9] Identification and delineation of primary lung, mediastinal, heart base, and pleural tumors is also superior with CT imaging.[1,3,4,7,10] However, as in human patients, no specific CT roentgen signs have been associated with neoplastic conditions in dogs and cats.[18,19] Possible exceptions to this include bronchioalveolar carcinoma in the cat[20,21] and histiocytic sarcoma in the dog.[22,23] Feline and human pulmonary bronchioalveolar carcinoma can present with cavitated pulmonary masses, bronchiectasis, and bronchial wall thickening (**Fig. 1**).[20,21,24] Canine pulmonary histiocytic sarcoma has been reported to present as a large mass with thoracic lymphadenopathy and an internal bronchus with a predilection for right middle or left cranial lung lobes.[22,23] Primary lung tumors generally metastasize to tracheobronchial lymph nodes (**Fig. 2**),[3,4,7] but dogs with histiocytic sarcoma also show involvement of craniomediastinal and sternal lymph nodes.[23]

Common mediastinal tumors in dogs and cats include thymoma, heart base tumors, and lymphoma.[25] Additional tumor types also include carcinoma, ectopic thyroid carcinoma, and mesothelioma.[26] CT evaluation of these tumors is generally nonspecific; however, thymoma tumors often have heterogeneous contrast uptake, and CT evaluation inconsistently detects vessel invasion (**Fig. 3**).[27,28]

COMPUTED TOMOGRAPHY FOR SURGICAL PLANNING: THORAX

Similar techniques are used for surgical CT planning. Smaller slice thickness through a particular area may be requested by the radiologist to better delineate margins and invasiveness.[28] Use of CT angiograms and three-dimensional reconstruction software improves diagnostic quality.

Table 1
CT techniques

Technique	Slice Thickness	Window/Level
Thorax CT		
120 kVp/150–250 mA	1.25–2.5 mm	Mediastinum: W = 400/L = 40
		Lung: W = 1500/L = −700
Skull CT		
120 kVp/100–150 mA	0.625–1.25 mm	Soft tissue: W = 400/L = 40
		Bone: W = 2000/L = 300
Neck CT		
120 kVp/100–150 mA	1.25–2.5 mm	Soft tissue: W = 400/L = 40
Abdomen CT		
120 kVp/150–300 mA	1.25–2.5 mm	Soft tissue: W = 400/L = 40

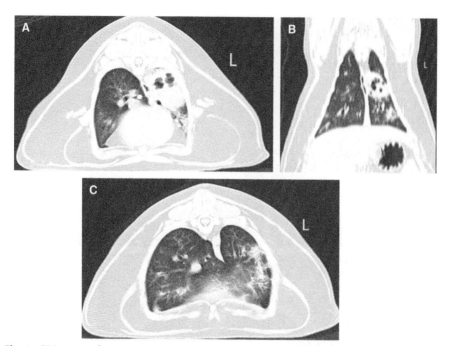

Fig. 1. CT images of a 15-year-old cat with fine-needle aspirate diagnosis of pulmonary carcinoma with CT features consistent with bronchoalveolar carcinoma. On the transverse and dorsal plane reconstructed lung window CT images (*A, B*) note the large soft tissue attenuating lung mass with several gas attenuating cavitations in the dorsal left cranial lung. Bronchial wall thickening and severe soft tissue attenuating peribronchial infiltrates are present in the left lung (*B, C*). This ill-defined infiltrate, best seen on the transverse lung window image (*C*), may represent bronchial metastasis from the primary tumor (*A, B*). L, left side of patient.

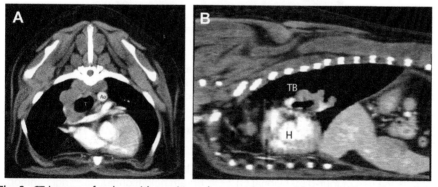

Fig. 2. CT images of a dog with a primary lung carcinoma with metastasis to the tracheobronchial lymph nodes. On the transverse, postcontrast CT image at the carina region in a mediastinal window (*A*) note the large soft tissue attenuating masses surrounding the trachea (T) and aorta (Ao). The metastatic lymph nodes are also seen on the sagittal reconstructed CT image in a mediastinal window (*B*). Note the irregular-shaped soft tissue attenuating masses dorsal to the heart (H) and air-filled carina. TB, tracheobronchial lymph nodes.

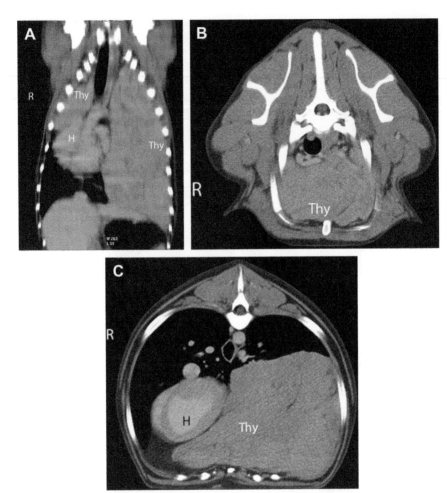

Fig. 3. CT images of a mixed breed MC dog with a confirmed thymoma tumor. All images are postcontrast administration and in a mediastinal window. On the dorsal plane reconstructed CT image (*A*) note the large soft tissue attenuating mass that is primarily on the left side, but is on the right side cranial to the heart (H). The mass is homogeneously, mildly contrast enhancing with small hypoattenuating areas (*B, C*). (*B*) is cranial to the heart. Note that the mass encompasses the entire cranial mediastinum. (*C*) The heart (H) is deviated to the right by the large tumor. R, right side of thorax; Thy, thymoma tumor.

COMPUTED TOMOGRAPHY SIMULATION FOR RADIATION THERAPY PLANNING: THORAX

Immobilization and motion control is paramount to treating thoracic tumors. In human patients the use of four-dimensional CT,[29–31] breath hold techniques,[32] rigid immobilization, and new technologies, such as dynamic contrast-enhanced imaging[33,34] and ViewRay (ViewRay, Oakwood, OH) real time imaging,[35] are used.

A simplified definition of breathing management in radiotherapy is putting the beam where the target volume is located, but in reality requires knowledge of where the target is at all times.[30] Any helical CT scanner can be outfitted with four-dimensional CT capabilities, but the cost of software, camera, and work station can range from \$165,000 to \$200,000. Motion management in veterinary radiotherapy is primarily documented through virtual studies evaluating immobilization devices,[36] daily image guidance,[37–39] adaptive radiotherapy (ART) techniques,[40] and contrast-enhanced CT images.[41] Motion management and accountability is essential when using intensity-modulated radiotherapy (IMRT)[36] techniques and becomes even more critical when treating tumors of the thorax and abdomen and using intensity-modulated stereotactic body radiotherapy planning.[38,40,41] At our institution we are currently investigating slow CT scans, where slice acquisition is prolonged to represent average organ motion,[30] as a cost-effective strategy to manage motion in radiotherapy planning.

COMPUTED TOMOGRAPHY FOR CANCER STAGING: HEAD AND NECK

CT imaging of tumors of the nasal and oral cavities and of the neck is important in the staging process of these cancers. Delineation and extent of the primary tumor along with imaging of regional lymph nodes guide clinicians for tissue sampling and treatment options.

Equipment and Technique

At our institution all the nasal, mandible, maxilla, and skull imaging that have neoplasia as a differential are placed in an immobilization device consisting of a Vac-Lok mattress (Med-Tec, Orange City, IA) and bite-block system (**Fig. 4**).[36,37] Our imaging protocol is 120 kVp, 150 to 250 mA, with 1.25 mm contiguous slices for most patients and 2.5 mm for large dogs (see **Table 1**). The window/level for soft tissues and precontrast and post-contrast evaluation is W = 400/L = 40 and for bone is W = 2000/L = 300. Dorsal and sagittal plane reconstructions are obtained in bone window and soft tissue window postcontrast administration. Imaging of tumors of the neck is performed with the patient in dorsal recumbency in a positioning mattress, using the same protocol as detailed previously.

Nasal, Oral, and Skull Tumors

Imaging the complex structures of the skull is well-suited for CT.[42] Although tissue sampling is paramount to obtaining an accurate diagnosis, some tumors have specific

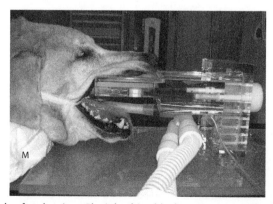

Fig. 4. Photograph of a dog in a Plexiglas bite block system. An individualized maxillary mold using dental material is made for each patient. This system is used when treating tumors of the sinonasal and oral cavity and skull. The edge of the positioning mattress (M) supports the dog's neck.

CT imaging characteristics, such as multilobular osteochondrosarcoma (**Fig. 5**)[43–45] and oral papillary squamous cell carcinoma.[46]

Common CT findings of nasal neoplasia include turbinate destruction, bony lysis of surrounding bones, soft tissue attenuating material within the nasal cavity and para-nasal sinuses with heterogeneous contrast enhancement, and a mass effect. Cribi-form plate lysis, contrast enhancement of adjacent brain with falx deviation away invading tumor, and facial deformities from tumor extension into soft tissues dorsal to incisive, nasal, frontal, and maxillary bones can be seen in advanced cases. As is the case with any neoplasia, histologic sampling is necessary. CT imaging with pre-contrast and postcontrast administration guides tumor and lymph nodes sampling.

Tumors of the nasal passage and paranasal sinuses in dogs and cats[47] account for approximately 1% to 2% of all neoplasms, with most being carcinoma (60%) and sarcoma (30%) histologies in dogs. Further breakdown of histology includes adenocar-cinoma, squamous cell carcinoma, fibrosarcoma, chondrosarcoma, and osteosar-coma.[48,49] Intranasal lymphoma occurs, with a higher prevalence in cats (**Fig. 6**).[47,49] A CT staging system has been reported for dogs that was correlated with treatment out-comes and tumor histology. In this paper, the authors found that cribiform plate lysis and aggressive tumors of the following histologies squamous cell carcinoma, anaplastic carcinoma, and undifferentiated carcinoma have a poorer treatment outcome.[50]

In dogs and cats, a common tumor of the oral cavity is squamous cell carcinoma (**Fig. 7**). Fibrosarcoma, malignant melanoma, and periodontal ligament tumors are common in dogs, but rare in cats.[51–53] CT imaging of oral cavity tumors has been described in the literature with descriptions of dental neoplasms (**Fig. 8**)[54] and squa-mous cell carcinoma.[46,55] Tumors of the nasopharynx occur in dogs and cats, and CT is the best imaging modality. Tumor types include lymphoma, tonsillar and nontonsillar squamous cell carcinoma, carcinoma, adenocarcinoma, fibrosarcoma, and mela-noma; the latter two tumor types are more common in dogs. A recent paper describes CT features in 25 dogs with nasopharyngeal masses.[56] The authors concluded that CT is appropriate for staging nasopharyngeal masses, but biopsy is needed to determine tumor type.

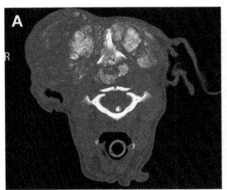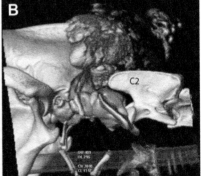

Fig. 5. CT images of a dog with a multinodular osteochondrosarcoma (MLO). On the trans-verse image at the level of caudal occipital bone in a bone window (*A*) note the distortion and enlargement of the right side of the head, destruction of the bony occiput, and the irregular "popcorn" bone attenuation of the MLO. On the three-dimensional reconstruction in a bone window (*B*) a more global view of the mass is seen. C2, spinous process of second vertebra; R, right side of the head.

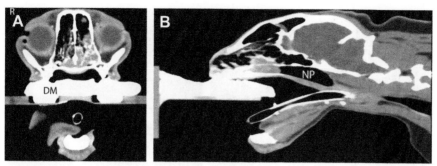

Fig. 6. CT images of a cat with nasal lymphoma in a soft tissue window. The soft tissue attenuating tumor is primarily left sided (*A*), but is also seen in the nasopharynx (*B*). A is a transverse image at the level of the eyes; the asymmetry of the eyes is caused by slight obliquity of the head. B is a reconstructed sagittal view of the head. Note the soft tissue attenuating material in the cranial nasopharynx. DM, dental material for maxillary mold; NP, nasopharynx; R, right side of head.

Neck Tumors

Canine thyroid tumors are the most common tumor imaged in the neck. Thyroid tumors can occur from the base of the tongue to the base of the heart. There are reports of ectopic thyroid tumors.[57,58] Generally thoracic CT imaging is performed at the same time because neck tumors and thyroid tumors metastasize to the lungs.

Esophageal tumors are uncommonly reported. Esophageal tumors secondary to *Spirocerca lupi* occur in endemic areas[59]; dogs present with regurgitation and caudal mediastinal masses. Because the parasite migrates through the thoracic aorta to the esophagus, changes to the aorta are seen and best identified on CT.[60] Reports of leiomyoma, leiomyosarcoma, adenocarcinoma, and carcinoma tumors of the esophagus exist[61–63] and are best imaged by CT.

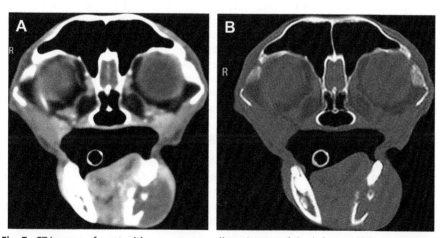

Fig. 7. CT images of a cat with a squamous cell carcinoma of the left mandible. On postcontrast transverse CT image in a soft tissue window (*A*) there is bony destruction of the left mandible with a hypoattenuating mass lateral to the mandible. The mass has only rim contrast enhancement. On the transverse CT image in a bone window (*B*) note the bony destruction of the alveolar bone and tooth root. R, right side.

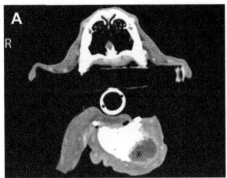
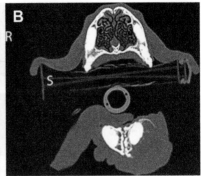

Fig. 8. Transverse CT images of a cystic acanthomatous ameloblastoma of the left rostral mandible in a dog. On the transverse image postcontrast in a soft tissue window (*A*) note the cystic component of the mass (*asterisk*). On the transverse image in a bone window (*B*) there is lysis of the alveolar bone of the rostral aspect of left mandibular canine tooth (304). R, right side of head.

COMPUTED TOMOGRAPHY FOR SURGICAL PLANNING: HEAD AND NECK

Similar techniques are used for surgical planning. Smaller slice thickness through a particular area may be requested by the radiologist to better delineate margins and invasiveness. Postcontrast images are especially helpful to delineate tumor extension.

COMPUTED TOMOGRAPHY SIMULATION FOR RADIATION THERAPY PLANNING: HEAD AND NECK

Immobilization of any tumor treated with radiation[64] including head and neck[65,66] is paramount to accurate delivery of radiotherapy, especially IMRT.[36,37] At our institution all suspected nasal, skull, and oral tumors that may be treated with radiation therapy are imaged in a bite block system and Vac-Lok mattress (see **Fig. 4**). Neck tumors are placed in dorsal recumbency with the head and neck to the shoulder region in a Vac-Lok mattress. Many tumors of the oral and nasal cavity, such as canine oral malignant melanoma, may have positive draining lymph nodes resulting in inclusion in the radiation treatment field or if normal on fine-needle aspiration undergo prophylactic treatment. The importance of expanding planning target volume (PTV) when including draining lymph nodes has been studied in dogs and cats using daily image-guided radiation therapy (IGRT) and bite block systems. PTV expansions to account for the unfixed nature of lymph nodes have been studied in dogs and cats with recommended PTV expansions.[67]

COMPUTED TOMOGRAPHY FOR CANCER STAGING: ABDOMEN

Often CT imaging of the abdomen replaces ultrasound for cancer staging and is added to the request for thoracic CT and primary tumor imaging. Abdomen CT is also used to stage a primary abdominal tumor looking for lymph node and other organ metastasis. At our institution we often use a portable ultrasound machine to perform fine-needle aspiration of suspected metastasis identified on CT imaging.

Equipment and Technique

If there is a potential for radiotherapy for an abdominal tumor, animals are placed in a Vac-Lok mattress for CT imaging. Patient positioning depends on tumor location. Patients may be in dorsal or lateral recumbency. Our imaging protocol is 120 kVp, 150 to

300 mA, with 1.25 mm contiguous slices for most patients and 2.5 mm for large dogs (see **Table 1**). The window/level for soft tissues and precontrast and postcontrast evaluation is W = 400/L = 40.

Abdominal Tumors

CT imaging for abdominal organs and potential metastasis is routine in veterinary medicine. Often patients that present to emergency with an abdominal mass have thoracic and abdominal CT (**Fig. 9**). Papers evaluating liver masses using triple-phase contrast CT imaging and dynamic liver CT imaging in dogs have reported differentiation among hepatocellular carcinoma, benign nodular hyperplasia, and hepatic metastasis,[68,69] and differentiation between hepatocellular carcinoma and benign nodular hyperplasia.[70] Similar techniques are being used to evaluate pancreatic insulinomas[71] and splenic masses,[72] and is commonly used in human medicine for renal masses.[73] CT imaging of adrenal masses in dogs has detected adjacent tumor vascular invasion,[56,74] but is not capable of delineating tumor type.[56]

COMPUTED TOMOGRAPHY FOR SURGICAL PLANNING: ABDOMEN

The ability to detect vascular invasion and to differentiate between malignant and benign lesions in the presurgical setting is of great benefit.[56,68,71,72,74] CT imaging provides an unobstructed view of abdominal organ anatomy and with reconstructed views a global anatomy of tumor extension and invasiveness.

COMPUTED TOMOGRAPHY SIMULATION FOR RADIATION THERAPY PLANNING: ABDOMEN

Patient immobilization is a key to accurate radiotherapy treatment delivery. Vac-Lok mattress systems are used for abdominal radiotherapy immobilization. In a small study six dogs with inoperable hepatocellular carcinoma tumors were treated with hypofractionated three-dimensional conformal radiation therapy.[75] In this study five dogs had a partial response and one dog had stable disease; only one dog had

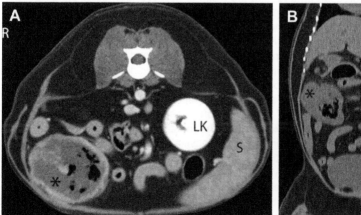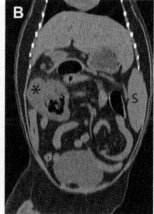

Fig. 9. CT images of gastrointestinal stromal mass. On transverse image postcontrast in a soft tissue window (*A*) the jejunal tumor (*asterisk*) is soft tissue attenuating with pockets of gas attenuation and a contrast-enhancing rim. On the dorsal plane reconstructed image (*B*) a global view of the tumor is seen (*asterisk*). The CT scan was useful for surgical planning. LK, left kidney; R, right side of abdomen; S, spleen.

radiation-related liver toxicity.[75] Three-dimensional conformal radiation therapy is the precursor to IMRT. Both have a multileaf collimator to shape the beam, but with IMRT the dose rate can be modulated during treatment. An additional necessity is daily IGRT. Studies have been done in veterinary medicine to look at IGRT in abdominal radiotherapy. Clinical veterinary radiation oncology researchers have studied urogenital tumors and evaluated interfraction motion using cone-beam CT,[67] and evaluated models of ART during treatment of urinary bladder tumors.[40] This same group looked at outcomes in a study of urogenital tumors treated with IMRT and IGRT and despite limitations of a small cohort and retrospective study, reported a well-tolerated treatment with good survival times.[76]

ART treatment is a feature of higher end linear accelerators and helical tomotherapy (Accuray, Madison, WI). First developed with helical tomotherapy, ART uses daily mega-voltage CT scan for daily IGRT and adapts the treatment plan if targets or organs at risk (OAR) change shape or size.[77,78] ART can be labor intensive to perform on a daily basis. At our institution we tend to use ART when there is PTV shrinkage or OAR moves into the PTV because of weight change rather than transient motion. Regarding urogenital malignancies, radiotherapy attempts should be made to treat the patient at the same time every day to have similar bladder and colon filling. Another study evaluated the use of contrast-enhanced CT images for treatment planning and delivery. This virtual study evaluated three tumor sites (nasal, appendicular, and pelvic) and looked at using contrast-enhanced CT for IMRT stereotactic body radiotherapy planning.[41] The goal of this study was to evaluate the dose to the gross tumor volume and OAR plans using noncontrast CT images, which is the gold standard, and contrast-enhanced CT. For all three sites there was less than 1% change in dose for gross tumor volume and OAR in both planning scenarios. The authors concluded that dose distribution between plans made on noncontrast and contrast-enhanced CTs was tolerable at all three treatment sites, but recommended caution when planning stereotactic body radiation therapy near areas of high contrast enhancement, such as the urinary bladder.[41]

MISCELLANEOUS TUMORS

Appendicular osteosarcoma tumors are a site of new research using stereotactic radiation therapy as a treatment modality. The gold standard treatment of appendicular osteosarcoma is amputation and chemotherapy. Radiation has been used in the palliative setting when amputation is either declined or not an option. Studies in the past looking at limb sparing used intraoperative radiotherapy and had mixed results.[79–81] In one small retrospective study, definitive radiotherapy and chemotherapy did not match standard of care therapy outcome.[80] Other studies used single large doses of intraoperative radiotherapy after en bloc resection of the tumor in the operating room. The irradiated section of tumorous bone was then reimplanted into the patient and stabilized using internal fixation.[79,81] The most difficult areas to salvage are the distal radius and tibia.[79] At our institution we have a current clinical trial evaluating stereotactic radiation therapy without surgery for appendicular osteosarcoma. Three doses of 8 Gy are given on a Monday, Wednesday, Friday schedule. We are finding the distal limbs the most challenging to plan because of the lack of soft tissues surrounding the tumor. It is important to spare a strip of skin that contains lymphatic drainage to maintain healthy tissue and prevent limb edema.

SUMMARY

This article presents some of the commonly treated tumors and the advances made in CT imaging and radiation therapy. With current CT technology, scans are obtained faster than many radiology sections can read them. The reliance of CT simulation for radiotherapy treatment planning has developed by leaps and bounds, and the existence of on-board kilovolt cone-beam CT and mega-voltage CT for IGRT has taken radiotherapy into the twenty-first century closing the gap to our medical colleagues. Omissions from this article deserve an article of their own and include brain tumors, feline injection site sarcomas, and canine sarcomas of the trunk and limbs.

REFERENCES

1. Prather AB, Berry CR, Thrall DE. Use of radiography in combination with computed tomography for the assessment of noncardiac thoracic disease in the dog and cat. Vet Radiol Ultrasound 2005;46(2):114–21.
2. Nemanic S, London CA, Wisner ER. Comparison of thoracic radiographs and single breath-hold helical CT for detection of pulmonary nodules in dogs with metastatic neoplasia. J Vet Intern Med 2006;20(3):508–15.
3. Paoloni MC, Adams WM, Dubielzig RR, et al. Comparison of results of computed tomography and radiography with histopathologic findings in tracheobronchial lymph nodes in dogs with primary lung tumors: 14 cases (1999-2002). J Am Vet Med Assoc 2006;228(11):1718–22.
4. Ballegeer EA, Adams WM, Dubielzig RR, et al. Computed tomography characteristics of canine tracheobronchial lymph node metastasis. Vet Radiol Ultrasound 2010;51(4):397–403.
5. Otoni CC, Rahal SC, Vulcano LC, et al. Survey radiography and computerized tomography imaging of the thorax in female dogs with mammary tumors. Acta Vet Scand 2010;52:20.
6. Eberle N, Fork M, von Babo V, et al. Comparison of examination of thoracic radiographs and thoracic computed tomography in dogs with appendicular osteosarcoma. Vet Comp Oncol 2011;9(2):131–40.
7. Marolf AJ, Gibbons DS, Podell BK, et al. Computed tomographic appearance of primary lung tumors in dogs. Vet Radiol Ultrasound 2011;52(2):168–72.
8. Alexander K, Joly H, Blond L, et al. A comparison of computed tomography, computed radiography, and film-screen radiography for the detection of canine pulmonary nodules. Vet Radiol Ultrasound 2012;53(3):258–65.
9. Armbrust LJ, Biller DS, Bamford A, et al. Comparison of three-view thoracic radiography and computed tomography for detection of pulmonary nodules in dogs with neoplasia. J Am Vet Med Assoc 2012;240(9):1088–94.
10. Reetz JA, Buza EL, Krick EL. CT features of pleural masses and nodules. Vet Radiol Ultrasound 2012;53(2):121–7.
11. Mattoon JS, Bryan JN. The future of imaging in veterinary oncology: learning from human medicine. Vet J 2013;197(3):541–52.
12. Oliveira CR, Mitchell MA, O'Brien RT. Thoracic computed tomography in feline patients without use of chemical restraint. Vet Radiol Ultrasound 2011;52(4): 368–76.
13. Oliveira CR, Ranallo FN, Pijanowski GJ, et al. The VetMousetrap: a device for computed tomographic imaging of the thorax of awake cats. Vet Radiol Ultrasound 2011;52(1):41–52.
14. Johnson EG, Wisner ER. Advances in respiratory imaging. Vet Clin North Am Small Anim Pract 2007;37(5):879–900, vi.
15. Johnson VS, Ramsey IK, Thompson H, et al. Thoracic high-resolution computed tomography in the diagnosis of metastatic carcinoma. J Small Anim Pract 2004; 45(3):134–43.

16. Joly H, d'Anjou MA, Alexander K, et al. Comparison of single-slice computed tomography protocols for detection of pulmonary nodules in dogs. Vet Radiol Ultrasound 2009;50(3):279–84.

17. Cardoso L, Gil F, Ramirez G, et al. Computed tomography (CT) of the lungs of the dog using a helical CT scanner, intravenous iodine contrast medium and different CT windows. Anat Histol Embryol 2007;36(5):328–31.

18. Scrivani PV, Thompson MS, Dykes NL, et al. Relationships among subgross anatomy, computed tomography, and histologic findings in dogs with disease localized to the pulmonary acini. Vet Radiol Ultrasound 2012;53(1):1–10.

19. Secrest S, Sakamoto K. Halo and reverse halo signs in canine pulmonary computed tomography. Vet Radiol Ultrasound 2014;55(3):272–7.

20. Ballegeer EA, Forrest LJ, Stepien RL. Radiographic appearance of bronchoalveolar carcinoma in nine cats. Vet Radiol Ultrasound 2002;43(3):267–71.

21. Lee KS, Kim Y, Han J, et al. Bronchioloalveolar carcinoma: clinical, histopathologic, and radiologic findings. Radiographics 1997;17(6):1345–57.

22. Barrett LE, Pollard RE, Zwingenberger A, et al. Radiographic characterization of primary lung tumors in 74 dogs. Vet Radiol Ultrasound 2014;55(5):480–7.

23. Tsai S, Sutherland-Smith J, Burgess K, et al. Imaging characteristics of intrathoracic histiocytic sarcoma in dogs. Vet Radiol Ultrasound 2012;53(1):21–7.

24. Gaeta M, Barone M, Caruso R, et al. CT-pathologic correlation in nodular bronchioloalveolar carcinoma. J Comput Assist Tomogr 1994;18(2):229–32.

25. Day MJ. Review of thymic pathology in 30 cats and 36 dogs. J Small Anim Pract 1997;38(9):393–403.

26. Pintore L, Bertazzolo W, Bonfanti U, et al. Cytological and histological correlation in diagnosing feline and canine mediastinal masses. J Small Anim Pract 2014; 55(1):28–32.

27. Yoon J, Feeney DA, Cronk DE, et al. Computed tomographic evaluation of canine and feline mediastinal masses in 14 patients. Vet Radiol Ultrasound 2004;45(6): 542–6.

28. Scherrer W, Kyles A, Samii V, et al. Computed tomographic assessment of vascular invasion and resectability of mediastinal masses in dogs and a cat. N Z Vet J 2008;56(6):330–3.

29. Chen GT, Kung JH, Rietzel E. Four-dimensional imaging and treatment planning of moving targets. Front Radiat Ther Oncol 2007;40:59–71.

30. Korreman SS. Motion in radiotherapy: photon therapy. Phys Med Biol 2012; 57(23):R161–91.

31. Moorrees J, Bezak E. Four dimensional radiotherapy: a review of current technologies and modalities. Australas Phys Eng Sci Med 2012;35(4):399–406.

32. Giraud P, Yorke E, Jiang S, et al. Reduction of organ motion effects in IMRT and conformal 3D radiation delivery by using gating and tracking techniques. Cancer Radiother 2006;10(5):269–82.

33. Cao Y. The promise of dynamic contrast-enhanced imaging in radiation therapy. Semin Radiat Oncol 2011;21(2):147–56.

34. La Fontaine MD, McDaniel LS, Kubicek LN, et al. Patient characteristics influencing the variability of distributed parameter-based models in DCE-CT kinetic analysis. Vet Comp Oncol 2015. [Epub ahead of print].

35. Saenz D, Bayouth J, Christensen N, et al. ViewRay real-time imaging of a motion phantom and in-vivo canine patients. Presented at the AAPM 2014 Innovation, 56th Annual Meeting & Exhibition. Austin (TX), July 20–24, 2014.

36. Kubicek LN, Seo S, Chappell RJ, et al. Helical tomotherapy setup variations in canine nasal tumor patients immobilized with a bite block. Vet Radiol Ultrasound 2012;53(4):474–81.

37. Deveau MA, Gutierrez AN, Mackie TR, et al. Dosimetric impact of daily setup variations during treatment of canine nasal tumors using intensity-modulated radiation therapy. Vet Radiol Ultrasound 2010;51(1):90–6.

38. Nieset JR, Harmon JF, Larue SM. Use of cone-beam computed tomography to characterize daily urinary bladder variations during fractionated radiotherapy for canine bladder cancer. Vet Radiol Ultrasound 2011;52(5):580–8.

39. Yoshikawa H, Harmon JF, Custis JT, et al. Repeatability of a planning target volume expansion protocol for radiation therapy of regional lymph nodes in canine and feline patients with head tumors. Vet Radiol Ultrasound 2012;53(6):667–72.

40. Nieset JR, Harmon JF, Johnson TE, et al. Comparison of adaptive radiotherapy techniques for external radiation therapy of canine bladder cancer. Vet Radiol Ultrasound 2014;55(6):644–50.

41. Yoshikawa H, Roback DM, Larue SM, et al. Dosimetric consequences of using contrast-enhanced computed tomographic images for intensity-modulated stereotactic body radiotherapy planning. Vet Radiol Ultrasound 2015;56(6):687–95.

42. Ghirelli CO, Villamizar LA, Pinto AC. Comparison of standard radiography and computed tomography in 21 dogs with maxillary masses. J Vet Dent 2013; 30(2):72–6.

43. Dernell WS, Straw RC, Cooper MF, et al. Multilobular osteochondrosarcoma in 39 dogs: 1979-1993. J Am Anim Hosp Assoc 1998;34(1):11–8.

44. Hathcock JT, Newton JC. Computed tomographic characteristics of multilobular tumor of bone involving the cranium in 7 dogs and zygomatic arch in 2 dogs. Vet Radiol Ultrasound 2000;41(3):214–7.

45. Lipsitz D, Levitski RE, Berry WL. Magnetic resonance imaging features of multilobular osteochondrosarcoma in 3 dogs. Vet Radiol Ultrasound 2001;42(1):14–9.

46. Soukup JW, Snyder CJ, Simmons BT, et al. Clinical, histologic, and computed tomographic features of oral papillary squamous cell carcinoma in dogs: 9 cases (2008-2011). J Vet Dent 2013;30(1):18–24.

47. Cox NR, Brawner WR Jr, Powers RD, et al. Tumors of the nose and paranasal sinuses in cats: 32 cases with comparison to a national database (1977-1987). J Am Anim Hosp Assoc 1991;27:339–47.

48. Madewell BR, Priester WA, Gillette EL, et al. Neoplasms of the nasal passages and paranasal sinuses in domesticated animals as reported by veterinary colleges. Am J Vet Res 1976;37:851–6.

49. Bright RM, Bojrab MJ. Intranasal neoplasia in the dog and cat. J Am Anim Hosp Assoc 1967;12:806.

50. Adams WM, Kleiter MM, Thrall DE, et al. Prognostic significance of tumor histology and computed tomographic staging for radiation treatment response of canine nasal tumors. Vet Radiol Ultrasound 2009;50(3):330–5.

51. Hoyt RF, Withrow SJ. Oral malignancy in the dog. J Am Anim Hosp Assoc 1984; 20:83–92.

52. Stebbins KE, Morse CC, Goldschmidt MH. Feline oral neoplasia: a ten-year survey. Vet Pathol 1989;26:121–8.

53. Dubielzig RR. Proliferative dental and gingival diseases of dogs and cats. J Am Anim Hosp Assoc 1982;18:577–84.

54. Amory JT, Reetz JA, Sanchez MD, et al. Computed tomographic characteristics of odontogenic neoplasms in dogs. Vet Radiol Ultrasound 2014;55(2):147–58.

55. Gendler A, Lewis JR, Reetz JA, et al. Computed tomographic features of oral squamous cell carcinoma in cats: 18 cases (2002-2008). J Am Vet Med Assoc 2010;236(3):319–25.

56. Carozzi G, Zotti A, Alberti M, et al. Computed tomographic features of pharyngeal neoplasia in 25 dogs. Vet Radiol Ultrasound 2015;56(6):628–37.

57. Liptak JM, Kamstock DA, Dernell WS, et al. Cranial mediastinal carcinomas in nine dogs. Vet Comp Oncol 2008;6(1):19–30.

58. Rossi F, Caleri E, Bacci B, et al. Computed tomographic features of basihyoid ectopic thyroid carcinoma in dogs. Vet Radiol Ultrasound 2013;54(6):575–81.

59. Ranen E, Lavy E, Aizenberg I, et al. Spirocercosis-associated esophageal sarcomas in dogs. A retrospective study of 17 cases (1997-2003). Vet Parasitol 2004;119(2–3):209–21.

60. Kirberger RM, Stander N, Cassel N, et al. Computed tomographic and radiographic characteristics of aortic lesions in 42 dogs with spirocercosis. Vet Radiol Ultrasound 2013;54(3):212–22.

61. Arnell K, Hill S, Hart J, et al. Persistent regurgitation in four dogs with caudal esophageal neoplasia. J Am Anim Hosp Assoc 2013;49(1):58–63.

62. Farese JP, Bacon NJ, Ehrhart NP, et al. Oesophageal leiomyosarcoma in dogs: surgical management and clinical outcome of four cases. Vet Comp Oncol 2008;6(1):31–8.

63. Ranen E, Dank G, Lavy E, et al. Oesophageal sarcomas in dogs: histological and clinical evaluation. Vet J 2008;178(1):78–84.

64. Green EM, Forrest LJ, Adams WM. A vacuum-formable mattress for veterinary radiotherapy positioning: comparison with conventional methods. Vet Radiol Ultrasound 2003;44(4):476–9.

65. Charney SC, Lutz WR, Klein MK, et al. Evaluation of a head-repositioner and Z-plate system for improved accuracy of dose delivery. Vet Radiol Ultrasound 2009;50(3):323–9.

66. Harmon J, Van Ufflen D, Larue S. Assessment of a radiotherapy patient cranial immobilization device using daily on-board kilovoltage imaging. Vet Radiol Ultrasound 2009;50(2):230–4.

67. Harmon J Jr, Yoshikawa H, Custis J, et al. Evaluation of canine prostate intrafractional motion using serial cone beam computed tomography imaging. Vet Radiol Ultrasound 2013;54(1):93–8.

68. Fukushima K, Kanemoto H, Ohno K, et al. CT characteristics of primary hepatic mass lesions in dogs. Vet Radiol Ultrasound 2012;53(3):252–7.

69. Kutara K, Seki M, Ishikawa C, et al. Triple-phase helical computed tomography in dogs with hepatic masses. Vet Radiol Ultrasound 2014;55(1):7–15.

70. Taniura T, Marukawa K, Yamada K, et al. Differential diagnosis of hepatic tumor-like lesions in dog by using dynamic CT scanning. Hiroshima J Med Sci 2009; 58(1):17–24.

71. Fukushima K, Fujiwara R, Yamamoto K, et al. Characterization of triple-phase computed tomography in dogs with pancreatic insulinoma. J Vet Med Sci 2016;77:1549–53.

72. Fife WD, Samii VF, Drost WT, et al. Comparison between malignant and nonmalignant splenic masses in dogs using contrast-enhanced computed tomography. Vet Radiol Ultrasound 2004;45(4):289–97.

73. Prasad SR, Dalrymple NC, Surabhi VR. Cross-sectional imaging evaluation of renal masses. Radiol Clin North Am 2008;46(1):95–111, vi–vii.

74. Schultz RM, Wisner ER, Johnson EG, et al. Contrast-enhanced computed tomography as a preoperative indicator of vascular invasion from adrenal masses in dogs. Vet Radiol Ultrasound 2009;50(6):625–9.
75. Mori T, Ito Y, Kawabe M, et al. Three-dimensional conformal radiation therapy for inoperable massive hepatocellular carcinoma in six dogs. J Small Anim Pract 2015;56(7):441–5.
76. Nolan MW, Kogan L, Griffin LR, et al. Intensity-modulated and image-guided radiation therapy for treatment of genitourinary carcinomas in dogs. J Vet Intern Med 2012;26(4):987–95.
77. Kupelian P, Langen K. Helical tomotherapy: image-guided and adaptive radiotherapy. Front Radiat Ther Oncol 2011;43:165–80.
78. Welsh JS, Lock M, Harari PM, et al. Clinical implementation of adaptive helical tomotherapy: a unique approach to image-guided intensity modulated radiotherapy. Technol Cancer Res Treat 2006;5(5):465–79.
79. Liptak JM, Dernell WS, Lascelles BD, et al. Intraoperative extracorporeal irradiation for limb sparing in 13 dogs. Vet Surg 2004;33(5):446–56.
80. Walter CU, Dernell WS, LaRue SM, et al. Curative-intent radiation therapy as a treatment modality for appendicular and axial osteosarcoma: a preliminary retrospective evaluation of 14 dogs with the disease. Vet Comp Oncol 2005;3(1):1–7.
81. Boston SE, Duerr F, Bacon N, et al. Intraoperative radiation for limb sparing of the distal aspect of the radius without transcarpal plating in five dogs. Vet Surg 2007; 36(4):314–23.

PET-Computed Tomography in Veterinary Medicine

Elissa K. Randall, DVM, MS

KEYWORDS

- PET/CT • FDG • Veterinary • Staging • SUV

KEY POINTS

- PET/computed tomography (CT) is used in veterinary medicine to diagnose and stage patients with cancer, using the glucose analogue 2-deoxy-2-18F-fluorodeoxyglucose (F-18 FDG).
- FDG-PET/CT is good at detecting areas of increased glucose metabolism and can detect primary tumors or metastatic lesions that are missed on routine examination and staging.
- Hypermetabolic areas (areas of increased glucose metabolism) are not specific for neoplastic tissue and may also represent physiologic variation or benign variation, including inflammation.
- Evaluation of the CT images may provide the information needed to determine the most likely diagnosis for a visualized hypermetabolic area, but cytology or histopathology is often needed for definitive diagnosis.

INTRODUCTION

Advanced imaging modalities, such as computed tomography (CT) and MRI, have been in use for decades in veterinary medicine. They provide images with superior anatomic information compared with radiographs and ultrasound. PET/CT is an advanced imaging modality that is becoming more commonly used in veterinary medicine. Special imaging equipment and appropriate nuclear medicine facilities are required to perform the studies, which are most commonly performed on patients with cancer.

WHAT IS PET/COMPUTED TOMOGRAPHY?

PET/CT was previously performed by acquiring a PET scan and CT scan on different machines at different times; but more recently, new machines acquire images on a dual PET/CT scanner as part of one imaging examination (**Fig. 1**). Combined

Disclosure statement: The author has nothing to disclose.
Department of Environmental and Radiological Health Sciences, Veterinary Teaching Hospital, Colorado State University, ACC 135, 300 West Drake Road, Fort Collins, CO 80523-1620, USA
E-mail address: elissa.randall@colostate.edu

vetsmall.theclinics.com

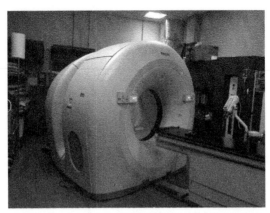

Fig. 1. A dual PET/CT scanner. The ring toward the front is the CT scanner. The ring in the back is the PET scanner. The table moves patients into the appropriate position for each phase of the PET/CT study. (*Courtesy of* Philips Healthcare. All rights reserved.)

PET/CT scanners provide automatic image fusion, whereas PET and CT studies obtained independently require appropriate software for fusion.

PET is a form of nuclear medicine that uses radiopharmaceuticals that are positron emitters. Positrons are positively charged particles, also called beta+ particles or β+. These particles travel a short distance (1–2 mm) before colliding with a negatively charged electron. When the two collide, 2 annihilation gamma photons are created and travel 180° from each other (coincident photons). The special detectors in a PET scanner detect and register these coincident photons, which arrive within a few nanoseconds of each other. The annihilation photons have energy of approximately 511 keV, which is higher than the 140 keV energy of technetium 99m, the radiopharmaceutical used for bone scans, glomerular filtration rate studies, and thyroid scans.[1]

CT is more familiar to the veterinary community. CT provides images based on x-ray attenuation, similar to radiography. However, images are acquired in slices and superimposition of structures is eliminated. CT images also have better contrast resolution than radiographs. The result is excellent anatomic depiction of patients. Multi-planar or 3-dimensional (3D) reformatting of images can provide more complete assessment.[2]

WHAT RADIOPHARMACEUTICALS ARE USED IN PET/COMPUTED TOMOGRAPHY?

The most commonly used PET radiopharmaceutical is 2-deoxy-2-18F-fluorodeoxyglucose (F-18 FDG). FDG is a glucose analogue that is labeled to F-18, a radioactive positron emitter. F-18 FDG is transported into the cell by glucose transporter proteins. In the cell, it is phosphorylated, similar to glucose. Glucose is then transported into mitochondria to be converted into energy or stored as glycogen. However, F-18 FDG undergoes no further reaction after this step and is effectively trapped in the cell. This mechanism allows F-18 FDG to be used to map glucose metabolism in the body.[3,4] Tumor cells often use more glucose than normal cells, making F-18 FDG an excellent tool to detect neoplastic tissue. However, some normal tissues use more glucose than other normal tissue and show high FDG uptake, so are hypermetabolic, or have higher FDG avidity, on PET images (**Fig. 2**). In addition, inflammatory lesions often use more glucose and are hypermetabolic on PET images. Knowing the appearance of variations of normal is key to image interpretation.

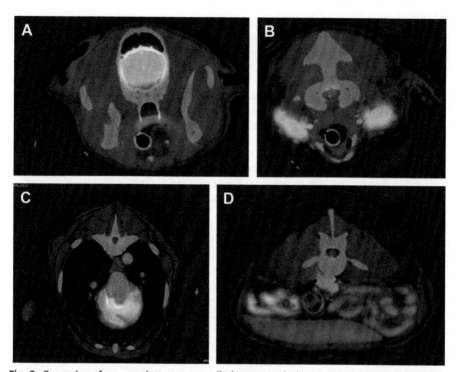

Fig. 2. Examples of organs that are normally hypermetabolic on FDG-PET/CT scans. All images are transverse fused PET/CT images. (*A*) The brain is diffusely hypermetabolic, with a standardized uptake value (SUV) maximum (max) of between 7.7 and 9.3 in this patient. (*B*) Salivary glands are generally hypermetabolic, though the degree varies with different salivary glands. Both mandibular salivary glands are visualized as ovoid hypermetabolic structures in this patient, with an SUV max of 5.7. (*C*) Cardiac muscle is variably hypermetabolic. This patient has several levels of metabolic activity in the heart, with the most hypermetabolic area of muscle having an SUV max of 7.7 to 9.3. (*D*) Intestines show variable metabolic activity. The patient has more hypermetabolic segments of small intestine on the left side of the image, with an SUV max of 5.0. Other, less hypermetabolic segments of small intestine on the right side of the images have an SUV max of 2.5.

F-18 FDG is excreted by the kidneys and eliminated in the urine. The half-life of F-18 FDG is 110 minutes, so approximately 50% of the given dose is present in the urine 2 hours after administration.[1] Because of this, patients typically have a urinary catheter placed while anesthetized in order to prevent radioactive contamination due to urine leakage.

Other PET radiopharmaceuticals used in clinical cases or clinical research in veterinary medicine include F-18 sodium fluoride (NaF), used to image bone and in particular osteoblastic activity; F-18 fluorothymidine (FLT), used to image DNA synthesis; and F-18 fluoromisonidazole and Cu-60,62,64 diacetyl-bis-N4-methylthiosemicarbazone (Cu-ATSM), used to study tumor hypoxia.[5–9] The focus of this article is F-18 FDG-PET/CT.

HOW IS A PET/COMPUTED TOMOGRAPHY STUDY ACQUIRED?

Protocols vary at different institutions. The protocol described is the one followed at Colorado State University, where images are obtained on a dual PET/CT scanner. Because a radiopharmaceutical is involved, having a clear understanding of the nuclear medicine radiation safety protocol, in addition to the CT radiation safety protocol, is important for all those involved. Appropriate facilities for the intake and storage of radiopharmaceuticals are necessary, as are appropriate facilities for housing radioactive patients.

Patients are fasted overnight before the PET/CT scan. Serum glucose is measured the morning of the scan. In humans, a moderate to severely elevated glucose (more than 200 ng/dL with a normal range 70–110 ng/dL, according to one reference) usually results in the scan being postponed until glucose levels are better regulated because high serum glucose can compete with F-18 FDG for uptake into the cell and affect the quality of the scan.[1] The normal range for glucose at this institution is 75 to 130 mg/dL for dogs and 69 to 136 mg/dL for cats. The author's institution does not abide by a strict cutoff for glucose values because this is an area of controversy, even in human medicine. However, uncontrolled diabetic patients do not undergo FDG-PET/CT scanning.

Patients are anesthetized according to the protocol determined by the anesthesia section. Patients are then transported to the PET/CT suite and positioned in dorsal or sternal recumbency. FDG is injected intravenously (0.14–0.17 mCi/kg), after which there is a 1-hour uptake period. This period is to allow FDG to distribute throughout the body and be transported into cells and trapped in those cells. Human patients are asked to sit quietly and silently in a room during the uptake period to limit physiologic uptake of FDG in skeletal muscle secondary to muscle use, which can make interpretation more difficult.[1] Because veterinary patients at this institution are anesthetized during the 1-hour uptake period, they have limited skeletal uptake from motion during this period. A preintravenous and postintravenous contrast whole-body CT scan is performed during the 1-hour uptake period. After 1 hour, PET images are acquired with patients in the same position. Whole-body PET images are obtained in 5 to 12 bed positions (2–3 minutes each) depending on the size of the patient. After the PET images are acquired, patients are transported to a special nuclear medicine ward (isolated from other hospital patients and personnel) and recovered there. Because of the short half-life of FDG (110 minutes), patients are typically scanned in the morning and released to go home the same evening, after their radiation level reaches the institutional safety level. Because of urinary excretion, patients are catheterized during the scan and eliminate in a specific nuclear medicine area after they have recovered from anesthesia.

In veterinary medicine, whole-body PET/CT scans typically include the entire patient, from the tip of the nose to beyond the caudal soft tissues of the pelvis, including all 4 limbs through the digits. Limbs may be positioned in extension or flexion. In comparison, most whole-body human PET/CT scans cover the base of the skull to the midthigh.[1]

IMAGE PROCESSING

Non–attenuation-corrected (NAC) PET images are reconstructed using the line-of-response row-action maximum likelihood algorithm method, which is a 3D reconstruction technique. CT attenuation-corrected (CTACs) images of PET are based on the precontrast CT dataset. PET images are available as CTAC and NAC images. CTAC images are the most commonly viewed of the PET images. The CT data provide information about the degree of photon attenuation by different tissues or structures. This information helps to provide proper scaling of the PET data by taking different tissue densities into account when interpreting the degree of PET photon emission and detection. However, when there are metallic implants or other very hyperattenuating structures, these can be overinterpreted and depicted as hypermetabolic areas on PET and potentially misinterpreted as malignant or inflammatory. Therefore, NAC images are also available. They will show normal FDG uptake in such areas and help the interpreter realize when a hypermetabolic region is artifactual.[10] Images are reviewed as CT-only images, PET-only images, and fused PET/CT images. PET images are fused with postcontrast CT images.

STANDARDIZED UPTAKE VALUE

Standardized uptake value (SUV) is a semiquantitative method of evaluating FDG uptake. It indicates the degree of FDG uptake in a measured structure, and SUV is directly proportional to metabolic activity. In simplified terms, if there were even distribution of the radiopharmaceutical throughout the body, the SUV would be 1. Therefore, a lesion with an SUV of 7 has 7 times the average uptake.[3] SUV maximum (max), SUV minimum, SUV average, and SUV total can be measured; but SUV max is the most commonly used in lesion analysis.[1] Examples of SUV max of normal structures in dogs are included in **Table 1**. SUV measurements have to be interpreted with caution because factors, such as body weight, time between injection and imaging, and serum glucose levels, affect SUV. In addition, comparison of SUV between institutions is difficult because of the different protocols, PET/CT equipment, and image acquisition settings.[8]

Although SUV measurements can be helpful, there is literature that suggests that visual inspection of a lesion is as reliable as SUV measurements in determining malignancy.[11] In human medicine, threshold values are used for some lesions to determine a benign from malignant nature. An example of this is solitary pulmonary nodules in people. A nodule greater than 1 cm with an SUV max equal to or greater than 2.5 is considered malignant.[1] However, no specific thresholds or specific cutoffs have been established in veterinary medicine. In addition, there is significant overlap in SUVs of benign and malignant lesions. Large numbers of PET/CT cases of specific tumor types would be necessary to establish SUV malignancy thresholds in veterinary medicine, a difficult task in this field.

WHAT INFORMATION DOES A PET/COMPUTED TOMOGRAPHY STUDY PROVIDE?

The CT images provide excellent anatomic depiction of normal and abnormal structures. The PET images show areas of high glucose metabolism. CT and PET images

Table 1 SUV max of normal organs in dogs	
Organ	**Typical SUV Max**
Brain	4–7
Salivary glands	2–6
Liver	1–3
Spleen	1–3
Skeletal muscle	0.5–1.5
Bone	0.5–2.0
Spinal cord	0.5–2.0
Intestines	0.5–8.0
Heart (myocardium)	0.5–9.0
Lymph nodes	0.5–2.0

are compared, side by side and fused, to determine if areas of noticeably high metabolic activity are normal or abnormal on CT. For example, the brain is normally markedly hypermetabolic because of its high glucose metabolism. Cardiac muscle is variably hypermetabolic because of the variation in myocardial metabolism relative to fasting and individual variation.[12,13] Salivary glands are hypermetabolic because of excretion of FDG in the saliva.[12] When a hypermetabolic area is noted, the CT will be used to determine what specific structure is hypermetabolic. Then knowledge of normal FDG uptake, and comparison with the contralateral structure if present, is used to determine if the degree of uptake is normal or abnormal for that structure. If a structure or area is deemed to be abnormally hypermetabolic, CT images provide a better picture of what is occurring locally and determine if a mass, inflammation, or other abnormalities are present.

FDG-PET/CT is used primarily to image patients with cancer. The ability to detect lesions with increased glucose use is helpful in identifying primary neoplastic lesions, determining the extent of known lesions, detecting metastatic lesions, and overall staging of patients with cancer. PET/CT aids in the detection, staging, treatment planning, and response to treatment of human and veterinary patients with cancer. In humans, the list of tumors covered for FDG-PET/CT by Medicare and Medicaid as of June 11, 2013 included colorectal, esophageal, head and neck (not thyroid or central nervous system) lymphoma, non–small cell lung, ovary, brain, cervix, small cell lung, soft tissue sarcoma, pancreas, testes, thyroid, breast, melanoma, and myeloma; a few of those have exceptions. Also listed as covered are *all other solid tumors* and *all other cancers not listed*. One tumor type not covered for initial diagnosis and staging is prostate cancer.[14] This long list of covered tumors underscores the importance of PET/CT in human oncology.

The normal distribution of FDG in cats and dogs has been described.[4,12,13] Physiologic variants, benign processes, and artifacts have also been described for FDG-PET/CT in dogs and cats.[15] The normal distribution of other radiopharmaceuticals has been investigated, including F-18 FLT in cats and F-18 NaF in dogs.[9,16] These studies pave the way for clinical investigation of disease processes in veterinary patients (**Fig. 3**).

PET/CT of the following tumor types have been reported on, or are currently being studied, in veterinary medicine: lymphoma, feline oral squamous cell carcinoma, osteosarcoma (OSA), mast cell tumor (MCT), plasma cell tumor, primary lung tumor, nasal tumors, mammary carcinoma, anal sac adenocarcinoma, pancreatic neuroendocrine carcinoma, soft tissue sarcoma, fibrosarcoma, hemangiopericytoma, squamous cell carcinoma, histiocytic sarcoma, Sertoli cell tumor, and gastrointestinal stromal tumor.[5,6,17–24] Some tumors have been studied as part of a coordinated series of cases of the same tumor type, and others have been cases that were part of a selection of multiple tumor types.

INITIAL DIAGNOSIS AND STAGING OF PATIENTS WITH CANCER

PET/CT is most often used to stage patients with a suspected or known primary tumor. It provides in-depth anatomic and metabolic information about the primary lesion and can detect metastatic lesions or diagnose unknown second neoplasms. PET/CT can also be used to look for the unknown primary lesion when metastasis is the first detected lesion.

PET/CT provides a way to achieve whole-body staging in one imaging procedure. The CT data are acquired in sufficiently small slices to provide excellent evaluation of the thorax and abdomen as well as of all bony structures. Charges vary by institution; but at this institution, the charge for a PET/CT is actually slightly less expensive

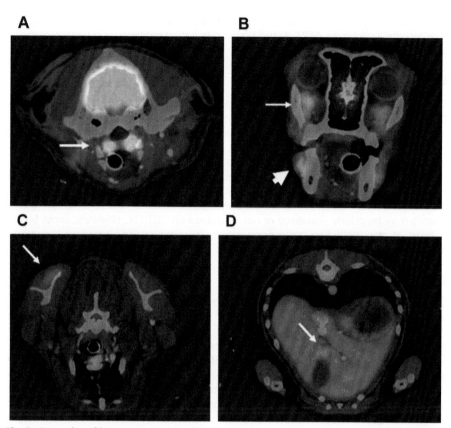

Fig. 3. Examples of benign variants in dogs: regions that may be hypermetabolic because of physiologic variation or inflammation, which may be subclinical. (*A*) A normal hypermetabolic brain is visible. Ventral to the brain are 2 rounded, hypermetabolic structures, which represent tonsils (*arrow*). Tonsils are frequently hypermetabolic, which may be because of physiologic variation or secondary to oral or dental inflammation. (*B*) Ventral to the eyes are mild to moderately hypermetabolic structures, which are normal zygomatic salivary glands (*small arrow*). Also, lateral to the mandible bilaterally are focal hypermetabolic areas, which may represent muscle uptake secondary to recent use or stretching during intubation, uptake in vasculature or local soft tissues, or salivary pooling (*large arrow*). (*C*) Focal uptake in the supraspinatus muscle (*arrow*), which may be due to altered weight bearing from known lameness or other focal muscle injury or recent use. (*D*) The liver can show patchy, mild to moderate hypermetabolic activity, as in this patient. This activity is seen is patients with no known hepatic disease and is considered a normal variant. There is also focal hypermetabolic uptake in the gallbladder (*arrow*), which is also considered a normal variant. Clinically silent hepatobiliary disease could be responsible for these changes.

than the combination of charges for a 3-view thoracic radiographic study + abdominal ultrasound + single-region CT. This charge does not include the cost of anesthesia, which is longer for PET/CT than CT alone. However, full-body staging is provided, with a more detailed evaluation of the lungs (for metastasis or other lesions), abdomen, head and neck, and spine/limbs.

The veterinary PET/CT literature up to this point has included a variety of tumor types, often single case reports or small numbers of the same tumor type. The tumor types with the greatest representation in veterinary FDG-PET or FDG-PET/CT literature include lymphoma, MCT, feline squamous cell carcinoma, and fibrosarcoma (5 cases or more of each).

LYMPHOMA AND MAST CELL TUMORS

Lymphoma and MCTs are neoplastic processes than are often disseminated to multiple organs and can involve liver, spleen, and lymph nodes. Patients with MCTs commonly have multiple cutaneous nodules. PET/CT has been shown to be similar to better than routine staging at detecting disease in lymph nodes. However, diffuse disease of the liver and spleen has been variably detected with PET/CT, being sometimes hypermetabolic and sometimes normal on PET images.[17,19] This data included a study that involved FDG-PET only.[19] Bone marrow infiltration has also been correctly diagnosed by PET/CT.[17] MCTs are variably hypermetabolic, and small or low-grade lesions may be poorly visualized or not visualized on PET/CT. However, most MCTs imaged at this institution have been visibly hypermetabolic, including low-grade MCTs (**Fig. 4**).

OSTEOSARCOMA

The tumor type most commonly staged with FDG-PET/CT at this institution is OSA, with approximately 60 cases having been imaged. Primary tumors are mildly to severely hypermetabolic, with SUV max ranging from 1.8 to 24.9 in one report; but an SUV max up to 34.9 has been seen.[25] Metastatic disease has been detected in patients with OSA; but many patients show no other evidence of disease, making the decision to pursue treatment more reasonable to owners. If metastasis is detected, those sites may be included in the radiation treatment planning process, if radiation therapy is pursued. Patients with a primary bone tumor often have areas of hypermetabolic activity in muscles of the contralateral limb, or multiple limbs, attributed to altered weight bearing (**Fig. 5**).

METASTASIS

When staging patients with cancer, primary lesions are usually hypermetabolic and well visualized on PET/CT. Metastatic lesions are also typically hypermetabolic and well visualized. One major benefit of PET/CT is in detecting metastatic lesions that were not detected on physical examination or lesions that do not appear abnormal on CT (**Fig. 6**). These lesions include lymph nodes that are normal on palpation and CT but hypermetabolic on PET. It is important to remember that these hypermetabolic lymph nodes may be reactive or metastatic, so cytology or histopathology should be attempted when possible (**Fig. 7**).

QUESTIONABLE LESIONS

One difficulty of PET/CT is that it is possible to also see lesions that are mildly to moderately hypermetabolic on PET but benign in appearance on CT. These lesions may be difficult to access for aspirates or biopsies, making confirmation of the benign or malignant nature difficult. Occasionally, repeat PET/CT can shed light on such lesions.

NON-NEOPLASTIC LESIONS

Many types of non-neoplastic lesions can be hypermetabolic and can range from mildly to severely hypermetabolic. If the lesions are superficial or related to known

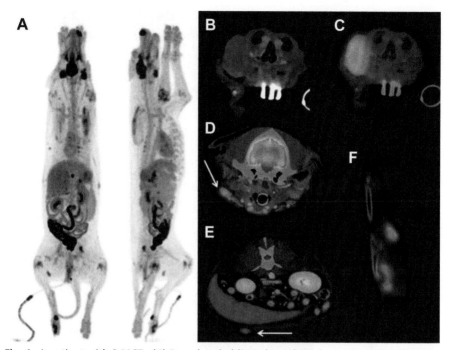

Fig. 4. A patient with 2 MCTs. (*A*) Dorsal and oblique lateral maximum intensity projection (MIP) images. These images show the FDG uptake throughout the body and allow the interpreter to identify hot spots that need to be investigated further on CT, PET, and fused PET/CT images. (*B*) CT image of a high-grade MCT on the right side of the nasal planum, which is mildly contrast enhancing. (*C*) Fused PET/CT image of the high-grade MCT of the nasal planum, which had an SUV max of 5.6. This mass is seen as a distinct hot spot on the nose on both MIP images. (*D*) Fused PET/CT image of a mildly enlarged and mildly hypermetabolic mandibular lymph node (*arrow*). This lymph node had an SUV max of 3.4, compared with the contralateral mandibular lymph nodes, which had an SUV max of 1.6. The right lymph node was considered possibly metastatic on imaging. It was interpreted as metastatic mast cell disease on cytology but reactive on histopathology. (*E*) Fused PET/CT image of a low-grade MCT on the abdominal body wall (*arrow*). This tumor had an SUV max of 1.8 and could be visualized on MIP images when viewed in a straight lateral position. (*F*) Sagittal fused PET/CT image of the left hind paw, which had multifocal areas of hypermetabolic activity, with an SUV max of 5.0 to 6.3. These areas are also well visualized on the MIP images. The paw was inspected, and multiple grass awns were removed.

procedures, it may be obvious to the interpreter why the lesion is hypermetabolic, decreasing the chance of misinterpretation of malignancy. Examples include hygromas, lick granulomas, feeding tube placement sites, and other superficial wounds or sites of infection. Unfortunately, some lesions that are not ascribable to a benign process or procedure, such as sclerotic, hypermetabolic lesions in vertebral bodies, are difficult to access for sampling; the clinician will have to decide the best treatment plan with the presumption of metastasis. Lesions that are logically diagnosed as metastatic disease, such as hypermetabolic lung nodules in a patient with a known primary tumor, may be proven to be malignant based on cellular sampling or follow-up imaging. However, some suspect metastatic lesions are proven to be benign on histopathology or follow-up imaging (**Fig. 8**). These cases again underscore the importance of obtaining histopathology of suspect metastatic lesions whenever possible.

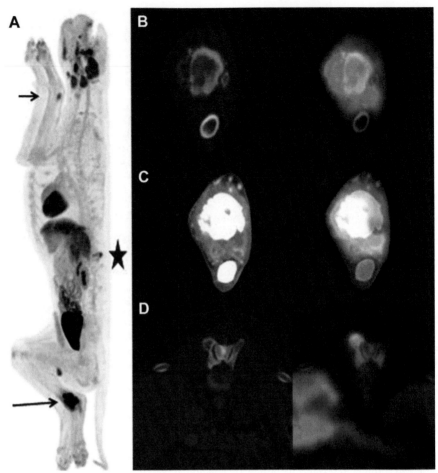

Fig. 5. Patient with OSA. (*A*) Oblique lateral maximum intensity projection image that shows the primary OSA in the left tibia (*long arrow*), a metastatic lesion to the left radius (*short arrow*), and a metastatic lesion to the articular facet of the first lumbar vertebra (*star*). The left popliteal lymph node was hypermetabolic and can be seen as a hot spot proximal to the primary lesion in the tibia. (*B*) Transverse CT image in a bone window, showing marked lysis and periosteal reaction of the primary tumor on the tibia. The image on the right is a fused PET/CT image at the same location showing the hypermetabolic activity of the tumor, which had an SUV max of 34.9. (*C*) Transverse CT image in a soft tissue window, showing the contrast-enhancing soft tissue swelling surrounding the mass. The image on the right is a fused PET/CT image at the same location showing the hypermetabolic activity of the bone and soft tissue abnormalities. (*D*) Transverse CT image in a bone window, showing lysis and expansion of the articular facet of the first lumbar vertebra and sclerosis of the pedicle. The image on the right is a fused PET/CT image at the same location showing the hypermetabolic activity in the articular facet, which had an SUV max of 6.2.

RADIATION TREATMENT PLANNING AND PET/COMPUTED TOMOGRAPHY AVID TUMORS
Oral Squamous Cell Carcinoma

PET/CT is valuable for guiding radiation treatment planning and can also be used to assess the response to radiation treatment. Cats with oral squamous cell carcinoma

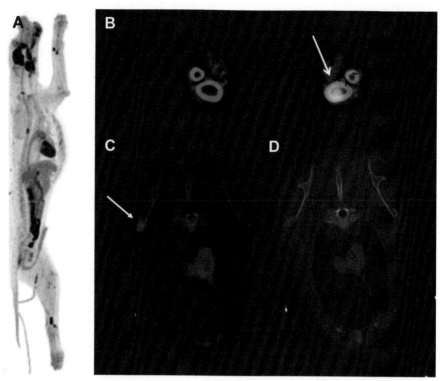

Fig. 6. (A) Patient with a recently excised plasmacytoma of the mandible who returned for staging after cutaneous nodules were noted. The PET/CT showed the cutaneous nodules along the dorsum (seen on the maximum intensity projection), plus multiple bone lesions that were new, surprising findings. The most hypermetabolic new bone lesions were in both distal radii, both distal tibias, and the right scapula. (B) Fused PET/CT image of the distal radii. At this level, the lesion in the left radius is visualized as a hypermetabolic area in the medullary cavity that was contrast enhancing on CT (*arrow*). The SUV max was 2.2. (C) Fused transverse PET/CT image showing a mildly hypermetabolic lesion in the right scapula (*arrow*). The SUV max was 2.8. (D) Transverse CT image in a bone window, showing mild, ill-defined lysis at the same location. Following the PET/CT, the cutaneous soft tissue nodules were biopsied and the diagnosis was changed to multiple myeloma.

were studied; PET/CT provided more extensive margins for soft tissue tumors than CT alone, whereas CT volume was greater than PET/CT volume in some cats, especially those with bone involvement. PET/CT also detected metastatic lesions that were equivocal on CT.[23] The end result was a larger gross tumor volume for radiation therapy treatment planning. Although it was not proven whether the hypermetabolic areas were entirely neoplastic tissue or also included inflammatory tissue, the greater tumor volume seen on PET/CT versus CT alone was used for radiation treatment to decrease the chances of missing tumor cells (geographic miss), which may decrease local tumor control.[18]

NASAL TUMORS

Similar conclusions were reached in a study of dogs with nasal tumors. PET/CT showed different tumor margins than CT alone, with CT often showing a larger overall

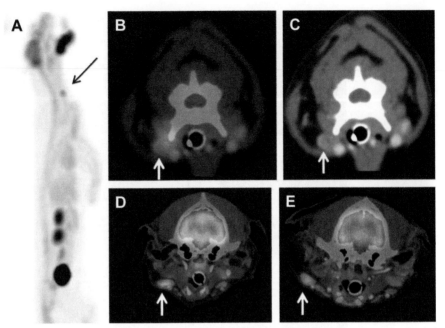

Fig. 7. (*A*) Lateral maximum intensity projection of a cat with an oral squamous cell carcinoma, seen as a large hypermetabolic area in the caudal mandibular region. The arrow is pointing to a focal area of mild hypermetabolic activity in the ventral cervical region. This area was further investigated on transverse images (*B, C*) and determined to be a deep cervical lymph node. (*B*) Transverse fused image showing the mild hypermetabolic activity in the area of the deep cervical lymph node. The SUV max was 3.6. (*C*) Transverse CT image in a soft tissue window at the same level as image (*B*). The right deep cervical lymph node (*arrow*) is mildly rounded and slightly larger than the left but is somewhat ill defined and difficult to identify as abnormal. Cytology of the right deep cervical lymph node revealed metastatic squamous cell carcinoma. (*D*) Fused transverse PET/CT image of a mildly enlarged and hypermetabolic mandibular lymph node (*arrow*) in dog with nasal squamous cell carcinoma. The SUV max was 4.1. Cytology revealed a reactive lymph node. (*E*) Fused transverse PET/CT image of a mildly enlarged and hypermetabolic mandibular lymph node (*arrow*) in dog with MCT. The SUV max was 3.5. Histopathology revealed a reactive lymph node.

volume. However, PET/CT detected hypermetabolic tissue outside the primary tumor that was normal on CT; in some dogs, the PET/CT volume was substantially greater than the CT volume. The conclusion was that PET/CT offers the best chance of depicting the maximal tumor volume, or potential areas of tumor, which would direct radiation therapy better than CT alone[26] (**Fig. 9**).

EVALUATING TREATMENT RESPONSE

PET/CT is valuable for evaluating the treatment response in human oncology patients and can be used to determine if a patient is responding to a treatment protocol or if the protocol needs to be altered. Evaluating the treatment response has also been investigated in veterinary medicine. FLT-PET/CT has been shown to depict the biological tumor response to chemotherapy in dogs with lymphoma. The SUV max of lymphoid tissues was significantly lower on the posttreatment scan compared with pretreatment

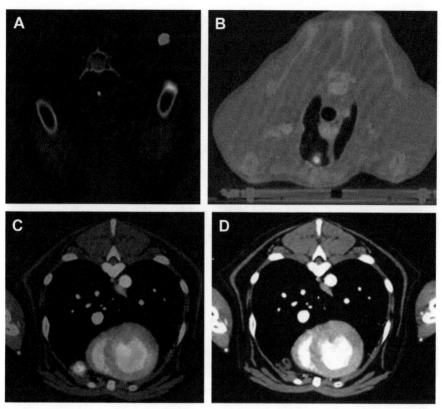

Fig. 8. (*A*) Fused transverse PET/CT image of a patient with OSA of the distal right femur. This image shows a focal hypermetabolic area in the cortex of the left humerus (SUV max 5.0.) There were no abnormalities on CT images, and repeat PET/CT performed 2 weeks later showed resolution of the hypermetabolic activity and a normal CT. The diagnosis was presumed focal trauma to the humerus before the first PET/CT. The repeat PET/CT helped rule out metastasis to the humerus. (*B*) Fused PET/CT image using a lung window. The patient had a previously resected adrenal gland carcinoma and a current presumed meningioma. There were multiple soft tissue nodules in the lungs that were mild to moderately hypermetabolic. The nodule shown was 10 mm in diameter and had an SUV max of 3.7. Histopathology of the nodules revealed benign granulomas. (*C, D*) Transverse fused PET/CT and soft tissue window CT images of a dog with a maxillary hemangiosarcoma. There is a small, hypermetabolic mass in the midventral mediastinum, adjacent to the heart. The SUV max was 6.3. The CT images shows that the mass is a mix of soft tissue and fat attenuating tissue and is heterogeneously contrast enhancing. Histopathology of the mass revealed focal granulomatous steatitis.

scans. This finding correlated with the patient clinical response. PET/CT also correctly detected tumor recurrence before it was diagnosed clinically.[5] FDG-PET/CT was used to evaluate the response to toceranib phosphate (Palladia) in 6 dogs. There were discordant findings between anatomic changes and metabolic changes on PET/CTs performed at least 4 weeks after the initiation of Palladia treatment, and lack of histopathology makes it difficult to determine whether the metabolic information from the PET or the anatomic information from the CT better reflected the disease process in the patients. However, the study supports the use of PET/CT to evaluate the treatment

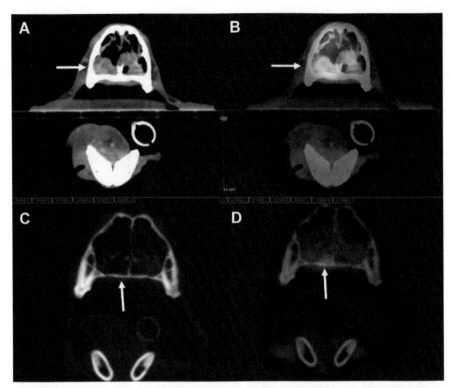

Fig. 9. (*A, B*) Transverse CT and fused PET/CT images of a dog with nasal squamous cell carcinoma. The arrow is pointing to a portion of the large, mainly right-sided mass. The SUV max was 13.5. There is also evidence of hyperattenuating soft tissue attenuating material in the left nasal cavity at the same level. (*C, D*) Transverse CT and fused PET/CT images of the midnasal cavity in the same dog, caudal to the large mass. PET/CT revealed hypermetabolic activity in a small area of soft tissue attenuating material close to midline (*arrows*). Based on the PET information, both the hypermetabolic area in the left nasal cavity and the focal area in the midright nasal cavity were included in the radiation field in order to prevent a geographic miss.

response or to restage patients and the need for histopathology of metabolic lesions when possible (**Fig. 10**).

OTHER USES OF 2-DEOXY-2-18F-FLUORODEOXYGLUCOSE–PET/COMPUTED TOMOGRAPHY

FDG-PET/CT can also be used to detect the source of fever of unknown origin (FUO) in veterinary patients. It has a moderate success rate in humans (40%–60%), but the degree of success in veterinary patients is still to be determined.[27,28] One example of a successful study is a patient with FUO in which hypermetabolic intrathoracic lymph nodes, pulmonary granulomas, and pulmonary interstitial disease were detected, guiding aspirates that led to a diagnosis of fungal disease (**Fig. 11**).

FDG-PET/CT can also be used to find a source of lameness in patients that are difficult to diagnose. The study may detect muscular injury, joint abnormality, infection, or neoplasia.

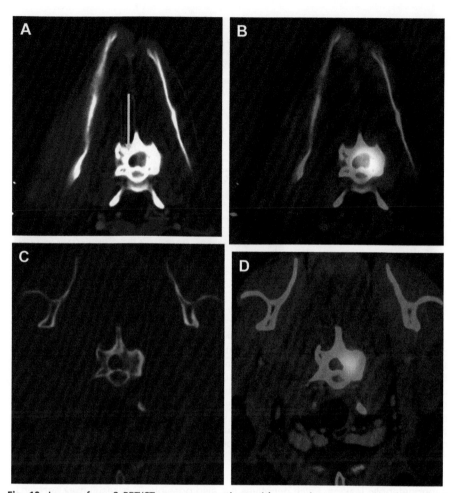

Fig. 10. Images from 2 PET/CT scans on a patient with a previous amputation for a tibial OSA. (*A*) Transverse CT image in a soft tissue window showing a soft tissue mass in the left side of the spinal canal, which is severely compressing the spinal cord. The spinal cord (*arrow*) is displaced to the right. There is lysis and bone production associated with the left pedicle of C7. (*B*) Fused PET/CT image at the same location as image (*A*) showing the hypermetabolic activity of the mass and abnormal bone, with an SUV max of 4.5. (*C*) Transverse CT image in a bone window from a follow-up PET/CT performed 3 months after radiation therapy for the presumed metastatic lesion of C7. The soft tissue component of the mass is greatly reduced in size, and the compression of the cord has improved. Compression is now mild and due to the smoothly mineralized portion of the mass that extends from the pedicle. (*D*) Transverse fused PET/CT image at the same level as (*C*). The SUV max decreased to 3.6. The patient's clinical signs related to the C7 lesion (tetraparesis) also significantly improved after stereotactic radiation therapy.

PITFALLS OF 2-DEOXY-2-18F-FLUORODEOXYGLUCOSE–PET/COMPUTED TOMOGRAPHY

As previously mentioned, there is overlap in the degree of hypermetabolic activity between benign, inflammatory lesions and malignant lesions. Therefore, cytology or histopathology should be performed when possible to confirm malignancy of

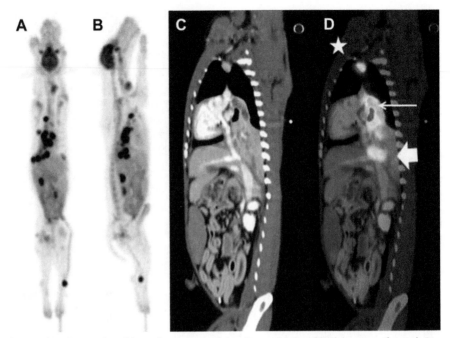

Fig. 11. (*A, B*) Dorsal and lateral maximum intensity projection (MIP) images of a Jack Russell terrier with a FUO. There are multiple areas of hypermetabolic activity in the thorax. (*C, D*) Sagittal CT and fused PET/CT images. The study revealed hypermetabolic pulmonary nodules (*star*), hypermetabolic, enlarged lymph nodes (*small arrow* pointing to tracheabronchial lymph nodes), and consolidated areas within multiple lung lobes (*large arrow* is pointing to right caudal lung lobe). Disease was confined to the thoracic cavity and was diagnosed as fungal disease (coccidioidomycosis). The hypermetabolic area in the cervical region seen on MIP images is inflammation at the site of esophageal feeding tube placement.

hypermetabolic lesions. False negatives are also possible. This result may happen in tumors that are small, low grade, necrotic, have large amounts of mucin, or are simply not as metabolically active.[1]

Aspirates of lesions that are detected before PET/CT should not be performed within 1 to 2 days before the scan because the procedure can cause local inflammation that may be hypermetabolic on PET/CT images, which can confound interpretation. In addition, care must be taken when obtaining aspirates that are diagnosed on PET/CT images. Ideally, aspirates should be performed on a separate day, when patient radioactivity is at background levels. Occasionally aspirates are obtained immediately after PET/CT, while patients are still anesthetized, for lesions that would be difficult to aspirate without anesthesia. In this case, only personnel with appropriate radiation safety training should obtain the samples, as patients are still radioactive. The samples also must be stored until they reach background levels of radioactivity and patients reach institutional release levels.

PET/CT has lower spatial resolution compared with CT and MRI, related to the annihilation process and technical factors of the PET/CT machine.[8] PET technology can detect lesions that are approximately 5 to 8 mm or greater. Therefore, lesions that are in the range of 5 to 8 mm or less may be missed on visual or quantitative inspection of images because of the lack of hypermetabolic activity.

There are many physiologic variants and artifacts that can complicate PET/CT interpretation. Physiologic variants include variable uptake in intestines, variable heterogeneity in liver and spleen, and muscle uptake. Artifacts include misregistration due to motion and vascular hypermetabolic activity upstream from the injection site. Other areas that commonly have increased metabolic activity due to presumed physiologic variation or inflammation include tonsils, gallbladder, nasal cavity, and a region of linear activity lateral to the mandible.[15] Experience reading canine and feline PET/CTs allows the interpreter to recognize these areas of normal variation.

SUMMARY

PET/CT is an imaging modality that is becoming increasingly available at veterinary or human referral imaging sites. PET/CT scans typically include whole-body imaging of patients with cancer and provide excellent anatomic and metabolic information for diagnostic and staging purposes. FDG-PET/CT has the ability to detect metabolic changes before anatomic change is evident. Good candidates for PET/CT are oncology patients who are healthy enough to undergo anesthesia for 2 to 3 hours. It is important to remember that, although FDG-PET/CT is good at detecting areas of increased metabolic activity, it is not specific for neoplasia, and cytology or histopathology of hypermetabolic lesions should be pursued when possible. In addition, strict cutoff values for SUV max have not been determined for specific malignancies in veterinary medicine; SUV max, although used to guide the degree of suspicion for malignancy, cannot be used to definitively diagnose a malignant lesion.

REFERENCES

1. Workman R, Coleman RE. PET/CT essentials for clinical practice. In: Workman R, Coleman RE, editors. New York: Springer; 2006. p. 1–22, 33–54.
2. Thrall D. Textbook of veterinary diagnostic imaging. 6th edition. St Louis (MO): Elsevier; 2013.
3. Lynch TB. PET/CT in clinical practice. In: Lynch TB, editor. London: Springer-Verlag; 2007. p. 1–15.
4. LeBlanc AK, Jakoby B, Townsend DW, et al. Thoracic and abdominal organ uptake of 2-deoxy-2-[18F] fluoro-D-glucose (18FDG) with positron emission tomography in the normal dog. Vet Radiol Ultrasound 2008;49:182–8.
5. Lawrence J, Vanderhoek M, Barbee D, et al. Use of 3'-deoxy-3'-[18F] fluorothymidine PET/CT for evaluating response to cytotoxic chemotherapy in dogs with non-Hodgkin's lymphoma. Vet Radiol Ultrasound 2009;50:660–8.
6. Ballegeer EA, Forrest LJ, Jeraj R, et al. PET/CT following intensity-modulated radiation therapy for primary lung tumor in a dog. Vet Radiol Ultrasound 2006;47:228–33.
7. Bruehlmeier M, Kaser-Hotz B, Achermann R, et al. Measurement of tumor hypoxia in spontaneous canine sarcomas. Vet Radiol Ultrasound 2005;46:348–54.
8. Lawrence J, Rohren E, Provenzale J. PET/CT today and tomorrow in veterinary cancer diagnosis and monitoring: fundamentals, early results and future perspectives. Vet Comp Oncol 2010;8:163–87.
9. Valdes-Martinez A, Kraft SL, Brundage CM, et al. Assessment of blood pool, soft tissue, and skeletal uptake of sodium fluoride F 18 with positron emission tomography-computed tomography in four clinically normal dogs. Am J Vet Res 2012;73:1589–95.

10. Visvikis D, Costa DC, Croasdale I, et al. CT-based attenuation correction in the calculation of semi-quantitative indices of [18F] FDG uptake in PET. Eur J Nucl Med Mol Imaging 2003;30:344–53.

11. Boland GW, Blake MA, Holalkere NS, et al. PET/CT for the characterization of adrenal masses in patients with cancer: qualitative versus quantitative accuracy in 150 consecutive patients. AJR Am J Roentgenol 2009;192:956–62.

12. LEE MS, LEE AR, JUNG MA, et al. Characterization of physiologic 18F-FDG uptake with PET-CT in dogs. Vet Radiol Ultrasound 2010;51:670–3.

13. LeBlanc AK, Wall JS, Morandi F, et al. Normal thoracic and abdominal distribution of 2-deoxy-2-[18F] fluoro-d-glucose (18FDG) in adult cats. Vet Radiol Ultrasound 2009;50:436–41.

14. Jacques L, Jensen TS, Rollins J, et al. The Centers for Medicare and Medicaid Services. Decision memo for positron emission tomography (FDG) for solid tumors (CAG-00181R4). Baltimore (MD): United State Government; 2013.

15. Randall E, Loeber S, Kraft S. Physiologic variants, benign processes, and artifacts from 106 canine and feline FDG-PET/computed tomography scans. Vet Radiol Ultrasound 2014;55:213–26.

16. Rowe JA, Morandi F, Wall JS, et al. Whole-body biodistribution of 3′-deoxy-3′-[18F] fluorothymidine (18FLT) in healthy adult cats. Vet Radiol Ultrasound 2013;54:299–306.

17. Ballegeer EA, Hollinger C, Kunst CM. Imaging diagnosis—multicentric lymphoma of granular lymphocytes imaged with FDG PET/CT in a dog. Vet Radiol Ultrasound 2013;54:75–80.

18. Yoshikawa H, Randall EK, Kraft SL, et al. Comparison between 2-18F-fluoro-2-deoxy-D-glucose positron emission tomography and contrast-enhanced computed tomography for measuring gross tumor volume in cats with oral squamous cell carcinoma. Vet Radiol Ultrasound 2013;54:307–13.

19. Leblanc AK, Jakoby BW, Townsend DW, et al. 18FDG-PET imaging in canine lymphoma and cutaneous mast cell tumor. Vet Radiol Ultrasound 2009;50:215–23.

20. LeBlanc AK, Miller AN, Galyon GD, et al. Preliminary evaluation of serial 18FDG-PET/CT to assess response to toceranib phosphate therapy in canine cancer. Vet Radiol Ultrasound 2012;53:348–57.

21. Hansen AE, McEvoy F, Engelholm SA, et al. FDG PET/CT imaging in canine cancer patients. Vet Radiol Ultrasound 2011;52:201–6.

22. Lee AR, Lee MS, Jung IS, et al. Imaging diagnosis—FDG-PET/CT of a canine splenic plasma cell tumor. Vet Radiol Ultrasound 2010;51:145–7.

23. Randall EK, Kraft SL, Yoshikawa H, Larue SM. Evaluation of 18F-FDG PET/CT as a diagnostic imaging and staging tool for feline oral squamous cell carcinoma. Vet Comp Oncol 2013. [Epub ahead of print].

24. Seiler SM, Baumgartner C, Hirschberger J, et al. Comparative oncology: evaluation of 2-deoxy-2-[18F] fluoro-D-glucose (FDG) positron emission tomography/computed tomography (PET/CT) for the staging of dogs with malignant tumors. PLoS One 2015;10:e0127800.

25. Mann K, Kraft SL, Hauke SM, et al. Quantitative analysis of 18F-fluorodeoxyglucose standardized uptake values in pretreatment PET/computed tomography imaging of canine osteosarcomas. Proceedings, American College of Veterinary Radiology Annual Scientific Conference. St Louis, MO, October 21–24, 2014. (Available from Veterinary Radiology and Ultrasound).

26. Loeber SJ, Custis JT, Randall EK, et al. Incorporation of FDG-PET/CT into radiation therapy planning to improve treatment of canine nasal tumors. Proceedings,

American College of Veterinary Radiology Annual Scientific Conference, St Louis, MO, October 21–24, 2014. (Available from Veterinary Radiology and Ultrasound).

27. Kei PL, Kok TY, Padhy AK, et al. [18F] FDG PET/CT in patients with fever of unknown origin: a local experience. Nucl Med Commun 2010;31:788–92.

28. Pelosi E, Skanjeti A, Penna D, et al. Role of integrated PET/CT with [(1)(8)F]-FDG in the management of patients with fever of unknown origin: a single-centre experience. Radiol Med 2011;116:809–20.

Interventional Radiology
Equipment and Techniques

Brian A. Scansen, DVM, MS

KEYWORDS

- Canine • Feline • Stent • Balloon • Embolization • Catheterization
- Minimally invasive

KEY POINTS

- Interventional radiology (IR) is the field of medicine that affects a therapeutic outcome via minimally invasive catheterization of peripheral blood vessels or body orifices guided by imaging.
- Fluoroscopy and specialized equipment are required to perform most procedures.
- Access needles, guide wires, sheaths, catheters, embolic agents, and devices are the tools used to treat many diseases in most organ systems; their design and use are discussed in this article.
- The field of veterinary IR is relatively new but rapidly expanding and offers new treatment paradigms for dogs and cats.

INTRODUCTION

Catheterization of internal organs and imaging were combined in the early 1900s for visualization of the gastrointestinal, renal, and cardiovascular systems in both animals and people.[1–3] Radiology and catheterization further evolved in the latter half of the twentieth century to yield the field of IR, defined as the area of medicine that affects a therapeutic outcome via minimally invasive catheterization of peripheral blood vessels or body orifices, guided by imaging. This may include balloon dilation of stenoses; particle, coil, or device occlusion of abnormal vasculature; stent implantation for narrowed lumens; biopsy or extraction of tumors, stones, or foreign material; placement of drainage or infusion catheters for medicinal or nutritional support; and so forth. In human medicine, the birth of IR as a specialty is widely attributed to Charles Dotter[4] in 1963, greatly facilitated by the description of percutaneous vascular access by

Disclosure Statement: The author has nothing to disclose.
Department of Clinical Sciences, College of Veterinary Medicine & Biomedical Sciences, Colorado State University, 1678 Campus Delivery, Fort Collins, CO 80523-1678, USA
E-mail address: brianscansen@yahoo.com

Vet Clin Small Anim 46 (2016) 535–552
http://dx.doi.org/10.1016/j.cvsm.2015.12.009   vetsmall.theclinics.com
0195-5616/16/$ – see front matter © 2016 Elsevier Inc. All rights reserved.

Sven Seldinger a decade prior.[5] The field of IR grew from fewer than 100 practicing physicians in the early 1970s to more than 4000 by 2003.[4]

The origin of IR in veterinary medicine is less clearly defined because image-guided interventions had been performed for decades by both cardiologists and radiologists prior to routine use of this term. The first stand-alone veterinary IR service and the first training fellowship in veterinary IR began, however, under the direction of Chick Weisse at the Ryan Veterinary Hospital of the University of Pennsylvania in 2005. In the 10 years since this beginning, veterinary IR has gained broad recognition as a viable treatment option for animals with myriad diseases and is practiced by veterinary surgeons, internists, criticalists, cardiologists, and radiologists. The intent of this article is to offer a brief overview of the equipment and techniques routinely performed in veterinary IR.

EQUIPMENT

Interventional radiologic procedures may be guided by radiography, fluoroscopy, ultrasound, or cross-sectional imaging. Most veterinary IR procedures utilize fluoroscopy or ultrasonography to guide therapy. Access to the site of intervention is occasionally facilitated by a surgical or hybrid approach or by videoendoscopic guidance, known as interventional endoscopy. Interventional procedures are preferably executed in a clean operating room or catheterization laboratory. The catheterization laboratory should ideally function as a sterile space, with storage for commonly used equipment. High-quality fluoroscopic imaging is needed and desirable equipment includes portable ultrasound for needle guidance or transesophageal echocardiography; a power injector for rapid delivery of iodinated contrast; anesthetic and hemodynamic equipment for patient monitoring and recording of intravascular pressures; sufficient monitors for visualization of real-time images and monitoring parameters; the capacity to bring in endoscopic equipment; and a crash cart for stocking of supplies required for emergent intervention, including a cardioverter-defibrillator.

Fluoroscopy

Most veterinary IR procedures require fluoroscopic guidance, with certain advanced features desired. The fluoroscopic system should allow digital archiving, provide high resolution, generate sufficient energy to penetrate the abdomen of a large dog, be capable of displaying and recording fast frame rates (25–30 frames per second or higher), and have electronic magnification, digital subtraction, and road-mapping capabilities.

The rapid heart rates of dogs and cats cause contrast filling of vascular structures to be temporally brief and a frame-by-frame review of a recorded angiographic run is needed to visualize the anatomy and perform measurements. Fast frame rates prevent an operator from "missing" the lesion during contrast injection into a high-flow organ. Digital subtraction angiography (DSA) is a technique whereby a fluoroscopic image is stored and then digitally subtracted from the remainder of the cine run prior to administration of contrast (**Fig. 1**). This facilitates visualization of the radiographic contrast in finer detail by removing overlying anatomy. Road mapping is similar in that a previously recorded angiogram can be overlaid onto a live fluoroscopic image, and guide wires or catheters can be directed and manipulated toward structures of interest without requiring additional contrast administration.

Fluoroscopic systems may be portable, requiring only a standard electrical outlet, or large fixed systems. Higher-quality imaging and advanced capabilities are available on the fixed systems, albeit at higher cost. Fluoroscopes use either an analog image

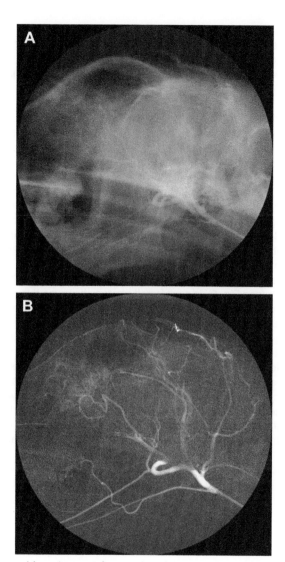

Fig. 1. External carotid angiograms from a dog. (*A*) Bony structures obscure intravascular contrast in standard fluoroscopic images, (*B*) but better detail of vasculature can be obtained when DSA is used, masking all structures in the image prior to contrast injection.

intensifier or a digital flat panel detector to generate an image. Advantages of flat panel detectors include lack of geometric distortion, a uniform response across the field of view, and a smaller footprint detector, improving access to the patient.[6] Most veterinary fluoroscopic systems today are image intensifier–based systems; however, flat panel detector technology can now be found in select academic and tertiary care centers.

Many human catheterization laboratories use biplane fluoroscopic systems that provide real-time imaging of 2 orthogonal views to improve anatomic guidance. New-generation fluoroscopic systems can also perform rotational angiography to circumferentially record a single injection from all angles and create a 3-D reconstruction of the anatomy. Finally, some systems have the capability of importing anatomic land-marks from cross-sectional imaging studies (CT or MRI) or real-time echocardio-graphic imaging onto the live 2-D fluoroscopic image to improve guidance during the intervention. Although desirable, many of these features are cost prohibitive in vet-erinary medicine.

Needles, Sheaths, Catheters, and Wires

For many interventions, access to a vessel or organ lumen is accomplished by place-ment of an introducer sheath through which catheters, wires, or devices may be safely advanced (**Fig. 2**). The sheath is placed over a wire, which has been directed into the organ or vessel lumen through an access needle or over-the-needle (OTN) catheter. Sheaths have an inner dilator, which tapers to a known wire diameter, allowing for a smooth transition from wire, to dilator, to outer sheath diameter. Traditionally, 18-gauge or 19-gauge access needles were used in combination with wires of 0.035-in or 0.038-in diameter to achieve access. Whether using an access needle or an OTN catheter, the operator should verify the desired wire passes easily prior to gaining access to the vessel or organ.

In small animals, access with a microintroducer, a 4F or 5F sheath that tapers to a 0.018-in guide wire (see **Fig. 2**), is a preferred strategy because this allows for use of a smaller-gauge access needle (typically 21-gauge or 22-gauge) and lessens trauma to the target. The needle is placed into the organ lumen via palpation or ultrasound guid-ance and verified by a "flash" of bodily fluid (eg, urine from the renal pelvis or blood from a femoral artery). When the access needle is within the lumen, a wire is advanced to provide a scaffold over which the introducer sheath can be directed. Once a micro-introducer is placed, a larger diameter wire can be placed in the vessel lumen through the microintroducer and exchanged for a conventional sheath of the desired size. A sheath may be short or long and of variable shape and typically has a hemostatic valve at the end as well as a side port. The size of a sheath is given by its internal diameter (eg, an 8F sheath has an inner diameter of 8F), in contrast to catheter sizing, as described later.

Catheters are tubes of variable shape and size that are manipulated in the body un-der fluoroscopic guidance (**Fig. 3**). They are radiopaque and have a Luer adaptor on

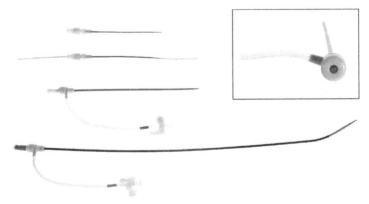

Fig. 2. Examples of introducer sheaths for vascular access. From the top to bottom are 5F microintroducer, 5F microintroducer with 0.018-in wire showing the taper from sheath to dilator to wire, 7F × 13-cm sheath with side port, and 7F × 45-cm Ansel sheath with angled tip and side port. The inset in the upper right corner shows the hemostatic valve at the back of most sheaths used for vascular access.

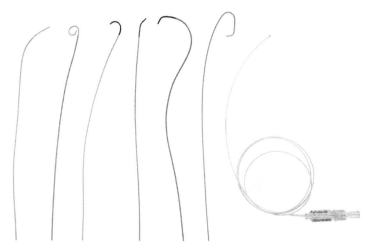

Fig. 3. Examples of catheter shapes and sizes used during interventional procedures. From left to right are 6F NIH, 5F pigtail marker catheter, 5F RIM, 5F Cobra hydrophilic catheter, 4F Kempe, 4F Judkins left, and 3F microcatheter.

the end, which allows connection to syringes and other medical devices. Although dozens of catheter shapes exist to facilitate a variety of procedures, most laboratories stock a limited selection of frequently used shapes and sizes, such as an angled tip of approximately 45° (examples include Berenstein, Kumpe, NIH, and multipurpose catheters), a reverse curve catheter (examples include Chung, left Judkins, RIM, Simmons, and visceral catheters), a double-curve catheter (examples include Cobra and right Judkins catheters), flow-directed catheters with an inflatable balloon (examples include balloon wedge pressure and Swan-Ganz catheters) and angiographic catheters (examples include Berman and pigtail catheters). Most procedures are performed using 4F or 5F catheters, although larger-bore catheters up to 8F may be desired for angiographic studies to allow rapid administration of contrast. Catheters that are smaller than 3F are termed *microcatheters* and are very flexible, allowing for access to tortuous small vessels.

Catheter stiffness varies by the catheter design, material, and manufacturer; some catheters have a hydrophilic coating, providing a lubricious and atraumatic surface when advanced into the body. Catheter size is determined by the outer diameter of the catheter, in contrast to sheaths. A 5F catheter can be passed through a 5F sheath because the inner diameter of the sheath and outer diameter of the catheter are equivalent. In practice, choosing a sheath 1 size larger than the desired catheter size allows for greater technical ease. Specialized catheters include balloon dilation catheters and drainage catheters.

Advancing a catheter into a body structure is performed over a guide wire in almost all circumstances. Manipulating a guide wire to the desired site for imaging or intervention is safer than direct advancement of a catheter; once a guide wire is positioned, catheters can be advanced to the target using the wire as a guide. Like catheters, there are numerous guide wires of variable shape, diameter, stiffness, taper, and composition (**Fig. 4**). Standard guide wires have a 0.035-in diameter and lengths of 150 cm or 180 cm; microwires are those that have a 0.018-in or smaller diameter. Exchange-length guide wires are 260 cm or longer, allowing replacement of a catheter without losing the position of the guide wire in the body.

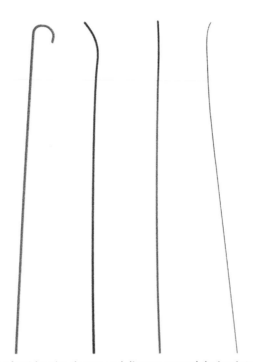

Fig. 4. Examples of guide wire shapes and diameters used during interventional procedures. From left to right are 0.038-in Teflon-coated stainless steel wire with 3-mm J-tip, 0.035-in hydrophilic guide wire with angled tip, 0.032-in hydrophilic guide wire with straight tip, and 0.014-in stainless steel guide wire with angled tip.

Traditional guide wires have a stainless steel core of variable stiffness around which lies a stainless steel spring coil, the entirety of which is coated in polytetrafluoroethylene (Teflon); additional heparin coatings are common to reduce thrombogenicity. Newer guide wires have a nitinol core, which is a superelastic alloy that provides good torque control with greater flexibility and maneuverability compared with stainless steel. Hydrophilic guide wires are commonly used that have a highly lubricious coating when wet, reducing friction and lessening the force required to advance the guide wire and allowing atraumatic catheterization of tortuous anatomy.

The end of a guide wire is preformed by the manufacturer into various shapes that facilitate catheterization, including straight, angled, complex curvature, and J-tipped. Other guide wires have a shapeable tip that can be manipulated into any desired shape. Guide wires with a 45° angulation are commonly used to select vascular branches; J-tipped guide wires provide an atraumatic tip within an organ lumen and avoid selection of branch points during advancement. The tip of a guide wire also has a variable taper, meaning the portion of the wire that is floppy prior to reaching the stiff core. Many wires have a short taper of 1 cm to 3 cm, whereas others are made with a 10-cm or longer taper. Greater flexibility at the tip can assist in the access of tortuous anatomy, whereas the stiff core is required to provide a sufficient scaffold to advance a catheter over the wire. Core stiffness may vary from standard to superstiff or even ultrastiff, with indications for each representing a compromise between stability for advancement of catheters or devices and stress on the structure catheterized.

Drainage Catheters

Drainage catheters are placed in a hollow viscous, abscess, or potential space within the body to allow efflux of bodily fluids (eg, nephrostomy tube) or to facilitate drainage from a pathologic process (eg, peritoneal abscess). Most drainage catheters are a pigtail or locking-loop configuration, which maximizes drainage while minimizing dislodgement of the system. They are placed over a wire using a stiff stylet to straighten the catheter. The locking-loop catheter maintains its pigtail configuration by use of a string that is tightened and secured at the external end of the catheter once the stylet is removed. Release of this string is required prior to removal; removal should be performed over a wire to straighten the curved end and avoid trauma to the tissue tract.

TECHNIQUES
Vascular Access – Venous

Venous access for interventional procedures is achieved percutaneously using the external jugular vein or femoral vein in dogs and cats (**Fig. 5**). The skin over the vein is clipped, scrubbed, and draped in a sterile fashion. A 1-mm to 2-mm skin incision

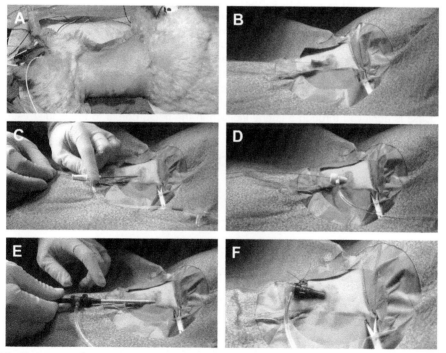

Fig. 5. Images of percutaneous venous access to the canine external jugular vein. (*A*) The neck is clipped and sterilely scrubbed. (*B*) After draping and a 2-mm skin incision, access is obtained with a 22-gauge catheter and a 0.018-in guide wire is directed into the lumen. (*C*) A 4F microintroducer is advanced over the guide wire. (*D*) A 0.035-in guide wire is advanced through the microintroducer, allowing a stronger scaffold for the sheath. (*E*) The microintroducer is removed and the sheath (9F in this case) is advanced over the guide wire. (*F*) The introducer sheath is sutured to the skin of the neck and the procedure can proceed. The use of a microintroducer is optional but preferred in small dogs or cats to limit damage to the vessel.

is made with a #11 blade and an access needle or OTN catheter is advanced into the vein. Ultrasound is useful to guide needle access, although palpation of the vein is often sufficient. For the femoral vein, the puncture is made 2 mm to 3 mm medial to the palpable arterial pulse because the femoral vein lies medial to the femoral artery and nerve (**Fig. 6**). The vein should bleed back through the hub, confirming position within the vessel lumen, and a guide wire is then advanced through the needle. Pressure is placed on the vein as the access needle or catheter is removed and wire position maintained. A sheath is then advanced into the vein over the wire and sutured to the proximate skin. A 0.035-in guide wire is used with an 18-gauge OTN catheter for large dogs versus a microintroducer and a 0.018-in guide wire through a 22-gauge OTN catheter for small dogs and cats.

Vascular Access – Arterial

Percutanous femoral arterial access can be performed and is the standard of care in people, with manual compression and reduced mobility prescribed after sheath removal to provide hemostasis of the arteriotomy. Manual compression was found to provide insufficient hemostasis in dogs after percutaneous arterial access and therefore most arterial interventions involve surgical exposure of the femoral artery. The inguinal region is clipped, scrubbed, and draped. A 3-cm to 4-cm incision is made distal to the inguinal ring along the long axis of the limb over the femoral pulse. Dissection isolates the femoral artery and vein (see **Fig. 6**). Suture is passed proximal and distal to the site of puncture and an access needle or OTN catheter is advanced into the artery. Pressure is greater in the artery than vein and back-bleeding can be significant. Rapid exchange and pressure at the site during wire manipulation and sheath placement are required to minimize blood loss.

Carotid arterial access is similar, although the surgical approach is deeper. Carotid access is achieved through a lateral incision in the neck, dorsal to the jugular vein.

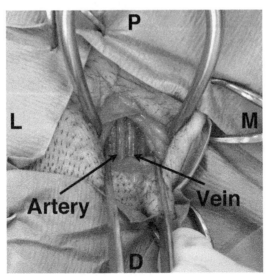

Fig. 6. Intraoperative image of the canine right femoral vasculature. After dissection, the femoral artery is seen lateral (cranial) to the vein. Not shown is the femoral nerve, which lies lateral to the artery and has been retracted in this image. D, distal; L, lateral; M, medial; P, proximal.

Alternatively, the carotid artery can be approached from the ventral neck with an incision lateral to the trachea. The carotid artery is found within the vagosympathetic trunk at the dorsolateral border of the trachea; the vagus nerve should be gently dissected from the carotid artery prior to vascular access.

The femoral or carotid artery is ligated above and below the access site or surgically repaired. Animals have substantial collateral circulation, allowing ligation of the common femoral or carotid artery, although this limits ability to re-intervene and is suboptimal for a procedure meant to be minimally invasive. The author has published successful use of a vascular closure device in a coagulopathic dog after percutaneous femoral arterial access,[7] which has become a common strategy in human medicine to minimize complications from manual compression. Several devices are available and result in effective hemostasis, allow for preservation of the vessel, and avoid a surgical approach to the artery, thereby reducing pain/discomfort in recovery. Their use in veterinary medicine is untested but may gain in popularity in the future if safety and efficacy can be proved in animals.

Biopsy, Snare, and Extraction Techniques

Several devices can be inserted through a sheath that provide the ability to grasp structures of interest, biopsy areas of suspected disease, or extract foreign bodies from within the patient. Such devices allow for the minimally invasive removal of ingested, inhaled, or embolized foreign material (**Fig. 7**). A commonly used device is a gooseneck snare, which is a loop of variable size positioned 90° to a wire and inserted to the intended site through a delivery catheter.[8,9] As the snare is exteriorized from the catheter, the loop releases and is manipulated around the target. The snare is retracted into the catheter, which tightens the loop around the target, capturing it and allowing its removal. It is usually best to pass the snare beyond the target and then draw it back to facilitate capture. Common indications for a snare in the cardiovascular system include heartworm retrieval and vascular foreign body retrieval.[10,11]

In the gastrointestinal or respiratory system, endoscopic delivery of a wire snare connected to an electrocautery device is used to facilitate polypectomy or to biopsy and debulk intraluminal masses.[12,13] Other devices include biopsy or retrieval forceps, the Ishihara flexible forceps commonly used for heartworm extraction, retrieval baskets of numerous design, and so forth. Depending on the desired target, some or all of these devices may be used under fluoroscopic or endoscopic visualization within the vascular system, heart, respiratory tree, or gastrointestinal tract.

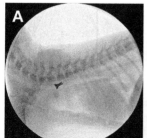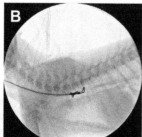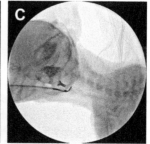

Fig. 7. Interventional removal of an esophageal foreign body (peripheral venous catheter) in a 2-month-old, 400-g kitten. (*A*) The object is visualized within the esophagus. (*B*) A snare catheter was introduced into the esophagus over a hydrophilic guide wire and a gooseneck snare advanced beyond the catheter and tightened. (*C*) Retraction of both snare and snare catheter results in retrieval of the foreign body.

Targeted Therapeutics, Sclerosants, and Embolics

Drugs, particles, or occlusive substances can be delivered selectively to target disease or obstruct anomalous vasculature. Examples include intra-arterial chemotherapy, arterial embolization for intractable epistaxis, transarterial chemoembolization (TACE) for nonresectable tumors, glue embolization for arteriovenous malformations or fistulae, and sclerotherapy for venous and lymphatic malformations.

Particles come in several sizes depending on the target vascular bed (**Fig. 8**). Particles are preferable to arterial ligation for vascular occlusion because upstream ligation (eg, common carotid artery ligation for intractable epistaxis) does not prevent collateral vessel development; selective particulate embolization limits the capacity of the vascular bed to revascularize. Small particles (less than 300 μm) are likely to reach small arteriole and capillary beds, resulting in complete embolization, although leaving the potential for tissue necrosis. Larger particles (greater than 700 μm) may allow small artery collateral flow to develop, making large particles safer, although

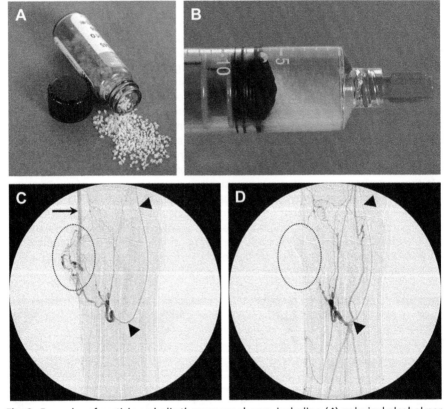

Fig. 8. Examples of particle embolic therapy are shown, including (A) polyvinyl alcohol particles and (B) calibrated microspheres of trisacryl cross-linked gelatin suspended in saline. (C, D) Injection of embolic particles is performed through superselective catheterization of a feeding vessel using a microcatheter (*arrowheads*). In this example, a small arteriovenous malformation (within *dotted circle*) on the lateral aspect of a canine tarsus is visualized (C) before and (D) after embolization, with polyvinyl alcohol hydrogel microspheres of 500 μm to 700 μm diameter. Note (D) the absence of flow to the lesion as well as absence of the draining vein (*arrow*) as compared with (C).

potentially less effective than small particles. Most procedures requiring particle embolization are successfully achieved with medium size particles (300–500 μm), although circumstances may dictate variation from this size.

Complete stasis is more likely to result in occlusion of the microvasculature and tissue necrosis than allowing persistent sluggish flow, although it carries a greater risk for complications. Early embolics included gelatin sponge and ground polyvinyl alcohol that were irregular in shape and inconsistent in size; newer calibrated microspheres are spherical, of consistent size, and less likely to form aggregates.[14] These newer agents have variable deformability and guidelines for use vary by proprietary agent.

Particle embolization can be combined with intra-arterial delivery of chemotherapeutics in a TACE procedure, which results in a first-pass effect of a chemotherapeutic agent through the tumor vasculature as well as occlusion of the tumor capillary bed. In humans, this provides a synergistic antineoplastic effect[15] and it has anecdotally been shown beneficial in dogs.[16] Delivery of standard chemotherapeutics without particle embolization directly to a tumor arterial bed may provide benefits beyond conventional intravenous chemotherapy. With intra-arterial delivery, the tumor capillary bed sees a full systemic dose of the medication. Although limited studies are available in veterinary patients, a preliminary study in dogs with urothelial malignancy suggested improved tumor response and fewer side effects.[17]

Glue embolization and sclerotherapy are performed to effect rapid occlusion of a vascular bed. Cyanoacrylate glue polymerizes in an ionic environment and special training is required prior to use because complications from nontarget glue embolization are likely. In veterinary medicine, glue embolization has been described for treatment of hepatic arteriovenous malformations.[18,19] Sclerotherapy involves injection of an irritant (such as ethanol or the sclerosing foam sodium tetraradecyl sulfate) into a vascular structure (venous or lymphatic malformation), which results in endothelial irritation, thrombosis, and closure of the vessel. Although not reported in animals, the author has used sodium tetraradecyl sulfate foam in a dog to sclerose an orbital varix with excellent results.

The approach for embolic procedures involves superselective catheterization of the vascular bed of interest. This means arterial access with an introducer sheath, upstream placement of a 4F or 5F catheter, and superselection of the arterial branch feeding the malformation or tumor with a microcatheter (see **Fig. 8**). Particles are mixed with contrast to allow visualization and are gently injected under fluoroscopic imaging, with monitoring for reflux that may cause nontarget embolization and to assess the degree of blood stasis.[20] A microcatheter that was used to deliver embolics should never be flushed unless the flush is monitored under fluoroscopic guidance and release of further embolic agent that remains within the catheter lumen is acceptable. Injection of glue or a sclerotic agent is more complicated and its discussion is beyond the scope of this article.

Coil or Device Occlusion

The intent of coils and occlusion devices is to obstruct larger diameter vessels, defects in intracardiac septae, or fistulous communications (**Fig. 9**). Coils come in numerous sizes, are fabricated from wires of comparable diameter to guide wires (eg, 0.018-in and 0.035-in), and are extruded through catheters by advancement of a guide wire behind the coil (**Fig. 10**). Coils have variable shape, diameter, and length and induce thrombosis either via a complex shape, synthetic fibers placed on the wire, or a hydrogel coating that swells on deployment.[21] First-generation coils were stainless steel, although platinum and nickel alloy (Inconel) coils are more commonly available today

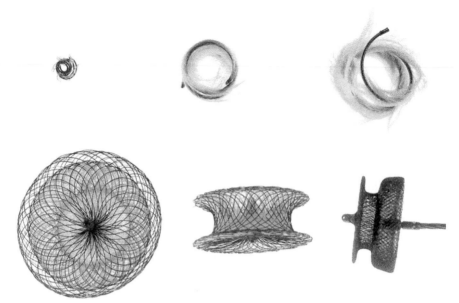

Fig. 9. Images of coils and devices used in veterinary IR. The top row shows different coil sizes, including (from left to right) a 0.018-in, 4-mm diameter platinum coil with a vortex shape; a 0.038-in, 6-mm diameter stainless steel coil; and a 0.038-in, 12-mm diameter stainless steel coil. Devices of woven nitinol are shown in the bottom row, including (from left to right) a 14-mm Amplatzer Septal Occluder, a 14-mm Amplatzer Muscular VSD Occluder, and a 7-mm Amplatz Canine Duct Occluder mounted on delivery cable.

related to improved MRI compatibility. Some coils are attached to a delivery system, allowing for careful positioning or reconstraint into the catheter; they are released either mechanically with an interlocking mechanism or via an electrolytic reaction. Coils are used in veterinary medicine primarily for the closure of congenital shunts (eg, patent ductus arteriosus or portosystemic communications [see **Fig. 10**]) and less commonly for aneurysms or fistulae.[22,23]

Many devices have been developed that are made from nitinol, allowing for compression into a catheter and reformation once deployed within the body. Vascular plugs, atrial and ventricular septal occluders, and devices optimized for closure of the canine patent ductus arteriosus are all examples of devices utilized in veterinary IR (see **Fig. 9**).[24–26]

Balloon Dilation

Several IR therapies rely on balloon dilation of a stenotic orifice, lumen, or valve (**Fig. 11**). There are many balloon dilation catheters available on the market, with varying profiles, materials, sizes, and maximal pressure. Most balloons are made from a thermoelastic polymer that is expanded when filled with air or saline/contrast. Specialized balloon dilation catheters include cutting balloons, which incorporate microblades that are exposed during inflation, and drug-eluting balloons, which deposit antiproliferative agents at the site of inflation.

The ideal balloon is made of a noncompliant material that expands solely to its stated size; is of a low profile, meaning it folds tightly over the catheter shaft; accommodates an appropriately sized guide wire; and offers good tracking and pushability.

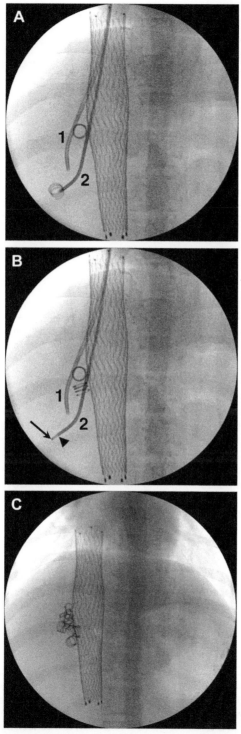

Fig. 10. Coil deployment during percutaneous transjugular coil embolization of canine right-divisional intrahepatic portocaval shunt. Two catheters (1 and 2) were advanced from the jugular

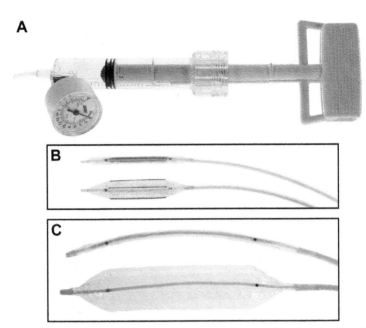

Fig. 11. Images of balloon dilation catheters used in veterinary IR. When inflating a balloon dilation catheter, (A) a controlled inflation device with a pressure gauge should be used. Many balloon varieties exist, including (B) cutting and (C) conventional balloon dilation catheters.

Because some of these traits are contradictory, the balloon chosen is always a trade-off of characteristics and all aspects should be considered in evaluating the target to be dilated and a patient's size and anatomy. Higher inflation pressure increases the radial force that the balloon applies to a stenosis; however, higher-pressure balloons are typically stiffer and have a larger profile necessitating a larger introducer.

A balloon dilation catheter is delivered to a stenosis over a guide wire and positioned with the center of the balloon engaging the stenosis to maximize radial force (**Fig. 12**). An inflation device with pressure gauge (see **Fig. 11**) is used to monitor inflation pressures to confirm nominal pressure – the pressure at which the balloon reaches the manufactured diameter, without exceeding burst pressure – the pressure at which the balloon's integrity cannot be guaranteed.

Stents

Stents are devices implanted to hold open a narrowed lumen or to provide a scaffold for coiling or other embolic therapies. Stents come in numerous designs and are composed of variable materials (**Fig. 13**). An example of a nonmetallic stent is the plastic double-pigtail ureteral stent.[27] Ureteral stents are fenestrated and

---

vein, to caudal vena cava, and passed between the interces of a caval SEMS. Catheter 1 provides portal pressure monitoring, with coils delivered through catheter 2. (A) A straight, floppy-tipped guide wire is advanced behind a coil and the coil partially extruded. (B) With further advancement, the tip of the guide wire (arrow) can be seen beyond the end of the catheter (arrowhead) and the coil released. (C) Additional coils are delivered until a targeted rise in portal pressure is documented; in this case, 8 coils were used.

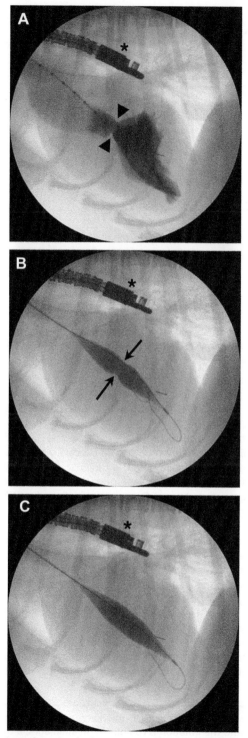

Fig. 12. Balloon dilation of a subvalvular stenotic ridge in canine subaortic stenosis. (*A*) A discrete ridge (*arrowheads*) is seen by left ventriculography. (*B*) A stenotic waist (*arrows*)

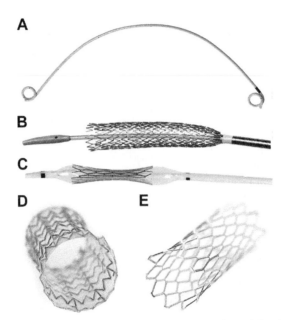

Fig. 13. Images of stents used in veterinary IR, including (*A*) plastic fenestrated double-pigtail ureteral stent, (*B*) SEMS, (*C*) BEMS, (*D*) covered stent, and (*E*) bare-metal stent.

implanted under fluoroscopic or cystoscopic guidance from an antegrade (via access to the renal pelvis) or retrograde (via access to the ureterovesicular opening) approach. Metallic stents include vascular, tracheal, biliary, nasopharyngeal, and uretheral stents.

Balloon-expandable metallic stents (BEMSs) and self-expanding metallic stents (SEMSs) exist; BEMSs are premounted onto a balloon dilation catheter and balloon inflation deploys the stent at the target. The BEMSs are typically made of stainless steel and used in veterinary IR for palliation of nasopharyngeal stenosis[28] or stenting of the right ventricular outflow tract.[29] Common indications for SEMSs in veterinary IR include tracheal, vena caval, and urethral stents.[30–32]

Woven and laser-cut SEMSs are used and differ in deployment characteristics. Woven SEMSs are composed of stainless steel or nitinol, compressed onto the delivery system, and unsheathed when at the target. Woven SEMSs display foreshortening, where the compressed stent is longer within the delivery system, and shortens in length as it expands to the final diameter. A benefit of woven SEMSs is reconstrainability, such that improper positioning can be corrected and the stent brought back onto the delivery system if less than 60% to 70% of the stent has been deployed. Laser-cut SEMSs are cut from a single tube of nitinol and utilize the thermal-phase transformation properties of this alloy.[33] Below its transformation temperature, nitinol can be deformed and crimped onto a delivery system, with an outer sheath preventing re-expansion. When warmed to body temperature, the crystal structure of the alloy

---

appears during initial balloon dilation. (*C*) With greater pressure generation in the balloon, the waist disappears and the inflation is completed. In all images, a transesophageal echocardiography probe (*asterisk*) is seen as well as a subcutaneous linear metallic foreign body overlying the heart.

changes and it returns to the original size. Laser-cut SEMSs are deployed by unsheathing the stent and have minimal foreshortening; however, the nature of their manufacture prevents reconstrainability.

Both BEMSs and SEMSs come in bare-metal forms with open interces, or covered forms, also called stent grafts. Covered stents help to constrain tissue proliferation and luminal restenosis, although, when placed in nonsterile areas, seem to have increased risk for infection. Last, drug-eluting stents are available in human medicine that limit tissue proliferation at the site of deployment, but these have not gained widespread acceptance in veterinary IR.

ACKNOWLEDGMENTS

The author gratefully acknowledges Tim Vojt and Marc Hardman of the Biomedical Media division in the College of Veterinary Medicine at The Ohio State University for assistance with photographic editing and artwork.

REFERENCES

1. Barrs TJ. Overview of radiopaque drugs: 1895-1931. Am J Health Syst Pharm 2006;63:2248–55.
2. Mueller RL, Sanborn TA. The history of interventional cardiology: cardiac catheterization, angioplasty, and related interventions. Am Heart J 1995;129:146–72.
3. Johnson V. Diagnostic imaging: reflecting on the past and looking to the future. Vet Rec 2013;172:546–51.
4. Rosch J, Keller FS, Kaufman JA. The birth, early years, and future of interventional radiology. J Vasc Interv Radiol 2003;14:841–53.
5. Seldinger SI. Catheter replacement of the needle in percutaneous arteriography; a new technique. Acta Radiol 1953;39:368–76.
6. Seibert JA. Flat-panel detectors: how much better are they? Pediatr Radiol 2006; 36:173–81.
7. Scansen BA, Hokanson CM, Friedenberg SG, et al. Use of a vascular closure device during percutaneous arterial access in a dog with impaired hemostasis. J Vet Emerg Crit Care, in press.
8. Gentile JM, Bulmer BJ, Heaney AM, et al. Endovascular retrieval of embolized jugular catheter fragments in three dogs using a nitinol gooseneck snare. J Vet Cardiol 2008;10:81–5.
9. Tan CA, Levi DS, Moore JW. Embolization and transcatheter retrieval of coils and devices. Pediatr Cardiol 2005;26:267–74.
10. Bove CM, Gordon SG, Saunders AB, et al. Outcome of minimally invasive surgical treatment of heartworm caval syndrome in dogs: 42 cases (1999-2007). J Am Vet Med Assoc 2010;236:187–92.
11. Culp WT, Weisse C, Berent AC, et al. Percutaneous endovascular retrieval of an intravascular foreign body in five dogs, a goat, and a horse. J Am Vet Med Assoc 2008;232:1850–6.
12. Yas E, Kelmer G, Shipov A, et al. Successful transendoscopic oesophageal mass ablation in two dogs with spirocerca lupi associated oesophageal sarcoma. J Small Anim Pract 2013;54:495–8.
13. Coleman KA, Berent AC, Weisse CW. Endoscopic mucosal resection and snare polypectomy for treatment of a colorectal polypoid adenoma in a dog. J Am Vet Med Assoc 2014;244:1435–40.
14. Osuga K, Maeda N, Higashihara H, et al. Current status of embolic agents for liver tumor embolization. Int J Clin Oncol 2012;17:306–15.

15. Facciorusso A, Licinio R, Muscatiello N, et al. Transarterial chemoembolization: evidences from the literature and applications in hepatocellular carcinoma patients. World J Hepatol 2015;7:2009–19.

16. Weisse C. Hepatic chemoembolization: a novel regional therapy. Vet Clin North Am Small Anim Pract 2009;39:627–30.

17. Culp WT, Weisse C, Berent AC, et al. Early tumor response to intraarterial or intravenous administration of carboplatin to treat naturally occurring lower urinary tract carcinoma in dogs. J Vet Intern Med 2015;29:900–7.

18. Chanoit G, Kyles AE, Weisse C, et al. Surgical and interventional radiographic treatment of dogs with hepatic arteriovenous fistulae. Vet Surg 2007;36:199–209.

19. Weisse C. Hepatic arteriovenous malformations (AVMs) and fistulas. Veterinary image-guided interventions. Ames (IA): John Wiley & Sons, Ltd; 2015. p. 227–37.

20. Weisse C. Liver tumors/metastases (TAE/cTACE/DEB-TACE). Veterinary image-guided interventions. Ames (IA): John Wiley & Sons, Ltd; 2015. p. 238–46.

21. Vaidya S, Tozer KR, Chen J. An overview of embolic agents. Semin Intervent Radiol 2008;25:204–15.

22. Singh MK, Kittleson MD, Kass PH, et al. Occlusion devices and approaches in canine patent ductus arteriosus: comparison of outcomes. J Vet Intern Med 2012;26:85–92.

23. McClellan NR, Mudge MC, Scansen BA, et al. Coil embolization of a palatine artery pseudoaneurysm in a gelding. Vet Surg 2014;43:487–94.

24. Hogan DF, Green HW, Sanders RA. Transcatheter closure of patent ductus arteriosus in a dog with a peripheral vascular occlusion device. J Vet Cardiol 2006;8: 139–43.

25. Gordon SG, Saunders AB, Achen SE, et al. Transarterial ductal occlusion using the Amplatz® canine duct occluder in 40 dog. J Vet Cardiol 2010;12:85–92.

26. Gordon SG, Miller MW, Roland RM, et al. Transcatheter atrial septal defect closure with the Amplatzer atrial septal occluder in 13 dogs: short- and mid-term outcome. J Vet Intern Med 2009;23:995–1002.

27. Berent AC. Ureteral obstructions in dogs and cats: a review of traditional and new interventional diagnostic and therapeutic options. J Vet Emerg Crit Care 2011;21: 86–103.

28. Berent AC, Weisse C, Todd K, et al. Use of a balloon-expandable metallic stent for treatment of nasopharyngeal stenosis in dogs and cats: six cases (2005-2007). J Am Vet Med Assoc 2008;233:1432–40.

29. Scansen BA, Kent AM, Cheatham SL, et al. Stenting of the right ventricular outflow tract in 2 dogs for palliation of dysplastic pulmonary valve stenosis and right-to-left intracardiac shunting defects. J Vet Cardiol 2014;16:205–14.

30. Weisse C. Intraluminal tracheal stenting. Veterinary image-guided interventions. Ames (IA): John Wiley & Sons, Ltd; 2015. p. 73–82.

31. Weisse C, Berent AC, Todd K, et al. Endovascular evaluation and treatment of intrahepatic portosystemic shunts in dogs: 100 cases (2001-2011). J Am Vet Med Assoc 2014;244:78–94.

32. Blackburn AL, Berent AC, Weisse CW, et al. Evaluation of outcome following urethral stent placement for the treatment of obstructive carcinoma of the urethra in dogs: 42 cases (2004-2008). J Am Vet Med Assoc 2013;242:59–68.

33. Stoeckel D, Pelton A, Duerig T. Self-expanding nitinol stents: material and design considerations. Eur Radiol 2004;14:292–301.

Interventional Oncology

William T.N. Culp, VMD

KEYWORDS

- Interventional radiology • Interventional oncology • Minimally invasive

KEY POINTS

- Interventional oncology (IO) has been established in veterinary medicine as a fourth major cancer treatment category along with surgery, chemotherapy, and radiation therapy.
- Locoregional therapies, such as intra-arterial chemotherapy, embolization/chemoembolization, and ablation, are used more regularly in veterinary patients and new treatments are emerging.
- Stenting of malignant obstructions has been described in several case series and initial results are promising.

OVERVIEW

The approach to the treatment of cancer in veterinary patients is constantly evolving. Whenever possible and practical, surgery is pursued because it provides the greatest opportunity for tumor control and, with certain tumor types, may result in a cure. Other cancer treatments, such as chemotherapy and radiation therapy, are commonplace in veterinary medicine, and the data outlining treatment regimens are growing rapidly. An absence of treatment options for veterinary cancer patients, however, has historically existed for some tumors. IO options, such as locoregional therapies or stenting of malignant obstructions, have opened the door to the potential for better therapeutic response and improved patient quality of life.

Prior to the use of IO techniques in veterinary medicine, tumors that were deemed nonresectable and chemotherapy resistant or radiation therapy resistant presented a therapeutic challenge. Although the evidence supporting the use of these treatments is scant in the veterinary literature, much has been accomplished in human medicine to suggest that IO options have efficacy. Additionally, for many nonresectable tumors, these techniques are the first-line therapy that is pursued. IO techniques that are emerging as possible primary treatment options, such as intra-arterial chemotherapy,

Disclosure Statement: Dr W.T.N. Culp has served as a laboratory instructor for a company that sells equipment that can be used to perform interventional radiology procedures.
Department of Surgical and Radiological Sciences, University of California-Davis, School of Veterinary Medicine, One Garrod Drive, Davis, CA 95616, USA
E-mail address: wculp@ucdavis.edu

Vet Clin Small Anim 46 (2016) 553–565
http://dx.doi.org/10.1016/j.cvsm.2015.12.010
0195-5616/16/$ – see front matter © 2016 Elsevier Inc. All rights reserved.
vetsmall.theclinics.com

embolization/chemoembolization, and tumor ablation, mirror procedures that are actively and regularly performed in human medicine.

ANATOMY

A thorough knowledge of the anatomy is essential for performing IO procedures effectively and safely. Introduction of instrumentation into and navigation through luminal structures requires an excellent understanding of anatomic landmarks and organ interaction. Additionally, the blood supply to various organs should be understood when transcatheter locoregional therapies are considered so that normal blood supply can be identified from tumoral blood supply, and complications, such as nontarget embolization, can be avoided. Recently, the arterial blood supply of the abdominal organs was described as a guide for performing intra-abdominal transcatheter therapies.[1]

Currently, vascular access in the majority of locoregional therapies in veterinary patients is arterial (eg, carotid and femoral arteries). If vascular stenting is performed, the jugular or femoral vein may also be used. Venous approaches do not require vascular repair postprocedure due to the low pressure in the venous system; however, arterial approaches generally require vessel ligation or repair. In humans, closure of an arteriotomy site is often performed with a vascular closure device[2,3]; vascular closure devices are generally not utilized in veterinary patients due to expense and the need for minimized postprocedure patient activity and because femoral and carotid arteries can be ligated.[4–6]

IMAGING DIAGNOSTICS

The use of imaging modalities allows for IO procedures to be performed in a minimally invasive fashion and improves a clinician's ability to access certain organs or regions of the body. Fluoroscopy is utilized during the majority of IO procedures in companion animals. The instrumentation used during IO procedures is radiopaque and contrast agents are often injected intraluminally (**Fig. 1**) or intravascularly, making fluoroscopy an excellent modality for performing real-time interventions.

Ultrasonography is regularly used as a means of cancer staging, specifically in the abdomen; furthermore, ultrasound guidance can provide crucial assistance in obtaining tissue samples via fine-needle aspiration or biopsy. Ultrasound can also be used to locate blood vessels for percutaneous vascular catheterization and is the most common imaging modality to be used to perform percutaneous tumor ablation.

Similar to ultrasound, CT and MRI are essential components of patient staging and preprocedural planning in veterinary medicine. These advanced imaging modalities are often combined with fluoroscopic imaging in human medicine to allow for real-time evaluation and treatment of lesions.[7,8] CT angiography and magnetic resonance angiography are utilized in the evaluation of veterinary patients regularly, but intraprocedural use of these diagnostics remains less common.

PATIENT SELECTION

When possible and appropriate, IO techniques should be considered in addition to more traditional options, such as surgery, chemotherapy, and radiation therapy. Because most patients diagnosed with cancer are older, procedures that cause the least amount of morbidity are ideal. In many scenarios in which IO options are offered, these techniques are the only available options. The overall goal of treatment is to improve quality of life after recovery from one of these procedures, and the benefit

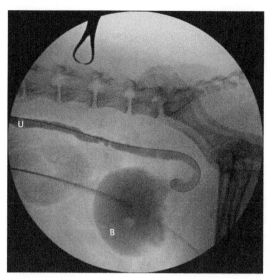

Fig. 1. A lateral fluoroscopic image has been obtained during a percutaneous ureteral stenting procedure performed to treat a ureteral obstruction secondary to lower urinary tract transitional cell carcinoma in an 8-year-old female spayed Beagle. A guide wire can be seen in the ureter (U) and an attempt is made to manipulate the guide wire into the bladder (B) past the malignant ureteral obstruction with fluoroscopic guidance.

of IO procedures is that these generally can be performed in a minimally invasive fashion with low initial negative impact on a patient's quality of life.

PROCEDURES

The areas of IO that have received the majority of attention thus far in veterinary medicine include locoregional therapies (intra-arterial chemotherapy, embolization/chemoembolization, and ablative therapies) and stenting of malignant obstructions. Other palliative treatments, such as the draining of malignant effusions and normal fluid accumulations, have also been performed.

Locoregional Therapies

Intra-arterial chemotherapy

The administration of chemotherapy in veterinary patients is generally performed intravenously. The intra-arterial delivery of chemotherapy, however, can provide some theoretic advantages over traditional administration. When a drug is delivered intra-arterially, the tumor receives a maximized dose thus allowing for a higher concentration to accumulate in the tumor.[9–11] Additionally, drugs that are administered intravenously have been shown to have higher systemic concentrations, and side effects of chemotherapy may occur more commonly.[9–11] Despite the proposed advantages, intra-arterial chemotherapy is still not universally used in human medicine, although some locations, in particular the head and neck regions, have shown promise. To perform the procedure, a sheath is placed within an artery (eg, femoral or carotid artery) that allows for access to the arterial supply of the tumor. Utilizing varying sizes and types of guide wires and catheters, the vascular supply of the affected organ is accessed via superselective catheterization. Once the desired vessel is selected (**Fig. 2**), chemotherapy can be administered, increasing the locally delivered dose

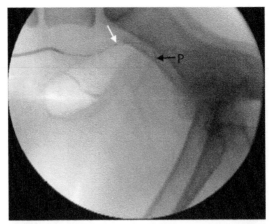

Fig. 2. A microcatheter (*white arrow*) has been advanced into the prostatic artery (P) during an intra-arterial chemotherapy procedure performed to treat a prostatic transitional cell carcinoma in a 12-year-old male castrated Labrador retriever.

and theoretically increasing the potential response of the tumor secondary to that particular chemotherapeutic drug.

A recent study evaluated the response to intra-arterial or intravenous administration of chemotherapy in the treatment of lower urinary tract neoplasia in dogs.[12] In the dogs of that study, there was a significantly greater decrease in tumor size in the dogs of the intra-arterial chemotherapy group compared with the intravenous chemotherapy group. Additionally, dogs in the intra-arterial group were less likely to develop side effects, such as anemia, lethargy, and anorexia.[12] This study only evaluated, however, the short-term response to these therapies and utilized ultrasound as the imaging modality for measurement, which has shown previous limitations.

Another use of intra-arterial chemotherapy in human patients is in combination with radiation therapy.[13–17] Drugs, such as platinum-based chemotherapy agents, can sensitize tumors to the effects of radiation therapy with the goal of combining therapies to maximize the efficacy. In veterinary patients, the use of radiation therapy in combination with intra-arterial chemotherapy has been evaluated in both osteosarcoma and bladder cancer patients.[18–21] In one of the appendicular osteosarcoma studies, the toxicity associated with chemotherapy administration and radiation side effects was rare, and median survival time in these dogs was 9.3 months.[21] In a study evaluating the combination of intra-arterial chemotherapy (cisplatin) with radiation therapy for treatment of bladder cancer, 2 dogs demonstrated an objective reduction in tumor size.[19] Side effects and toxicity were minimal in these 2 dogs.[19]

Embolization/Chemoembolization

Embolotherapy is an established treatment modality in human oncology and is considered standard of care for some tumors. The reasoning behind embolization is that localized, tumor-specific ischemia leads to tumor cell death. The addition of chemotherapy to embolization (chemoembolization) theoretically can increase the tumor response because tumor death from ischemia would be further improved by the cytotoxic effects of chemotherapy. On some occasions, the goal of embolization is to achieve temporary occlusion, which may allow for future treatments and prevent the development of collateral blood vessels to the tumor.[22]

Embolization performed without chemotherapy is often referred to as bland embo-lization. When chemoembolization is performed, chemotherapy can be delivered in conjunction with the embolic agent (conventional chemoembolization) or delivered via beads (drug-eluting bead chemoembolization) that have been loaded with chemo-therapy (eg, doxorubicin). Radioembolization is a developing embolotherapy in humans and involves the delivery of radioactive particles (eg, yttrium 90) directly to the arterial blood supply of a tumor.[23] This last option has not been pursued in clinical veterinary cases at this time.

Tumor embolization is generally performed via catheter delivery of embolic agents. Several embolic agents have been used to perform embolization, and these agents are available in temporary and permanent forms; generally, the temporary embolic agents (eg, gelfoam) are utilized for trauma or in situations when a permanent occlusion would cause unacceptable end-organ devascularization. Permanent agents commonly cho-sen for tumor embolization include particles, such as polyvinyl alcohol and acrylic spheres; other permanent agents, such as coils, glue (cyanoacrylate), and ethylene vi-nyl alcohol, are generally reserved for vascular anomalies.

The response of liver tumors to embolization/chemoembolization has been the most studied in both human and veterinary patients.[24–26] The liver has a unique blood sup-ply in that the majority of the blood supplying the liver comes from the portal vein, yet it has been established that tumors in the liver receive the majority of their blood supply from the hepatic arteries.[27,28] This allows for targeting of the major tumoral blood sup-ply while preserving blood flow to the normal liver.

To perform liver embolization/chemoembolization, the arterial blood supply is accessed from the femoral artery. Utilizing fluoroscopy and serial angiographic studies, the hepatic artery (branching from the celiac artery) is selected, and an angio-graphic map of the hepatic tumoral blood supply is obtained (**Fig. 3**). Once the hepatic artery (or arteries) that is supplying the tumor is identified, the embolic agent (with or

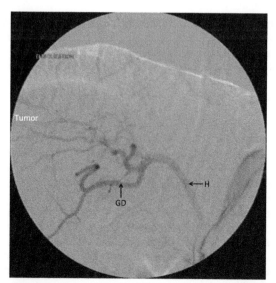

Fig. 3. A fluoroscopic image has been obtained during a liver embolization procedure in a 9-year-old female spayed chow chow. The hepatic artery (H) has been catheterized and iodinated contrast medium has been injected to map the tumoral blood supply and identify the gastroduodenal artery (GD).

without chemotherapy) can be delivered to the tumor. Because the outcome associated with traditional surgery in veterinary patients is considered good,[29] it is generally the first-line therapy, whereas embolization and chemoembolization are generally reserved for large masses in an unfavorable location or diffuse neoplasia of the liver.

Two studies have evaluated the use of liver embolization/chemoembolization in veterinary patients.[24,26] Several mixtures of chemoembolic agents were used. Survival times postprocedure were available in 3 dogs and ranged from 28 to 137 days. Stable disease or subjective decreases in tumor size were noted in several of the cases.[24,26] Selection of the hepatic artery with sparing of the gastroduodenal artery is important and was possible in all cases.

Recently, the response to embolization of nasal and prostate tumors has been evaluated at the author's clinic. Treatment of nasal tumors with radiation therapy is considered by most as the treatment of choice.[30–32] Euthanasia of patients with nasal tumors, however, is often a result of progression of the local disease, and other therapeutics need to be considered to more effectively treat nasal tumors. Because the blood supply to the nasal cavity can be isolated, embolization is a possibility. A majority of intranasal tumors are present bilaterally within the nasal cavity; the femoral artery is thus utilized as the entry point into the arterial system to allow for bilateral catheterization of the carotid arteries and, furthermore, the arteries supplying the nasal cavity. A thorough understanding of the vascular anatomy cranial to the heart is essential because nontarget embolization of nervous system structures is possible.

Recently, a study of 5 dogs undergoing prostatic artery embolization in the treatment of prostatic carcinoma was reported.[33] Prostatic artery embolization was successfully performed in all cases and no complications were encountered. Initial tumor response to the embolization was encouraging because all dogs demonstrated a decrease in tumor volume (comparing pre-CT and post-CT measurements) and the dogs still alive at the time of presentation were free of clinical signs.[33]

Ablation

Descriptions of the use of tumor ablation have been sparse in the veterinary literature, but the proven applications in human patients provide promise for possible uses in animals as well. Ablative techniques function via chemical or thermal destruction of tumor cells. Chemical ablation techniques generally involve the intratumoral injection of liquid agents, with ethanol the most described technique. Thermal ablation is based on the delivery of energy or freezing agents directly to a tumor to incite cell death.

The major thermal ablative techniques include radiofrequency ablation (RFA), cryoablation, microwave ablation, laser ablation, and high-intensity focused ultrasound (HIFU). With these techniques that generate heat, tumor death is caused by the transfer of heat to tumor cells with subsequent necrosis.[34–36] When performing cryoablation, varying freeze-thaw cycles result in the development of intracellular ice crystals and cellular dehydration, both of which lead to cellular damage and death.[35]

With RFA, cryoablation, and microwave ablation, probes are introduced into tumor tissue percutaneously or through a natural orifice. Guidance of the probes into the appropriate location is performed with image guidance, which may include fluoroscopy, CT, or MRI, although ultrasound is generally the most utilized imaging modality. These procedures can also be performed with direct access to the tumor, for example, after a celiotomy or with endoscopic-guidance.

RFA is commonly used in human patients in the treatment of hepatic malignancies.[36–38] Additionally, primary and metastatic bone tumors are often treated with RFA.[37,38] RFA has been utilized in the treatment of canine primary hyperparathyroidism[39] and feline hyperthyroidism[40]; investigation into the use of this modality in the treatment of malignant neoplasia is lacking.

The use of cryoablation in the treatment of prostate, kidney, liver, uterine, and bone tumors has been well reported.[38,41–43] Two reported cases of cryoablation in the treatment of nasal and maxillary tumors exist in the veterinary literature.[44,45] In a recent report of the use of cryoablation to treat a recurrent nasal adenocarcinoma, long-term tumor control was achieved.[44] In that case, probe placement was guided with fluoroscopy and CT, and tumor response was monitored by CT. Clinical signs were mild and included epiphora in the periprocedural period and mild chronic nasal discharge.[44] Combination therapy with transarterial embolization, systemic cyclophosphamide, and cryoablation was used to treat a dog with a maxillary fibrosarcoma; partial tumor remission was noted at a 4-week recheck examination.[45]

Microwave ablation, laser ablation, and HIFU have tremendous potential; although these techniques are considered relatively new, early results for many tumor types are promising.[34,46–48] In the author's clinic, a focal renal tumor has been treated successfully with microwave ablation. In that case, no long-term complications were encountered. MRI-guided HIFU has been reported in 1 dog with a hepatocellular adenoma.[49] The treatment was able to cause ablation of significant volumes of the tumor, and tumor necrosis was noted to correlate with the planned treatment region.[49]

Ethanol injection into neoplastic tissue is the major form of chemical ablation that has been described. Ethanol causes cellular necrosis through dehydration, vascular thrombosis, and ischemia. In a study evaluating dogs with hyperparathyroidism, 18 dogs underwent ethanol ablation, and, of those, 72% experienced control of hypercalcemia.[50]

Stenting of Malignant Obstructions

A stent is a tubelike device that recanalizes a luminal obstruction. Stents re-establish an opening to allow for the excretion of body fluids or waste as well as for the passage of food, liquid, air, or blood. Stents have provided a highly effective treatment option for opening malignant obstructions in companion animals. Additionally, stents can be placed intraluminally in a minimally invasive fashion and recovery is generally rapid.

Urethral stenting is likely one of the most common applications of IO in veterinary medicine. The importance of urethral stenting lies in the ability of the stent to palliate a condition that is immediately life threatening, specifically uretheral obstruction with resultant urine retention (**Fig. 4**). With many cases of urinary tract obstruction secondary to neoplasia (tumors of the prostate, bladder, and urethra), the cause of death is the severity of local disease as opposed to metastasis.

Three clinical studies have described the use of urethral stents in canine patients.[51–53] These studies found that urethral stents can be successfully placed in canine patients with lower urinary tract neoplasia and can effectively reestablish urine flow. Complications that were encountered included incontinence, stent obstruction, and stent migration; however, most dogs were considered to have an improved quality of life.[51–53]

Urethral stent placement to relieve malignant obstructions has also been described in 3 separate feline studies, including a total of 5 cases.[54–56] The results in the majority of those cases were considered good to excellent.[54–56] In female cats and male cats with a previous perineal urethrostomy, placement of urethral stents can be performed in a retrograde manner through the urethral opening. In unaltered male cats, a small cystotomy is likely necessary because the instrumentation is too large to fit through the typical penile urethral orifice.

Ureteral stenting of malignant obstruction in dogs is generally pursued when a lower urinary tract neoplasia (bladder, urethra, or prostate tumor) has grown into a position

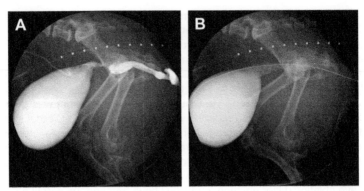

Fig. 4. (*A*) A retrograde contrast cystourethrogram is performed in a 12-year-old female spayed dachshund with urethral transitional cell carcinoma prior to urethral stent placement. Iodinated contrast medium has been injected and the area of urethral obstruction can be clearly identified. Additionally, a ureter can be identified because contrast has been introduced during the injection. (*B*) A urethral stent has been placed to relieve the obstruction.

where the ureteral orifice is unilaterally or bilaterally covered resulting in obstruction and secondary hydroureter and/or hydronephrosis (see **Fig. 1**). An incisionless technique for ureteral stents in dogs has been described[57] and involves an antegrade approach after nephrocentesis. In 1 study[57] evaluating outcomes in 12 dogs with ureteral obstruction, results were promising in that stents were able to be placed in all dogs and complications were rare; additionally, all dogs were discharged and in those that had follow-up ultrasound, hydronephrosis, and hydroureter were improved in all.

In the author's experience, ureteral stents placed for the treatment of malignant obstructions in cats are most effectively placed after a celiotomy; guide wire placement across the obstruction (prior to stent passage) is still performed most easily via an antegrade approach despite a celiotomy being performed.

Although surgical resection and anastomosis of tracheal neoplastic lesions has been historically pursued in companion animals, other options, such as radiation therapy, endoscopic debulking, and tracheal stenting, have developed.[58–60] The stenting of a feline tracheal carcinoma has been reported, and in this case a self-expanding stent was placed with fluoroscopic guidance.[58] The cat of this report was noted to develop pulmonary metastasis 6 weeks post–stent placement, and euthanasia was elected at that time.[58]

Colonic neoplasia is a common diagnosis in humans, and although surgical resection is generally considered the treatment of choice when possible, debate exists as to the recommended treatment in patients presenting with colonic obstruction. Three clinical cases of colonic stenting have been reported in the veterinary literature, including 2 cats and 1 dog.[61,62] In 1 cat, clinical signs of tenesmus were improved poststenting and the cat survived for 274 days post–stent placement.[61] A second cat underwent successful colonic stent placement to relieve an obstruction secondary to a colonic adenocarcinoma and maintained fecal continence after stenting. In that cat, however, euthanasia was pursued 19 days post–stent placement due to progression of abdominal effusion secondary to carcinomatosis.[61] In a single canine case report, successful stent placement was noted and clinical signs improved for just over 200 days.[62]

Approximately 50% of humans with esophageal neoplasia are diagnosed when local disease is at an advanced state, preventing the option of surgical resection.[63–65]

The use of esophageal stents has been shown to improve quality of life and improve clinical signs associated with esophageal neoplasia (eg, dysphagia).[64,65] One case of canine esophageal stent placement for a malignant obstruction (squamous cell carcinoma) has been described.[66] In that case, the placement of an esophageal stent relieved the obstruction and improved clinical signs.[66]

Vascular obstruction secondary to malignant obstructions is extremely rare, but stent placement can effectively open an obstructed vessel. The use of stents to relieve Budd-Chiari syndrome has been described in a case series of 3 dogs.[67] Procedural success and relief of clinical signs was achieved in all 3 dogs, and survival times varied from 7 to 20 months.[67]

Fluid Drainage

Interventional techniques can be utilized to drain both normal and malignant fluid accumulations. Percutaneous placement of tubes into the urinary bladder and gallbladder can allow for drainage of these organs when a malignancy results in obstruction. Stenting is generally preferred in the author's clinic because this provides a more permanent option for fluid drainage; however, temporary relief of obstructions with drainage tubes in these organs may stabilize these patients prior to stent placement.

Malignant effusions can develop secondary to thoracic or abdominal cavity neoplasia or after rupture of an organ secondary to a tumor. Drainage catheters can be placed simply with minimal sedation utilizing a minimally invasive percutaneous technique. These catheters are generally not effective long term but can allow for temporary stabilization of a patient until a more permanent option is elected. Additionally, a drainage catheter can be placed with IO techniques and connected to a subcutaneous port to allow for lifelong drainage (**Fig. 5**).

IO is an ever-growing field with many potential applications in veterinary medicine. Although other oncologic therapies, such as surgery, conventional chemotherapy, and radiation therapy, will always have their place as part of the treatment regimen in companion animals, available IO techniques have the potential to supplement or improve

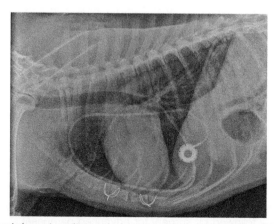

Fig. 5. A left lateral thoracic radiograph demonstrating a drainage catheter that has been placed intrathoracically and connected to a port in the subcutaneous space in an 8-year-old female spayed German shepherd dog. This dog was developing persistent pleural effusion secondary to intrathoracic mesothelioma and required drainage of the fluid on a regular basis.

potential outcomes. Overall, the goal of all these therapies will continue to be striving for an improved quality of life in the pets that are undergoing treatment.

REFERENCES

1. Culp WT, Mayhew PD, Pascoe PJ, et al. Angiographic anatomy of the major abdominal arterial blood supply in the dog. Vet Radiol Ultrasound 2015;56: 474–85.
2. Dauerman HL, Applegate RJ, Cohen DJ. Vascular closure devices: the second decade. J Am Coll Cardiol 2007;50:1617–26.
3. Hussain T, Al-Hamali S. Femoral artery occlusion with a percutaneous arterial closure device after a routine coronary angiogram: a case report and literature review. Ann R Coll Surg Engl 2011;93:e102–4.
4. Perkins RL, Edmark KW. Ligation of femoral vessels and azygous vein in the dog. J Am Vet Med Assoc 1971;159:993–4.
5. Clendenin MA, Conrad MC. Collateral vessel development, following unilateral chronic carotid occlusion in the dog. Am J Vet Res 1979;40:84–8.
6. Clendenin MA, Conrad MC. Collateral vessel development after chronic bilateral common carotid artery occlusion in the dog. Am J Vet Res 1979;40:1244–8.
7. Saeed M, Hetts SW, English J, et al. MR fluoroscopy in vascular and cardiac interventions (review). Int J Cardiovasc Imaging 2012;28:117–37.
8. Saybasili H, Faranesh AZ, Saikus CE, et al. Interventional MRI using multiple 3D angiography roadmaps with real-time imaging. J Magn Reson Imaging 2010;31: 1015–9.
9. Chen C, Wang W, Zhou H, et al. Pharmacokinetic comparison between systemic and local chemotherapy by carboplatin in dogs. Reprod Sci 2009;16:1097–102.
10. von Scheel J, Golde G. Pharmacokinetics of intra-arterial tumour therapy. An experimental study. Arch Otorhinolaryngol 1984;239:153–61.
11. von Scheel J, Krautzberger W, Foth B, et al. A special method of intra-arterial infusion for treatment of head and neck cancer. Recent Results Cancer Res 1983;86: 169–73.
12. Culp WT, Weisse C, Berent AC, et al. Early tumor response to intraarterial or intravenous administration of carboplatin to treat naturally occurring lower urinary tract carcinoma in dogs. J Vet Intern Med 2015;29:900–7.
13. Ikushima I, Korogi Y, Ishii A, et al. Superselective intra-arterial infusion chemotherapy for stage III/IV squamous cell carcinomas of the oral cavity: midterm results. Eur J Radiol 2008;66:7–12.
14. Korogi Y, Hirai T, Nishimura R, et al. Superselective intraarterial infusion of cisplatin for squamous cell carcinoma of the mouth: preliminary clinical experience. Am J Roentgenol 1995;165:1269–72.
15. Kovacs AF, Mose S, Bottcher HD, et al. Multimodality treatment including postoperative radiation and concurrent chemotherapy with weekly docetaxel is feasible and effective in patients with oral and oropharyngeal cancer. Strahlenther Onkol 2005;181:26–34.
16. Samant S, Robbins KT, Vang M, et al. Intra-arterial cisplatin and concomitant radiation therapy followed by surgery for advanced paranasal sinus cancer. Arch Otolaryngol Head Neck Surg 2004;130:948–55.
17. Wilson WR, Siegel RS, Harisiadis LA, et al. High-dose intra-arterial cisplatin therapy followed by radiation therapy for advanced squamous cell carcinoma of the head and neck. Arch Otolaryngol Head Neck Surg 2001;127:809–12.

18. Heidner GL, Page RL, McEntee MC, et al. Treatment of canine appendicular osteosarcoma using cobalt 60 radiation and intraarterial cisplatin. J Vet Intern Med 1991;5:313–6.

19. McCaw DL. Radiation and cisplatin for treatment of canine urinary bladder carcinoma. Vet Radiol 1988;29:264–8.

20. Powers BE, Withrow SJ, Thrall DE, et al. Percent tumor necrosis as a predictor of treatment response in canine osteosarcoma. Cancer 1991;67:126–34.

21. Withrow SJ, Thrall DE, Straw RC, et al. Intra-arterial cisplatin with or without radiation in limb-sparing for canine osteosarcoma. Cancer 1993;71:2484–90.

22. Gunven P. Liver embolizations in oncology: a review. Part I. Arterial (chemo)embolizations. Med Oncol 2008;25:1–11.

23. Henrie AM, Wittstrom K, Delu A, et al. Evaluation of liver biomarkers as prognostic factors for outcomes to Yttrium-90 radioembolization of primary and secondary liver malignancies. Cancer Biother Radiopharm 2015;30:305–9.

24. Cave TA, Johnson V, Beths T, et al. Treatment of unresectable hepatocellular adenoma in dogs with transarterial iodized oil and chemotherapy with and without an embolic agent: a report of two cases. Vet Comp Oncol 2003;1:191–9.

25. Facciorusso A, Licinio R, Muscatiello N, et al. Transarterial chemoembolization: Evidences from the literature and applications in hepatocellular carcinoma patients. World J Hepatol 2015;7:2009–19.

26. Weisse C, Clifford CA, Holt D, et al. Percutaneous arterial embolization and chemoembolization for treatment of benign and malignant tumors in three dogs and a goat. J Am Vet Med Assoc 2002;221:1430–6.

27. Breedis C, Young G. The blood supply of neoplasms in the liver. Am J Pathol 1954;30:969–77.

28. Zhou WP, Lai EC, Li AJ, et al. A prospective, randomized, controlled trial of preoperative transarterial chemoembolization for resectable large hepatocellular carcinoma. Ann Surg 2009;249:195–202.

29. Liptak JM, Dernell WS, Monnet E, et al. Massive hepatocellular carcinoma in dogs: 48 cases (1992-2002). J Am Vet Med Assoc 2004;225:1225–30.

30. Buchholz J, Hagen R, Leo C, et al. 3D conformal radiation therapy for palliative treatment of canine nasal tumors. Vet Radiol Ultrasound 2009;50:679–83.

31. MacEwen EG, Withrow SJ, Patnaik AK. Nasal tumors in the dog: retrospective evaluation of diagnosis, prognosis, and treatment. J Am Vet Med Assoc 1977; 170:45–8.

32. Theon AP, Madewell BR, Harb MF, et al. Megavoltage irradiation of neoplasms of the nasal and paranasal cavities in 77 dogs. J Am Vet Med Assoc 1993;202: 1469–75.

33. Culp WTN, Johnson EG, Palm CA, et al. Prostatic artery embolization: novel treatment of naturally-occurring prostate neoplasia in canine patients. Proceedings, 12th Annual Meeting, Veterinary Endoscopy Society. Santa Barbara, CA, April 13, 2015.

34. Carrafiello G, Lagana D, Mangini M, et al. Microwave tumors ablation: principles, clinical applications and review of preliminary experiences. Int J Surg 2008; 6(Suppl 1):S65–9.

35. Bhardwaj N, Strickland AD, Ahmad F, et al. Liver ablation techniques: a review. Surg Endosc 2010;24:254–65.

36. Ni Y, Mulier S, Miao Y, et al. A review of the general aspects of radiofrequency ablation. Abdom Imaging 2005;30:381–400.

37. Brown DB. Concepts, considerations, and concerns on the cutting edge of radiofrequency ablation. J Vasc Interv Radiol 2005;16:597–613.

38. Kurup AN, Callstrom MR. Ablation of skeletal metastases: current status. J Vasc Interv Radiol 2010;21:S242–50.

39. Pollard RE, Long CD, Nelson RW, et al. Percutaneous ultrasonographically guided radiofrequency heat ablation for treatment of primary hyperparathyroidism in dogs. J Am Vet Med Assoc 2001;218:1106–10.

40. Mallery KF, Pollard RE, Nelson RW, et al. Percutaneous ultrasound-guided radiofrequency heat ablation for treatment of hyperthyroidism in cats. J Am Vet Med Assoc 2003;223:1602–7.

41. Carrafiello G, Lagana D, Pellegrino C, et al. Ablation of painful metastatic bone tumors: a systematic review. Int J Surg 2008;6(Suppl 1):S47–52.

42. Callstrom MR, Kurup AN. Percutaneous ablation for bone and soft tissue metastases–why cryoablation? Skeletal Radiol 2009;38:835–9.

43. Nazario J, Tam AL. Ablation of bone metastases. Surg Oncol Clin N Am 2011;20: 355–68.

44. Murphy SM, Lawrence JA, Schmiedt CW, et al. Image-guided transnasal cryoablation of a recurrent nasal adenocarcinoma in a dog. J Small Anim Pract 2011; 52:329–33.

45. Weisse C, Berent A, Solomon S. Combined transarterial embolization, systemic cyclophosphamide, and cryotherapy ablation for "Hi-Lo" maxillary fibrosarcoma in a dog. Proceedings, 8th Annual Meeting, Veterinary Endoscopy Society. San Pedro, Belize, May 6, 2011.

46. Ji X, Bai JF, Shen GF, et al. High-intensity focused ultrasound with large scale spherical phased array for the ablation of deep tumors. J Zhejiang Univ Sci B 2009;10:639–47.

47. Padma S, Martinie JB, Iannitti DA. Liver tumor ablation: percutaneous and open approaches. J Surg Oncol 2009;100:619–34.

48. Rebillard X, Soulie M, Chartier-Kastler E, et al. High-intensity focused ultrasound in prostate cancer; a systematic literature review of the French association of urology. BJU Int 2008;101:1205–13.

49. Kopelman D, Inbar Y, Hanannel A, et al. Magnetic resonance-guided focused ultrasound surgery (MRgFUS). Four ablation treatments of a single canine hepatocellular adenoma. HPB (Oxford) 2006;8:292–8.

50. Rasor L, Pollard R, Feldman EC. Retrospective evaluation of three treatment methods for primary hyperparathyroidism in dogs. J Am Anim Hosp Assoc 2007;43:70–7.

51. Blackburn AL, Berent AC, Weisse CW, et al. Evaluation of outcome following urethral stent placement for the treatment of obstructive carcinoma of the urethra in dogs: 42 cases (2004-2008). J Am Vet Med Assoc 2013;242:59–68.

52. McMillan SK, Knapp DW, Ramos-Vara JA, et al. Outcome of urethral stent placement for management of urethral obstruction secondary to transitional cell carcinoma in dogs: 19 cases (2007-2010). J Am Vet Med Assoc 2012;241:1627–32.

53. Weisse C, Berent A, Todd K, et al. Evaluation of palliative stenting for management of malignant urethral obstructions in dogs. J Am Vet Med Assoc 2006; 229:226–34.

54. Brace MA, Weisse C, Berent A. Preliminary experience with stenting for management of non-urolith urethral obstruction in eight cats. Vet Surg 2014;43:199–208.

55. Christensen NI, Culvenor J, Langova V. Fluoroscopic stent placement for the relief of malignant urethral obstruction in a cat. Aust Vet J 2010;88:478–82.

56. Newman RG, Mehler SJ, Kitchell BE, et al. Use of a balloon-expandable metallic stent to relieve malignant urethral obstruction in a cat. J Am Vet Med Assoc 2009; 234:236–9.

57. Berent AC, Weisse C, Beal MW, et al. Use of indwelling, double-pigtail stents for treatment of malignant ureteral obstruction in dogs: 12 cases (2006-2009). J Am Vet Med Assoc 2011;238:1017–25.
58. Culp WT, Weisse C, Cole SG, et al. Intraluminal tracheal stenting for treatment of tracheal narrowing in three cats. Vet Surg 2007;36:107–13.
59. Jakubiak MJ, Siedlecki CT, Zenger E, et al. Laryngeal, laryngotracheal, and tracheal masses in cats: 27 cases (1998-2003). J Am Anim Hosp Assoc 2005; 41:310–6.
60. Queen EV, Vaughan MA, Johnson LR. Bronchoscopic debulking of tracheal carcinoma in 3 cats using a wire snare. J Vet Intern Med 2010;24:990–3.
61. Hume DZ, Solomon JA, Weisse CW. Palliative use of a stent for colonic obstruction caused by adenocarcinoma in two cats. J Am Vet Med Assoc 2006;228: 392–6.
62. Culp WT, Macphail CM, Perry JA, et al. Use of a nitinol stent to palliate a colorectal neoplastic obstruction in a dog. J Am Vet Med Assoc 2011;239:222–7.
63. Bona D, Laface L, Bonavina L, et al. Covered nitinol stents for the treatment of esophageal strictures and leaks. World J Gastroenterol 2010;16:2260–4.
64. Eroglu A, Turkyilmaz A, Subasi M, et al. The use of self-expandable metallic stents for palliative treatment of inoperable esophageal cancer. Dis Esophagus 2010;23:64–70.
65. Xinopoulos D, Dimitroulopoulos D, Moschandrea I, et al. Natural course of inoperable esophageal cancer treated with metallic expandable stents: quality of life and cost-effectiveness analysis. J Gastroenterol Hepatol 2004;19:1397–402.
66. Hansen KS, Weisse C, Berent AC, et al. Use of a self-expanding metallic stent to palliate esophageal neoplastic obstruction in a dog. J Am Vet Med Assoc 2012; 240:1202–7.
67. Schlicksup MD, Weisse CW, Berent AC, et al. Use of endovascular stents in three dogs with Budd-Chiari syndrome. J Am Vet Med Assoc 2009;235:544–50.

Interventional Radiology of the Urinary Tract

Allyson C. Berent, DVM

KEYWORDS

- Ureteral obstruction • Ureteral stenting
- Subcutaneous ureteral bypass device (SUB) • Nephrolithiasis
- Nephrostomy tube placement • Idiopathic renal hematuria • Sclerotherapy
- Cystostomy tube placement

KEY POINTS

- Minimally invasive treatment options using interventional radiology and interventional endoscopy for urologic disease have become more common over the past decade in veterinary medicine.
- Urinary tract obstructions and urinary incontinence are the most common reasons for urinary interventions in veterinary medicine.
- Ureteral obstructions are underdiagnosed and a common clinical problem in veterinary medicine.
- Ureteral obstructions should be considered an emergency, and decompression should be performed as quickly as possible.
- Diagnostic imaging is the mainstay in diagnosing a ureteral obstruction and has changed in the last few years, with ultrasound and radiographs being the most sensitive tools in making this diagnosis preoperatively.
- Concurrent hydroureter and hydronephrosis should be considered a ureteral obstruction until proven otherwise, regardless of the size of the dilation or the presence of a clear obstructive lesion on imaging.

Interventional radiology (IR) uses many image-guided techniques to diagnose and treat various disease of the body. There is a gamut of applications for the urinary tract in veterinary medicine.[1–23] This technology typically involves the use of fluoroscopy, endoscopy, +/− ultrasound to gain access to the kidney, ureter, bladder, and/or urethra in order to treat various ailments like urinary tract obstructions, stone disease, hemorrhagic lesions, urologic neoplasia, or urinary incontinence. Over the past decade, these therapeutic and diagnostic modalities have become increasingly more accessible in veterinary medicine, which has followed a similar trend of what is considered standard of care in human medicine.[1–23] The traditional types of therapies using IR techniques

Disclosure Statement: Dr A.C. Berent is a consultant for Norfolk Vet Products and Infiniti Medical, LLC, both of which distribute various medical devices that are discussed in this article.
Department of Interventional Radiology and Endoscopy, The Animal Medical Center, 510 East 62nd Street, New York, NY 10065, USA
E-mail address: Allyson.Berent@amcny.org

Vet Clin Small Anim 46 (2016) 567–596
http://dx.doi.org/10.1016/j.cvsm.2015.12.011
0195-5616/16/$ – see front matter © 2016 Elsevier Inc. All rights reserved.

are associated with relief of various urinary tract obstructions (ureteral stenting, nephrostomy tube placement, subcutaneous ureteral bypass device [SUB], urethral stenting, cystostomy tube placement), cessation of urinary tract bleeding (sclerotherapy, nephroscopy with electrocautery), and intra-arterial delivery of therapeutics to obtain higher local concentrations (chemotherapy or stem cell therapy).

There are many advantages to interventional techniques when compared with traditional surgical alternatives. The reduced perioperative morbidity and mortality rates, shorter hospital stays, and new therapeutic options being available when previously there were no treatments considered safe or available are the main benefits of this technology. The main disadvantages are the requirement for proper technical training, the need for specialized expensive equipment, and the steep learning curve in order to properly perform most of these highly technical procedures.

With the high incidence of upper and lower urinary tract disease, combined with the invasiveness and morbidity associated with traditional techniques, the use of minimally invasive techniques is attractive. This article reviews some of the most commonly performed interventional procedures in small animal veterinary patients in the area of urology.

KIDNEY
Interventional Approach to Nephrolithiasis

The need for nephrolith removal is rarely necessary in veterinary medicine, especially in cats. Nephroliths are considered problematic when they are (1) causing intractable pyelonephritis (despite appropriate medical and dietary management), (2) causing a ureteral outflow tract obstruction associated with hydronephrosis, or (3) enlarging and overtaking the renal parenchyma resulting in progressive renal damage. It is important to note that most nephroliths do not seem to cause pain or discomfort unless they are associated with pyelonephritis, pyonephrosis, or a ureteral outflow obstruction, so the need for removal is rarely necessary.

Traditional open surgical options to treat problematic nephroliths (nephrotomy or ureteronephrectomy) are associated with frequent complications, and high long-term morbidity.[24,25] In a study of normal cats in which a nephrotomy was performed,[24] there was a 10% to 20% decrease in the glomerular filtration rate (GFR) despite normal renal function to start. In clinical patients, with prior renal injury associated with uroliths, compensatory mechanisms are often exhausted before diagnosis, so similar surgical interventions could have a more detrimental effect on renal function, emphasizing that one must be careful extrapolating these surgery results to clinical patients with upper tract uroliths and pre-existing renal disease. In the author's opinion, open surgical nephrotomy is reserved for removal of large, obstructed nephroliths in dogs when other options, such as extracorporeal shock-wave lithotripsy (ESWL) or percutaneous nephrolithotomy (PCNL), are not available. Open nephrotomy for removal of nonobstructive nephroliths in cats is not recommended particularly because the data confirming any benefit from nephrolith removal are lacking, and data confirming a negative effect on renal function exist.[26]

Extracorporeal shock-wave lithotripsy

ESWL refers to fragmentation of stones into small pieces using shocks generated outside of the body (**Fig. 1**). It is typically used for nephroliths and ureteroliths in dogs and not currently recommended in cats[3–5] because of the small size of their native ureteral lumen (0.3 mm) and their stone type (calcium oxalate monohydrate) being resistant to ESWL fragmentation.[27] ESWL fragments stones into pieces that are typically 1 mm or bigger in diameter, making passage of all of the fragments in a

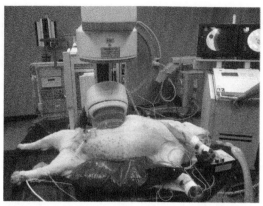

Fig. 1. An 8-year-old male castrated English bulldog during ESWL for nephroliths and ureteroliths.

cat highly unlikely. ESWL uses external shock waves that pass through a water medium and are then delivered through the soft tissues of a patient onto the stones; this is typically guided using fluoroscopy in various tangential views. The stone is shocked anywhere from 1000 to 3500 times at different energy levels to break up a stone into small fragments that are then allowed to pass down the ureter and into the urinary bladder. This debris can take weeks to pass. ESWL is thought to be very safe for the kidney, although subclinical intrarenal hemorrhage has been documented to occur.[3-5] Studies have shown minimal effect on the GFR after ESWL.[28,29] The availability of ESWL for veterinary patients in limited, and currently only available at Purdue University (Dr Larry Adams) and The Animal Medical Center, NYC (Dr Allyson Berent), to the author's knowledge.

In dogs, ESWL fragmentation is very successful, although up to 30% of dogs will require more than one treatment to achieve adequate fragmentation of nephroliths.[3-5] The mortality with ESWL is less than 1%, with the most common complication being the development of a transient ureteral obstruction in approximately 10% of cases.[3-5] The risk of ureteral obstruction may be minimized by placement of a ureteral stent before ESWL treatment to allow for passive ureteral dilation and to prevent obstruction during fragment passage.[30] Pancreatitis is another possible complication with ESWL, which was documented in 2% to 3% of cases.[31]

For stones larger than 1.5 cm, endoscopic nephrolithotomy (ENL) is often recommended over ESWL in both human and veterinary patients, because the risk for multiple procedures and for the development of a ureteral obstruction is high.

Endoscopic nephrolithotomy
ENL can either be performed percutaneously (PCNL) or surgically assisted (surgically assisted endoscopic nephrolithotomy, SENL) and is typically reserved in veterinary medicine for problematic nephroliths larger than 1.5 cm (of calcium oxalate, urate, or mixed composition), or problematic stones of cysteine composition, which are notoriously ESWL resistant (**Fig. 2**). This procedure has been shown to have minimal effect on renal function in both children and adults with large stone burdens, solitary kidneys, or renal insufficiency.[32] PCNL is considered highly renal-sparing when compared with alternatives like laparoscopic-assisted nephrotomy and traditional nephrotomy,[28,33,34] most likely due to this procedure causing renal parenchymal dilation, which spares functional renal tissue, rather than nephron transection.

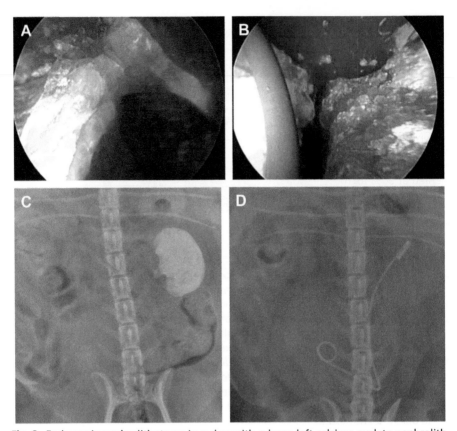

Fig. 2. Endoscopic nephrolithotomy in a dog with a large left calcium oxalate nephrolith. (*A*) Endoscopic image during intracorporeal nephroscopic-guided lithotripsy. (*B*) Broken stone in the renal pelvis during lithotripsy. A guidewire is within the renal pelvis to maintain access down the entire ureter. (*C*) Ventrodorsal radiograph of the dog before ENL. (*D*) Ventrodorsal radiograph after ENL and ureteral stent placement showing the full removal of all stone fragments during ENL.

ENL is done using both endoscopic and fluoroscopic guidance (see **Fig. 2**). For PCNL, ultrasound guidance is also needed. Renal access is obtained using an 18-gauge renal access trocar needle and directed onto the nephrolith from the lateral aspect on the greater curvature of the kidney. Once the needle punctures the renal pelvis, a contrast study is performed using a 50% mixture of iohexol and sterile saline for a pyeloureterogram. Then, a 0.035-inch hydrophilic guidewire is advanced through the needle, into the renal pelvis, down the ureter, into the urinary bladder, and out the urethra. This hydrophilic guidewire is considered the safety wire, which maintains through-and-through guidewire access.

Next, a balloon dilation catheter is advanced over the guidewire that is preloaded with a dilation sheath. This balloon is advanced from the skin, into the renal pelvis, guiding the location of the end of the balloon under fluoroscopic guidance. The balloon is then inflated to the predetermined size to allow for the access sheath to be smoothly advanced over the balloon and onto the nephrolith. This balloon dilation catheter is typically an 8-mm balloon and a 24-French access sheath. Once access is obtained, then the balloon is removed and the nephroscope is advanced into the renal pelvis through the sheath, and intracorporeal lithotripsy of the stone is performed until all stone fragments are successfully removed.

On completion of the procedure, a double pigtail ureteral stent is typically placed within the ureter over the guidewire in the event any ureteral spasm or small stone fragments remain and need to pass. The sheath is then removed. If this is done percutaneously, then a locking-loop pigtail nephrostomy tube is left in the stoma to allow a nephropexy to form, over approximately 4 to 6 weeks. If this is done surgically assisted, then the stoma is primarily closed with a mattress suture.

PCNL/SENL was recently reported in an abstract of 9 dogs and 1 cat.[7] Patient size was not seen to be a factor in success, but proper training and appropriate equipment are needed for a successful outcome. The success rate of PCNL has been documented at 90% to 100% in both the adult and the pediatric human populations, and the author has experienced the same in veterinary patients.

Idiopathic Renal Hematuria

Idiopathic renal hematuria (IRH) is a rare condition, most commonly seen in young, large-breed dogs, in which a focal area of bleeding in the upper urinary tract results in severe chronic hematuria, and the potential for iron deficiency anemia, blood clot formation, and a ureteral or urethral obstruction. In people, a hemangioma, angioma, or vascular malformation may be visualized ureteroscopically in the renal pelvis, and treatment via electrocautery can typically be easily accomplished.[25,35,36] This condition has been reported to occur bilaterally in 25% to 33% of affected canine patients, either at the time of diagnosis or in the future. Historically, when this condition was diagnosed, ureteronephrectomy was recommended in veterinary medicine. Because of the newer renal-sparing options, like sclerotherapy and ureteroscopy with electrocautery, and the risk for bilateral disease, nephrectomy should be considered contraindicated.

The diagnosis is typically made by cystoscopic imaging of urine jets from the ureterovesicular junction (UVJ). Urine is seen to be bright red from the bleeding side. IRH has also been diagnosed surgically by ureteral catheterization. Care should be taken in making this diagnosis with this approach because ureteral trauma and iatrogenic bleeding during catheterization can misdiagnose this condition. Cystoscopy should always be performed when possible.

Sclerotherapy

Sclerotherapy can be performed with the use of infusions of silver nitrate and/or povidone-iodine as cauterizing agents. These liquids can be infused into the renal pelvis and initiate cauterization of the bleeding lesion and can be done in any dog (male or female) regardless of size (**Fig. 3**). This procedure is done using cystoscopic and fluoroscopic guidance. Using an angle-tipped hydrophilic guidewire and open-ended ureteral catheter, a retrograde ureteropyelogram is performed to confirm that no lesions are seen within the lumen of the ureter or renal pelvis. Often a blood clot is seen in the renal pelvis. Then, the wire is coiled up in the renal pelvis and the ureteral catheter is removed over the wire.

Next, a ureteropelvic junction balloon dilation catheter is advanced over the wire under fluoroscopic guidance, and it is advanced to the proximal ureter. The balloon is inflated and a contrast study (50% saline and iohexol) is done to quantify the exact amount of fluid it takes to fill the renal pelvis without back-filling into the nephrons. Once this volume is recorded, the contrast agent is drained and the mixture of povidone-iodine, sterile water, and contrast, or liquid sterilized 0.5% silver nitrate, is used. Details of this protocol are published elsewhere.[8] Once the infusion is done,

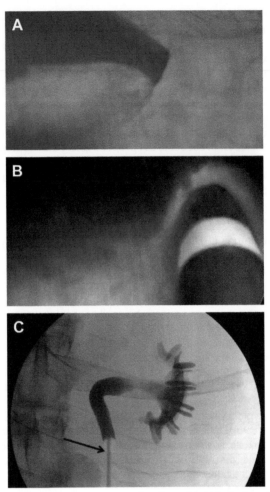

Fig. 3. Cystoscopic and fluoroscopic images of a dog with IRH. Patient is in dorsal recumbency. (*A*) Patient has blood visualized from the left ureteral opening. (*B*) A ureteral catheter up the ureter on the left side guided by both cystoscopic and fluoroscopic imaging. (*C*) Fluoroscopic image of a retrograde ureteropyelogram using a ureteropelvic junction balloon catheter (*arrow*) allowing for renal pelvic infusion of a sclerotherapeutic.

the material is left to dwell inside the renal pelvis for 20 minutes before being drained and repeated. Once completed, the guidewire is replaced and a double pigtail ureteral stent is placed within the ureteral lumen to prevent ureteritis. This stent is typically removed 2 weeks after the procedure as long as the bleeding has ceased.

In a recent study[8] in which sclerotherapy was used for the treatment of IRH, complete cessation of macroscopic hematuria occurred in 4 of 6 dogs within a median of 6 hours (range, postoperative to 7 days). Two additional dogs improved: one moderately and one substantially. None of the dogs required nephrectomy. To date, the author has performed this procedure in more than 25 dogs with success rates remaining at approximately 80% to 85%. Povidone-iodine alone was used in one patient by the author, and this too was successful. Further investigation of the necessity of the silver nitrate is underway.

Ureteroscopy

Ureteroscopy for electrocautery has only been performed in a small number of patients in the author's practice, and this is typically reserved for patients that have failed sclerotherapy. Ureteroscopy is also done using fluoroscopic guidance. There were no complications noted from the procedure when a stent was placed after the procedure (**Fig. 4**).

Intra-arterial Stem Cell Delivery for Chronic Kidney Disease/Protein-losing Nephropathy

Infusion of autologous and allogeneic mesenchymal stem cells, an adipose stromal component containing stem cells, is being investigated for the treatment of various feline and canine renal diseases (**Fig. 5**). The goals of multipotent stem cell therapy are to decrease the inflammatory reaction and fibrosis associated with both glomerulonephritis and interstitial nephritis through paracrine mechanisms, with the aim to slow the progression of the disease.[37] Tissue regeneration has not yet been proven, but studies are showing very promising results in various animal models.

With intravenous infusions, the first-pass extraction of the cells occurs in the lungs, which are the first capillary bed to encounter the cells. Using interventional radiologic techniques to direct delivery of the stem cells into the renal artery (via the femoral or carotid artery) using fluoroscopic guidance allows the glomeruli and vasa recta to be the first capillary bed to extract the cells, ultimately resulting in the highest engraftment rate.

The procedure is performed by doing a small cut down to either the femoral or the carotid artery to obtain vascular access. Using a 4-French vascular access introducer sheath, a guidewire and catheter are advanced into the aorta and the renal artery is cannulated. A contrast study using approximately 0.25 to 0.5 mL of iohexol is performed to confirm proper catheter placement into the proximal aspect of the renal artery, and then the catheter is flushed with saline. The aliquot of stem cells are then infused into the renal artery over about 5 minutes. In dogs, both kidneys are infused with an equal volume of cells. In cats, one kidney is typically used per treatment. On completion of the procedure, the catheter and sheath are removed and the artery is ligated.

A phase I clinical trial evaluating safety of intra-arterial delivery of autogenous cells in both dogs and cats is completed, and the procedure was shown to be technically possible and safe. A randomized, placebo-controlled study is currently underway

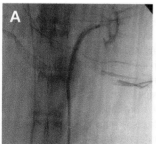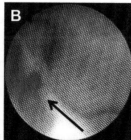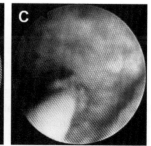

Fig. 4. Endoscopic and fluoroscopic images during ureteronephroscopy of a patient with renal hematuria. (*A*) Fluoroscopic image of a flexible ureteroscope up the ureter and into the renal pelvis. (*B*) An endoscopic image of a renal pelvic bleed causing the hematuria (*arrow*). (*C*) A Bugbee electrocautery probe during ablation of the bleeding lesion.

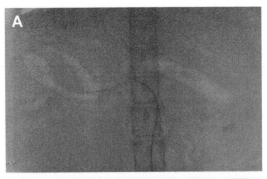

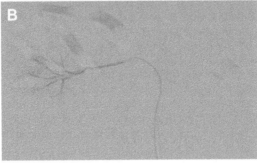

Fig. 5. Fluoroscopic imaging during intra-arterial renal stem cell delivery in a cat with chronic kidney disease in dorsal recumbency. (*A*) Guidewire and catheter advanced up the aorta from the femoral artery and into the right renal artery. (*B*) Contrast arteriogram confirming renal arterial infusion and proper catheter placement before stem cell delivery.

evaluating the efficacy of this approach in feline patients with International Renal Interest Society stage 3 chronic kidney disease. In the author's practice, more than 125 treatments have been performed in both dogs and cats. The efficacy to this point has been promising, although the studies are ongoing and the endpoints have not yet been met.

URETER

Ureteral diseases are occurring in small animal veterinary patients with increased frequency over the past decade, with ureteral obstruction being the most common condition in the upper urinary tract. The invasiveness and morbidity/mortality associated with traditional surgical techniques[38–40] make the use of endourologic alternatives highly appealing.

The physiologic response to a ureteral obstruction is very complex, with a rapid decrease in the GFR, resulting in progressive renal damage,[32,41] necessitating timely and successful intervention for the best ultimate outcome. The composition of most ureteroliths in dogs (50%–75%) and cats (>95%) are calcium based, making dissolution completely contraindicated in cats, and should not be considered in dogs without concurrent decompression.[9,16,17,38,39] With medical management being effective in some feline cases (8%–13%)[42] and traditional surgical interventions being associated with relatively high postoperative complication rates (31% in cats and ~7–15% in dogs)[38–40] and perioperative mortality (21% in cats and 6.25% in dogs),[38–40] short-term medical therapy should be considered before any intervention (24–48 hours) whenever possible.

In cases that are oliguric or anuric, hyperkalemic, overhydrated, or unstable, medical management may not be safe and immediate decompression is necessary. Interventional alternatives to traditional surgery are shown to result in immediate decompression, fewer perioperative complications, lower perioperative mortalities, successful treatments for all causes of obstruction (stone, stricture, tumor), and a decreased recurrence rate of future obstructions.[9-17] Diagnosis of a ureteral obstruction has been met with great controversy among internists, surgeons, and radiologists over the past decade. Traditional imaging modalities like intravenous pyelography (IVP), computed tomography (CT)-IVP, antegrade pyelography, and more recently, scintigraphy, have been found to be inconsistent, and often redundant, to simpler imaging like ultrasound and abdominal radiographs.[43-47] Ultrasound and abdominal radiography have been shown to be the most sensitive diagnostic tool for documenting a ureteral obstruction,[38,45] with the other more advanced imaging modalities offering very little additional information clinically, and risking the intravenous infusion of a nephrotoxic substance, like contrast material, in an already renal compromised patient. In more than 400 cases seen in the author's practice with ureteral obstructions in the past 10 years, the combination of ultrasound and abdominal radiographs most often accurately diagnoses the obstruction that is seen surgically or fluoroscopically using a ureteropyelogram.

The presence of renal pelvic dilation, regardless of the exact size, with concurrent hydroureter secondary to any obstructive lesion (stone, tumor, debris, and other) is diagnostic for a ureteral obstruction and should encourage decompression for the best return of renal function. At times, an obstructive lesion cannot be clearly visualized on ultrasound or radiographs, and this is often associated with a ureteral stricture or dried solidified blood calculi that do not shadow and/or are not radiopaque. When an obstructive lesion is not clearly seen on the ultrasound, regardless of hydronephrosis and hydroureter, a stone can often be seen radiographically, which was obscured by air in the bowel during the ultrasound examination (**Fig. 6**). This finding emphasizes why these 2 modalities are best used in combination. In addition, a recent report on circumcaval ureters[12] found that ureteral obstructions in cats without a clearly visualized obstructive lesion can often be associated with a ureteral stricture and a circumcaval ureter (17% of obstructed cats) and are found to be right-sided in about 80% of cases.

Another interesting finding diagnostically, and supported by an article by D'Anjou and colleagues,[43] was that renal pelvic size is not predictable of the cause of the dilation, and a minimally dilated renal pelvis can still be associated with ureteral obstruction. In this article, there was a trend to suggest that the larger the dilation, the more likely the cause was associated with an obstruction. In addition, it is appreciated in the author's practice that the severity of the postrenal azotemia is not associated with the size of the renal pelvis. Any degree of renal pelvic dilation (>1.5–2 mm) with concurrent hydroureter should be considered a ureteral obstruction until proven otherwise. When a clear obstructive lesion is not identified on ultrasound or radiographs (eg, stone), then a stricture, purulent plug, or dried solidified blood stones should be considered. Minimal hydroureter and hydronephrosis that taper gently within 1 to 2 cm of the renal pelvis have been associated with nonobstructive abnormality, and in these cases, ureterography can be helpful. Cases of a 3-mm renal pelvis with a 2-mm hydroureter in severely azotemic cats are seen, and renal pelvic decompression resolves the severe azotemia.

The pyelography at the time of intervention is shown to further support this diagnosis. In this article,[43] any renal pelvis greater than 13 mm was definitively associated with a ureteral obstruction, regardless of cause, and a renal pelvis greater than 7 mm

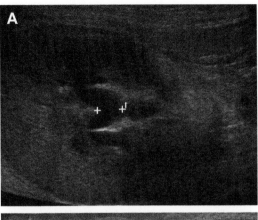

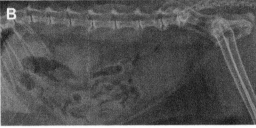

Fig. 6. Ultrasound and radiographic imaging in a cat with multiple ureterolithiasis. (*A*) Ultrasound image in transverse documenting hydroureter and renal pelvic dilation without evidence of stone disease. The calipers are measuring the renal pelvis diameter in transverse. (*B*) Lateral radiograph showing too numerous to count ureteroliths in the same cat, and the cause for the ureteral obstruction.

was most likely associated with a ureteral obstruction. Renal pelvises under 7 mm could also be associated with a ureteral obstruction, but other differentials given were pyelonephritis, intravenous fluid therapy, and chronic kidney disease/polyuria. One important detail of this article to note is that ureteral dimensions were not assessed, and there was no gold standard of diagnosis of a ureteral obstruction, like postmortem examination, surgery, or pyelography. Thus, there was no confirmation that the cases that were diagnosed with disease other than a ureteral obstruction were truly not obstructed and those that were diagnosed with a ureteral obstruction were truly obstructed. This finding likely underdiagnosed ureteral obstructions in this series.

Another important factor seen in using imaging for the diagnosis of a ureteral obstruction is to avoid prognosticating based on renal pelvic size, degree of renal parenchyma visible, severity of the dilation, and the assumed chronicity of the condition. It has been documented on multiple occasions in the author's practice that acute obstructions caused by ureteral ligations after an ovariectomy can have a severely dilated renal pelvis (>3 cm) with minimal visual parenchyma, and after decompression the kidney can return to looking normal within days. Similarly true is a severe dilation that is suspected to be present for weeks to months has been found to have a dramatic return to function and tissue decompression after a few weeks, termed the "no renal parenchyma syndrome," that is far too often diagnosed ultrasonographically. There are no data to support that the size of the renal pelvis is prognostic for the overall renal outcome, but rather the contrary is actually true.

A study by Horowitz and colleagues[13] showed that there was no prognostic factor found on any imaging modality, including renal pelvic size, kidney size, and laterality of the disease on ultrasound. Nothing was able to predict overall renal recovery after successful renal decompression, and more than 90% of cases had dramatic improvements in renal function at 3 months. In the author's practice, all ureteral obstructions, regardless of size of the pelvis, cause for obstruction, or the partial or complete nature of the obstruction, necessitate decompression on an emergent basis and should be recommended to the client.

Benign Ureteral Obstruction

Traditional ureteral surgery

Traditional ureteral surgery for obstructive ureterolithiasis is reported to include ureterotomy, neoureterocystostomy, ureteronephrectomy, or renal transplantation.[38–40] In a small study in dogs, results after a ureterotomy, pyelotomy, or ureteronephrectomy were associated with a surgical mortality of 6.25%, with 15% requiring an additional surgery for reobstruction within 30 days.[40] In addition, 43% of dogs in this study had evidence of recurrent urinary tract infections after surgery, 21% remained azotemic, and 15% had worsening azotemia. In cats, the procedure-associated complication and mortality rates are reported to be 30% and 21%, respectively. Most complications associated with surgery are due to ureterotomy site edema, nephroliths that pass from the renal pelvis to the surgery site, stricture formation, missed ureteroliths, and surgery-associated urine leakage.[38,39]

Percutaneous nephrostomy tube placement

One fast alternative for renal pelvis decompression in a more unstable patient is to place a nephrostomy tube (**Fig. 7**). A nephrostomy tube is typically considered a temporary solution but is highly effective. It may aid in stabilization and determination of renal function before a more expensive and lengthy invasive procedure. A nephrostomy tube is typically done with both ultrasound and fluoroscopic guidance using a modified Seldinger technique. In dogs, this is usually done percutaneously,

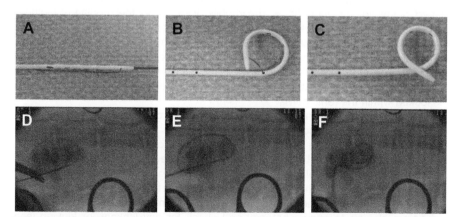

Fig. 7. Percutaneous nephrostomy tube placement. (*A*) Locking-loop pigtail catheter straightened out over a guidewire and hollow stiff trocar. (*B*) Once the wire and trocar are removed, the pigtail look is formed as the string is pulled. (*C*) The string is locked, creating a secure pigtail. (*D*) Pyelogram with a guidewire coiled within the renal pelvis. (*E*) Pigtail catheter advanced into the renal pelvis over the guidewire. (*F*) Locking-loop string pulled, creating a secured catheter within the renal pelvis for drainage.

and in cats, surgically assisted, due to their mobile small kidneys and need for a nephropexy.

Using ultrasound guidance, a renal access needle (18-gauge) is used to puncture the kidney into the renal pelvis for a pyelocentesis and pyelogram. The renal pelvis must remain relatively dilated so the amount of contrast infused is a 50% mixture of contrast and saline and is often equivalent to the amount retrieved on pyelocentesis; this is guided under concurrent fluoroscopy. The stylette of the access needle is removed and an angle-tipped hydrophilic guidewire is advanced into the renal pelvis through the trocar needle and coiled within the renal pelvis. Then, the locking-loop pigtail nephrostomy catheter is removed over the guidewire and the locking-loop nephrostomy catheter is advanced over the guidewire and coiled within the renal pelvis. The wire is withdrawn; the locking string is then secured, and the renal pelvis is drained. This catheter is carefully secured to the body wall using a purse-string and Chinese finger trap pattern.

Twenty cases using this type of locking-loop pigtail catheter were reported.[20] All catheters performed successfully by providing temporary urinary diversion and drainage for successful renal pelvis decompression. Only a few complications were reported.

Subcutaneous ureteral bypass device in cats

The development of an indwelling SUB device using a combination locking-loop nephrostomy catheter and cystostomy catheter connected to a subcutaenous shunting port has been used regularly in cats in some practices for the last 5 to 6 years with high success (**Fig. 8**). In humans, a similar device has been shown to reduce complications associated with externalized nephrostomy tubes and improve quality of life when compared with long-term ureteral stent exchanges as a long-term treatment modality.[20] The use of an SUB device has been described in abstract form in 25 cats and 2 dogs[10] and has been placed in more than 185 cats to date in the author's practice.

The SUB device is placed with surgical assistance using fluoroscopic guidance. The nephrostomy catheter is 6.5 French in diameter and is placed over a 0.035-inch "J"-shaped guidewire, or angle-tipped hydrophilic wire, using the modified-Seldinger technique (see **Fig. 8**). The caudal pole of the kidney is punctured using an 18-gauge catheter, and a pyelocentesis and antegrade pyelogram are performed, thus documenting the ureteral obstruction and allowing visualization of the renal pelvis for guidewire placement. Once the wire is coiled within the renal pelvis, the catheter is removed and the multifenestrated locking-loop nephrostomy catheter is advanced over the wire and locked within the renal pelvis.

Next, the cystostomy catheter is placed into the apex of the bladder and sutured in place. Each catheter is secured to the renal capsule and serosal surface of the bladder, respectively, using sterile cyanoacrylate glue to adhere the serosal surface of the kidney/bladder to a Dacron cuff, which is to prevent leakage and migration. Once the catheters are in place, they are passed through the ventral body wall, just lateral to the abdominal incision, and connected to the shunting port securely. Contrast material (50% iohexol and sterile saline) is infused through the shunting port before closure to ensure patency and check for any leakage or kinking (see **Fig. 8**).

With the commercially available device, 93% of patients survived to discharge, and no death was due to a ureteral obstruction or procedure associated complications.[10,12,13] The main short- and long-term complications were occlusion with stone material (~13%), occlusion with a blood clot (<3%), and kinking (<3%) of the tubing

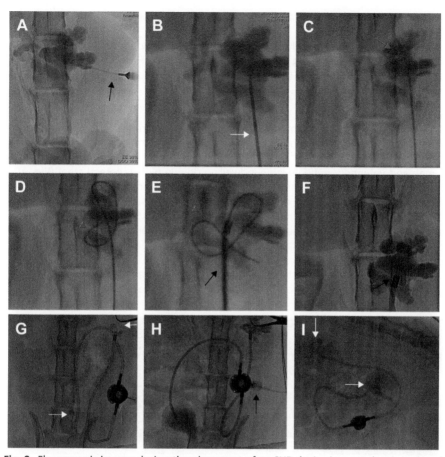

Fig. 8. Fluoroscopic images during the placement of an SUB device in a cat that is in dorsal recumbency during surgery. (*A*) Pyelocentesis using a 22-gauge intravenous catheter (*black arrow*) and antegrade pyelogram showing the dilated renal pelvis, dilated proximal ureter, and the location of the proximal ureteral stricture. (*B*) Caudal pole pyelocentesis with an 18-gauge catheter (*white arrow*) for SUB placement. (*C*) Guidewire (*red arrow*) advanced through the 18-gauge catheter and (*D*) coiled within the renal pelvis. (*E*) Nephrostomy catheter (*black arrow*) advanced over the guidewire (*red arrow*) and coiled within the renal pelvis. (*F*) Pigtail catheter locked within the renal pelvis (*black arrow*). (*G*) Connection of the nephrostomy and cystostomy catheters (*white arrows*) to the shunting port (*red arrow*) that is subcutaneous. (*H*) Contrast study done through the shunting port using a Huber needle (*black arrow*) showing filling of both the renal pelvis and the bladder. (*I*) Lateral fluoroscopic image of the SUB after placement. Red arrow shows the port and white arrows show the nephrostomy and cystostomy catheters within the lumen of the kidney and urinary bladder.

over a median follow-up period of 3.5 years (range, 1 month to >6 years). Leakage of urine through the device is a rare complication, and with the new commercially available device and appropriate training, this is very uncommon. All of these complications can be typically fixed with a catheter exchange/manipulation. Because of the subcutaneous shunting port available for flushing and sampling of the device, management and maintenance have helped to maintain high patency rates. Initially, the SUB device was reserved for feline patients with proximal ureteral strictures or ureteral stent failures, but more recently, it has been used for all causes of feline ureteral obstructions in certain practices, and stents are reserved for canine ureteral obstructions.

The SUB device is routinely flushed at 1 month postoperatively and then every 3 months thereafter. Flushing is done using a noncoring Huber needle through the subcutaneous shunting port, using ultrasound guidance to monitor the renal pelvis and bladder for flow (**Fig. 9**).

Feline ureteral stenting

Ureteral stents are used in humans to divert urine from the renal pelvis into the urinary bladder for obstructions secondary to ureterolithiasis, ureteral stenosis/strictures, malignant neoplasia, or trauma.[42,48–51] The main type of ureteral stents used in both human and veterinary patients is an indwelling double pigtail ureteral stent (**Fig. 10**). In human medicine, it is recommended that the stents be removed or exchanged after 3 to 6 months,[49,51,52] but this does not seem to be necessary in feline or canine patients because they have remained patent and in place for more than 6 years in some patients. Stent placement may be considered a long-term treatment option for various causes of ureteral obstructions; however, potential side effects and long-term complications can exist.[2,9,11–14]

Feline ureteral stents are typically placed surgically assisted in an antegrade approach using the modified Seldinger technique under fluoroscopic guidance

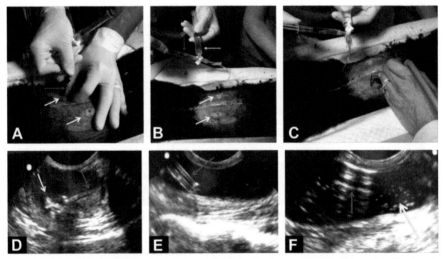

Fig. 9. Ultrasound-guided flushing of the SUB device in a cat with bilateral SUBs due to dried solidified blood stones. The cat is in dorsal recumbency. (*A*) Both ports (*white arrows*) are clipped and aseptically prepared. The Huber needle (*blue arrow*) is inserted into the shunting port. (*B*) Urine is withdrawn in the empty syringe. Notice the bloody urine (*red arrow*) that is withdrawn from the urinary tract, which is typical of cats with renal hematuria and dried solidified blood stones. A syringe of sterile saline (*yellow arrow*) is then infused into the system, while watching under ultrasound guidance. No more than 1 mL should be infused at a time, and it should never be infused if that amount was not able to be withdrawn. White arrows show the ports under the skin. (*C*) Similar procedure on the other side. (*D*) Monitoring the infusion during flushing of the renal pelvis to see bubbles (*yellow arrows*) forming within the system, which confirms patency. Red arrows are the lines of the nephrostomy tube. (*E*) Same confirmation in the urinary bladder. Red arrow shows the nephrostomy catheter entering the kidney. (*F*) Notice the bubbles (*yellow arrows*) within the urinary bladder coming from the cystostomy tube (*red arrows*).

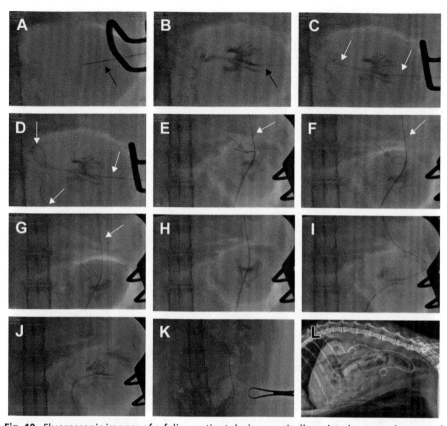

Fig. 10. Fluoroscopic images of a feline patient during surgically assisted antegrade ureteral stent placement. The patient is in dorsal recumbency, and the head is at the top of the fluoroscopic images. (*A*) Left renal pelvis being accessed with a 22-gauge over-the-needle catheter (*black arrow*). (*B*) Ureteropyelogram being performed. Notice the dilated and tortuous ureter proximal to the more distal ureteral obstruction. Black arrow shows the guide wire entering the renal pelvis. (*C*) Guidewire (*white arrows*) being advanced through the catheter, into the renal pelvis and down the proximal ureter. (*D*) Guidewire (*white arrows*) advanced around the tortuous ureter and down to the obstructive lesion. (*E*) The ureteral stent (*red arrow*) being advanced over the guidewire (*white arrow*) in an antegrade manner after the ureteral dilator ensured the stent would fit. The wire is passed out of one of the proximal holes of the stent so the loop is not over the wire (see **Fig. 11**). (*F, G*) The stent (*red arrow*) is pulled from the bladder distally, and the loop is pulled into the renal pelvis, keeping the through-and-through wire (*white arrow*) access out of the kidney. (*H*) The loop is formed within the renal pelvis, and the guidewire is then removed (*I*). (*J*) The ureteral stent is coiled with one loop in the renal pelvis (*red arrow*). (*K*) The entire stent (*red arrows*) is seen traveling from the renal pelvis, down the ureteral lumen, and into the urinary bladder. (*L*) Lateral radiograph showing a double pigtail ureteral stent bypassing multiple ureteroliths.

(see **Fig. 10**). Using a 22-gauge over-the-needle catheter, the renal pelvis is punctured through the greater curvature of the kidney and an antegrade ureteropyelogram is performed. Then, a 0.018-inch angle-tipped hydrophilic guidewire is used to negotiate around the obstruction from the renal pelvis, down the ureter, and into the urinary bladder. Then, the ureter is dilated over the wire using a 0.034-inch dilation catheter, and finally, the 2.5-French double pigtail ureteral stent is

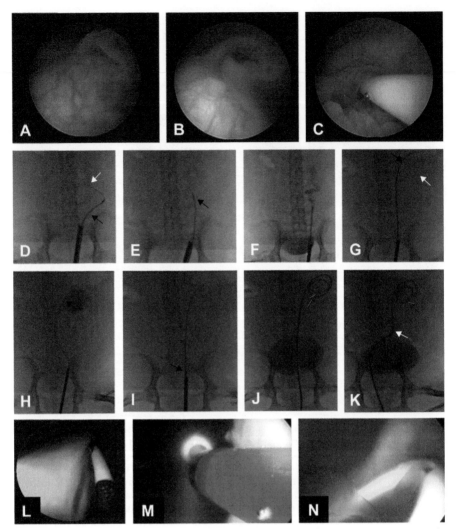

Fig. 11. Cystoscopic- and fluoroscopic-guided retrograde ureteral stent placement in a female dog. (A) Cystoscopic image of a dog in dorsal recumbency showing the left UVJ. (B) Guidewire being advanced into the ureteral lumen from the UVJ. (C) Open-ended ureteral catheter being advanced over the guidewire into the ureteral lumen. (D) Fluoroscopic image of the guidewire (*white arrow*) and open-ended ureteral catheter (*black arrow*) being advanced retrograde up the ureter. (E) The wire is removed, and the catheter remains in the ureter for a retrograde ureteropyelogram. Black arrow shows the open ended ureteral catheter. (F) Retrograde ureteropyelogram being performed outlining the ureteral obstruction. (G) Guidewire (*white arrow*) advanced back into the catheter and curled within the renal pelvis with the ureteral catheter (*black arrow*) advanced to the renal pelvis. (H) Contrast seen within the renal pelvis after a pyelogram was performed through the ureteral catheter (*black arrow*). (I) The ureteral catheter (*black arrow*) is pulled back over a guidewire from the UPJ in image (H) to the UVJ in image (I), allowing for measurement of the ureteral length for stent sizing. (J) The ureteral stent (*blue arrow*) is advanced over the guidewire and curled within the renal pelvis. The bladder is filled with contrast to be able to mark the UVJ under fluoroscopy. (K) Once the proximal loop of the stent (*blue arrow*) is within the renal pelvis, the guidewire is retracted (*white arrow*). (L) Endoscopic image of the

placed over the wire, allowing one loop to coil within the renal pelvis, and the other within the urinary bladder.

In a recent study in 69 cats (79 ureters),[9] with both stone- and stricture-induced obstructions, successful stent placement was achieved in 95% of ureters. More than 60% of the cases in this study were considered poor ureterotomy candidates based on stone number, stone location, stricture location, and presence of concurrent nephroliths. There was a median of 4 stones per ureter and 86% had concurrent nephroliths. About 25% of cats had a ureteral stricture (with or without a stone). After the stent was placed, 95% of cases had significant improvement in their azotemia, and there was a perioperative mortality of 7.5%, none of which died of surgical complications or a persistent/recurrent ureteral obstruction.[9] The main long-term complications reported were dysuria (38% reported and 2% persisted), stent occlusion (19%), stent migration (6%), and need for stent exchange (27%). Because of these long-term complications, the SUB device is routinely recommended in cats, improving these long-term complication rates dramatically.[1,2,9–13]

Canine ureteral stenting for benign disease

The use of double pigtail ureteral stents (**Fig. 11**) in dogs has been investigated as an alternative to traditional surgery, resulting in immediate ureteral decompression, stabilization of the associated azotemia, a decreased risk of ureteral stricture or ureteral leakage, and a decreased rate of ureteral obstruction recurrence. Placement of a double-pigtail ureteral stent, via either minimally invasive techniques (endoscopy and fluoroscopy or ultrasound and fluoroscopy), seems to have circumvented many of the complications of traditional surgery, avoiding the need for nephrotomy or ureteronephrectomy, and resulting in expedited stabilization and shorter hospital stays.[16,17,40] Ureteral dilation in dogs has been recently shown[21] to occur within 2 weeks of stent placement. In this study, 10 ureteral stents were placed and monitored with CT before and after placement over a 2- to 10-week interval, and passive dilation was documented in all dogs. In addition, this dilation was significant enough to allow for successful ureteroscopy in all ureters at the time of ureteral stent removal. This concept of passive ureteral dilation has been well documented in human medicine.[30]

The main concern with stents is typically seen months to years after placement. They are not usually life threatening and are relatively easy to address on an outpatient basis. These concerns include stent occlusion, stent compression with unsuccessful renal drainage, migration, encrustation, and proliferative tissue at the UVJ. These problems are relatively rare in dogs.[16,17]

In dogs with ureterolithiasis, ureteral stenting is almost always performed noninvasively with endoscopic and fluoroscopic guidance (see **Fig. 11**) by gaining access to the ureter through the UVJ cystoscopically. A guidewire and open-ended ureteral catheter are advanced up the ureter. A retrograde ureteropyelogram is performed documenting the obstruction and tortuosity of the ureter using a 50% contrast/saline mixture. The wire is then advanced around the obstruction and into the renal pelvis.

---

ureteral stent as it exits the UVJ. The black mark seen is an endoscopic marker to alert the endoscopist when the distal loop of the pigtail is beginning. (*M*) Endoscopic image of the junction of the ureteral stent and the pusher catheter as they both exit the working channel of the endoscope. Notice the guidewire is through the lumen of both catheters. (*N*) Once the stent is within the bladder, the pushing catheter and wire are completely removed and you can see fluid draining through the fenestrations of the stent ensuring patency.

Once the renal pelvis is catheterized, it is drained and lavaged, especially if it is associated with a pyonephrosis.[16] Then, the ureteral length is measured, and an appropriately sized ureteral stent is placed over the guidewire through the working channel of the cystoscope using fluoroscopic guidance. The patient is typically discharged the same day as the procedure.

This procedure has a reported mortality of less than 2%.[16,17] This minimally invasive procedure is successful in more than 90% of dogs. The main long-term issue in dogs is the risk of recurrent urinary tract infections (15%–59% after stent vs ∼60%–80% prestent),[16,17] which was also reported after traditional surgery. Recurrent urinary tract infections are likely not associated with the presence of the stent, but instead concurrent stone disease, established pyelonephritis, decreased renal function, and concurrent immune dysfunction. Careful monitoring of image findings, urinalysis, and cultures is required to avoid ascending pyelonephritis, and owners should be aware of the potential for stent occlusion, migration, and the need for stent exchange. Cystoscopic-assisted ureteral stent placement is technically challenging and should not be attempted without endourology training. For canine patients suspected of having struvite ureterolithiasis, successful dissolution after ureteral stent placement is documented, and dissolution diet and long-term antibiotic therapy should always be used as indicated in these cases (**Fig. 12**).

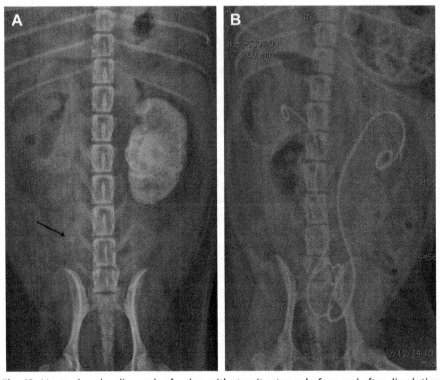

Fig. 12. Ventrodorsal radiograph of a dog with struvite stones before and after dissolution with diet and antibiotic therapy. (*A*) Left-sided staghorn nephrolith and right-sided ureterolith (*black arrow*) causing a ureteral obstruction. (*B*) Bilateral ureteral stents placed at the time of diagnosis; this radiograph shows dissolution of both the nephrolith and the ureterolith after 7 months of diet and antibiotic therapy.

Canine malignant ureteral obstruction

Ureteral stenting Ureteral stenting for the treatment of trigonal obstructive neoplasia is typically performed using both ultrasound and fluoroscopic guidance. The patient is placed in lateral recumbency, and an antegrade pyelogram is done percutaneously under ultrasound guidance, as described above (**Fig. 13**). Using fluoroscopic visualization, a guidewire is advanced down the ureter, through the tumor at the UVJ, and into the urinary bladder. The wire is then passed down the urethra, and through-and-through access is obtained, allowing for retrograde ureteral stent placement. In 2011, a study of 12 dogs (15 ureters)[18] that had ureteral stents placed for ureteral obstructive neoplasia, 1 dog required surgical conversion. All patients survived to discharge, and the median survival time from time of diagnosis was 285 days (range, 10–1571), and following stent placement was 57 days (range, 7–337). This procedure is typically performed on an outpatient basis.

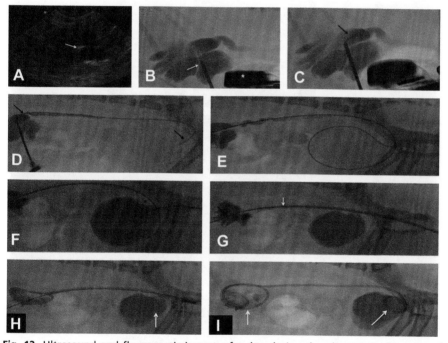

Fig. 13. Ultrasound and fluoroscopic images of a dog during the placement of a ureteral stent due to a malignant ureteral obstruction associated with TCC. This dog is in lateral recumbency. (*A*) Ultrasound image during pyelocentesis (*white arrow*) and pyelogram. (*B*) Fluoroscopic image during pyelogram through an 18-gauge renal trocar needle (*white arrow*). The ultrasound probe (*yellow asterisk*) is seen in the field. (*C*) Guidewire (*black arrow*) being advanced down the ureter through the trocar needle. (*D*) Guidewire (*black arrows*) down the ureter to the level of the UVJ as it nears the tumor. (*E*) Guidewire passed through the tumor and into the urinary bladder as it is aimed out of the urethra. (*F*) Tumor seen at the dorsal caudal bladder wall (*black asterisk*) and the wire is passed out the urethra. (*G*) The wire is pulled straight, and through-and-through access is obtained. A ureteral dilator sheath (*white arrow*) is advanced over the wire into the proximal ureter. Black arrow shows the guide wire. (*H*) A stent is being advanced up the ureter and coiled inside the renal pelvis. The caudal end of the stent is coiled in the urinary bladder (*yellow arrow*) with a pushing catheter (*blue arrow*). (*I*) Both ends of the stent are now in place (*yellow arrows*).

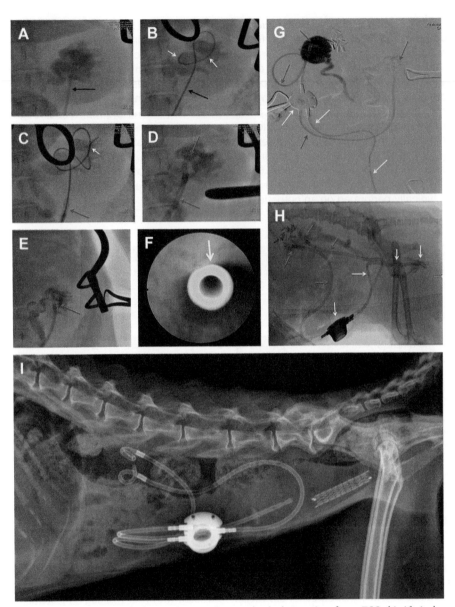

Fig. 14. Bilateral ureteral obstructions and a urethral obstruction from TCC. (*A–H*) A dog wherein bilateral SUBs were placed with a radical cystectomy to remove all gross disease. (*A*) Fluoroscopic images (*A–E, G*) are in dorsal recumbency during surgery. (*A*) Renal access using an 18-gauge catheter (*black arrow*) into the renal pelvis from the caudal pole of the kidney. (*B*) Guidewire (*white arrows*) coiling within the renal pelvis, advanced through the catheter (*black arrow*). (*C*) Nephrostomy catheter (*red arrow*) being advanced over the guidewire (*white arrow*). (*D*) Locking-loop pigtail nephrostomy tube (*red arrows*) within the renal pelvis. (*E*) Contrast study through the catheter (*red arrow*) during a pyelogram showing patency of the catheter and no leakage. (*F*) Cystoscopy image of the urethral catheter (*yellow arrow*) coming down the urethra after radical cystectomy. (*G*) Dorsoventral projection during a digital subtraction image while performing a contrast study through the 3-way shunting port (*white arrow*) showing both renal pelvises filling through the 2

A SUB system can be used for malignant ureteral obstructions as well, but requires surgical placement. For cases where the tumor is localized to the urinary bladder +/− proximal urethra, the entire bladder and urethra have been removed via a radical cystectomy and both renal pelvises have a SUB catheter placed. Then, both kidney catheters are then connected to a 3-way port (**Fig. 14**), and a third catheter is placed down the urethra or into the vagina. These dogs have been completely incontinent, but if done in the right cases, only microscopic disease will remain.

URINARY BLADDER AND URETHRA
Diagnostic Cystourethrography

Diagnostic cystourethrography is very important in IR because documentation of subtle urethral lesions can be difficult. The preferred method is to perform this procedure in lateral recumbency under fluoroscopic guidance to document in real time urethral dilation and spasm. Using still images, as with digital radiography, can easily misdiagnose a ureteral stricture for an area of transient urethral spasm during contrast injection. In dogs, a guidewire is used to catheterize the urethra and urinary bladder. Over the guidewire, a vascular access sheath (5–8 French, depending on the size and sex of the dog) is advanced over the wire and into the urethra. It is very important that the contrast study be done with appropriate bladder filling. It is easy to misinterpret an underfilled bladder and urethra for a urethral lesion, like a stricture, when it is really a result of poor urethral and bladder distension.

The bladder should be filled with a 30% to 50% mixture of sterile contrast and saline until it is palpably distended. Then, through the side arm of the sheath, the urethra is infused with contrast while the sheath is withdrawn caudally to maximally distend the urethra. This procedure is termed a "pull-out urethrogram." If the bladder is not full, then the urethra will typically not distend well. If an area of the urethra is suspicious for a lesion, then the sheath should be placed caudal to this lesion, and simultaneous manual expression of the bladder during infusion of the sheath should be done to maximally distend this region and fill the urethra. Care should be taken to magnify and collimate the fluoroscopic image to avoid excessive digital exposure. A bladder spoon/paddle can be used for this; this will further demarcate a lesion in the urethra or distend a urethra that is normal but spasming from the infusion and is particularly important in cats, who have a very long, narrow, and highly spastic urethral muscle. In male cats, a sheath cannot be used because it is too large for their penile urethra. In that case, a 3.5-French or 5-French urethral catheter is typically used (**Fig. 15**).

Cystostomy Tube Placement for Various Causes of Urethral Obstruction

Cystostomy tubes are often placed to bypass a urethral obstruction or buy time while a urethral, trigonal, or bladder lesion is healing; this can be secondary to malignant neoplasia, aggressive bladder surgeries, severe urethritis, detrusor reflex dyssynergia, urethral strictures, urethral tears, or urethral stones that are difficult to remove

---

nephrostomy catheters (*red arrows*) and the urethral catheter (*yellow arrows*). (*H*) Lateral fluoroscopy image showing the entire system with the red arrows outlining the 2 nephrostomy catheters and the yellow arrow outlining the urethroscopy catheter after the bladder was removed. The white arrow is the 3-way shunting port of the SUB device. (*I*) A lateral radiograph of a cat with bilateral ureteral and urethral obstructions secondary to TCC. This cat had bilateral SUB devices placed and a urethral stent. The SUB devices were placed to a 3-way subcutaneous access port.

A

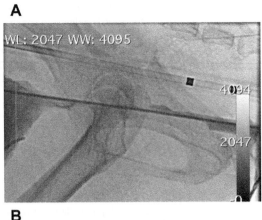

B

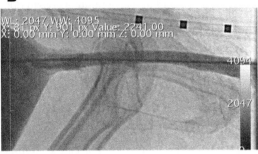

Fig. 15. Cystourethrogram of a cat in lateral recumbency. Notice the narrow urethra documented in image (*A*). (*B*) After a pullout urethrogram and concurrent bladder compression, the entire urethra distends, documenting a patent urethra without a stricture that was misdiagnosed on (*A*).

surgically. With the advent of urethral stents, the use of cystostomy tubes has declined in the author's practice, but the ease and success of placement of these tubes make them a viable option when necessary.

Cystostomy tubes can be placed either percutaneously or surgically. With the locking-loop pigtail catheter (**Fig. 16**), percutaneous cystostomy tube placement has become a fast, safe, and highly effective technique. Cystostomy tubes can be placed using either ultrasound or fluoroscopic guidance. The author prefers fluoroscopic guidance using the modified Seldinger technique. As described earlier for nephrostomy tubes, a stab incision is made through the skin and abdominal musculature over the area of puncture. Then, an 18-gauge over-the-needle catheter is advanced into the urinary bladder via cystocentesis (paramedian approach at the bladder body), until urine is draining. The stylet is removed, and a sterile urine sample is obtained for culture and analysis. Then, a cystogram is performed using a 50% mixture of contrast medium and sterile saline to fill the bladder (approximate total bladder volume is 5–15 mL/kg). Next, a 0.035-inch hydrophilic angle-tipped guidewire is advanced through the catheter and coiled within the urinary bladder. The guidewire can be advanced down the urethra using fluoroscopic guidance if antegrade catheterization is desired (see the following discussion), using this same technique.

For placement of the cystostomy tube, the locking-loop catheter is cannulated with the stiff hollow trocar and is advanced over the wire. This catheter is then punctured

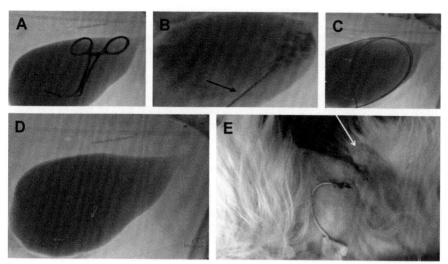

Fig. 16. Percutaneous modified Seldinger technique for the placement of the locking-loop pigtail cystostomy catheter. (*A*) Lateral recumbency shows the entire bladder and proximal urethra. Black arrow shows the 18 gauge over the needle catheter. (*B*) 18-gauge intravenous catheter (*black arrow*) placed within the urinary bladder for a cystogram. (*C*) Guidewire (*red arrows*) coiled in urinary bladder. (*D*) Fluoroscopy image of the locking loop cystostomy catheter (*red arrows*) as it is pulled toward the body wall and the wire is removed. (*E*) Male dog with a cystostomy tube exiting the abdominal wall. This dog is in dorsal recumbency, and the cystostomy tube (*red arrow*) is seen passing lateral to the prepuce (*white arrow*).

through the body and urinary bladder wall. Once it is well within the urinary bladder, the hollow trocar is withdrawn as the catheter is advanced over the guidewire to ensure that the entire distal end of the catheter is within the bladder lumen. Then, the locking string is engaged as the trocar and guidewire are removed, creating a loop of the pigtail catheter. The bladder is then drained and filled to ensure the entire pigtail is appropriately positioned in the bladder lumen and is functioning well. The loop of the catheter should be within the lumen of the bladder, extending approximately 1 to 2 cm from the wall, so that it is not too snug against the bladder wall; this allows movement when the bladder is both full and empty to prevent dislodgement. The catheter is then carefully secured to the body wall using a purse-string suture and Chinese finger trap suture pattern. Because there is no surgical cystopexy, this tube should remain in place for at least 2 to 4 weeks before removal.

Other tubes, such as latex mushroom-tipped catheters, Foley catheters, or low-profile tubes, can be placed surgically or with laparoscopic assistance.[53–55] These tubes are placed with a surgical cystopexy. Catheter care and cleanliness should be emphasized, because cystostomy tubes are commonly associated with secondary infections (86% in one study) because of the external nature of the tube. Additional complications with cystostomy tubes have been reported in as high as 49% of patients, involving inadvertent tube removal, ingestion of the tube by the patient, fistulous tract formation, and mushroom-tip breakage during removal.[55] Cystostomy tube placement is not ideal in circumstances wherein chemotherapy (for malignant obstructions) or immunosuppressive therapy (for immune-mediated proliferative urethritis) is being used and secondary infections and poor wound healing may occur. In addition, if a tube is removed prematurely and no cystopexy has been created, the risk of uroabdomen is possible.

Antegrade Urethral Catheterization

For animals that are difficult or too small to catheterize, have a urethral tear, or have a distal urethral obstruction, antegrade urethral catheterization can be performed (**Fig. 17**). This technique can be performed surgically or interventionally and should be done under general anesthesia or heavy sedation.[56] When performing the technique percutaneously, the patient is placed in lateral recumbency and an area in the caudal lateral abdomen over the bladder is clipped and the area as well as the vulva or prepuce is prepared aseptically. A cystocentesis is performed using an 18-gauge over-the-needle catheter directed toward the trigone of the bladder, as discussed in the section about percutaneous cystostomy tube placement. Urine (5–15 mL) is drained from the bladder and replaced with an equal amount of contrast material diluted 50% with sterile saline until the proximal urethra is identified.

A hydrophilic guidewire (0.018 inch for male cats and 0.035 inch for female cats) is advanced into the bladder and aimed toward the bladder trigone and urethra, using fluoroscopic guidance. Once the urethra is cannulated with the guidewire, it is advanced down the urethra antegrade, around the obstructive lesion or tear, and out of the distal urethra, prepuce, or vulva. When performed surgically, contrast enhancement and the use of fluoroscopy are not necessary, allowing for "through-and-through" guidewire access. Once the guidewire is outside the urethra, a urinary catheter (open-ended; red rubber [3.5–5.0 French for male cats and 5.0–8 French for female cats], a locking-loop pigtail catheter [5 French for male cats; 6–8 French for female cats], or a nonlocking pigtail catheter) is advanced over the wire in a retrograde manner, within the urethral lumen and into the urinary bladder.

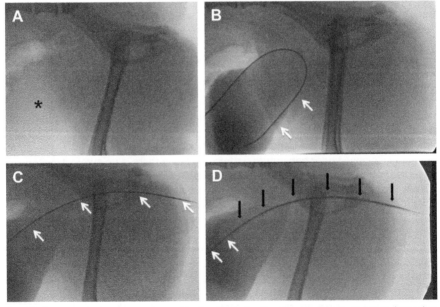

Fig. 17. Percutaneous antegrade urethral catheterization in a male cat. Cat is in lateral recumbency. (*A*) Urinary bladder (*black asterisk*). (*B*) Guidewire (*white arrows*) coiled within the urinary bladder. (*C*) Wire (*white arrows*) out of the urethra gaining through-and-through access. (*D*) Catheter (*black arrows*) advanced retrograde over the guidewire (*white arrows*).

This procedure is highly effective for male cats with urethral tears because the tear is typically made in a longitudinal retrograde direction, making antegrade passage easy. Longitudinal urethral tears will usually heal within 5 to 10 days without surgical intervention, and the catheter should be maintained for that length of time, using clean or sterile technique.[57]

Urethral Stenting for Urethral Obstructions

Urethral stents are most commonly used for the relief of benign or malignant obstructions in the trigone or urethra in dogs and cats.[58–61] The most common cause of malignant obstructions in dogs and cats are due to transitional cell carcinoma (TCC).[58,59] Benign obstructions are less common and are most typically associated with urethral strictures from either urethral tears, vehicular trauma, or chronic obstructive stone disease.[60,61]

When signs of obstruction occur, more aggressive therapy is indicated, with euthanasia commonly ensuing due to a lack of good alternative options. Placement of surgical cystostomy tubes, debulking surgery, and surgical diversionary procedures are invasive and often associated with undesirable outcomes.[62–66] Placement of self-expanding metallic stents under fluoroscopic guidance via a transurethral approach can be a fast, reliable, and safe alternative to establish urethral patency regardless of the benign or malignant nature and is an outpatient procedure.[58–61] Benign urethral strictures may resolve with balloon dilation alone and have been successful in a small number of patients as well.

To place a urethral stent, the patient is placed in lateral recumbency, and a marker catheter is placed inside the colon to allow for urethral measurement and determination of stent size. The bladder is maximally distended with contrast, and a pullout urethrogram is performed to allow for maximal distension of the urethra using a 50% mixture of contrast and saline. Measurements of the normal urethral diameter and the length of the associated obstruction are obtained, and an appropriately sized self-expanding metallic urethral stent is chosen (approximately 10%–15% greater than the normal urethral diameter and 3–5 mm longer than the obstruction on both the cranial and the caudal ends). The stent is deployed under fluoroscopic guidance, and a repeat contrast cystourethrogram is performed to document restored urethral patency.

The procedure is considered outpatient, and the animals are typically discharged the same day. In some cases with trigonal TCC, bilateral concurrent ureteral obstructions may be present so an ultrasound should be evaluated and followed regularly. When this is encountered, it is typically recommended to have bilateral SUBs or percutaneous antegrade ureteral stents placed (see above). These procedures can be highly successful when necessary (**Fig. 18**).

In a recent study evaluating the use of urethral stents for malignant obstructions in dogs, the median survival time after stent placement was 78 days, but for those patients treated with chemotherapy, median survival time was 251 days.[58] Resolution of urinary tract obstruction was achieved in 97.6% of dogs, and 26% were severely incontinent.[58] Another study evaluating urethral stents in 11 dogs for benign urethral obstructions found 100% of dogs had clinical relief of their urethral obstruction with a stent with only 12.5% of dogs being severely incontinent after stent placement, when not incontinent before stent placement.[60] Another study[61] evaluating 9 cats after urethral stent placement for benign and malignant obstruction also had a 100% success in obstruction relief, with a 25% severe incontinence rate following stenting. Palliative stenting for urethral obstructions in dogs and cats can provide a rapid, effective, and safe alternative to more traditional and invasive options, and long-term survival times can be achieved.

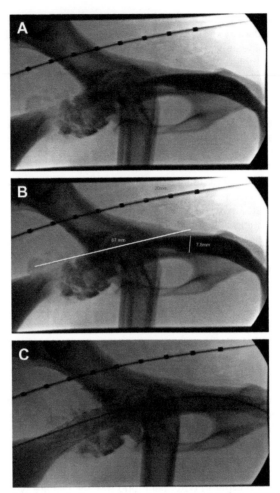

Fig. 18. Fluoroscopic images during urethral stent placement for prostatic TCC in a male dog. Dog is in lateral recumbency. Marker catheter is in the colon. (*A*) Cystourethrogram during a pullout study. (*B*) Measurements using the marker catheter (*red line*) to adjust for magnification. Measuring urethral diameter (*white line*) and length of stent desired (*yellow line*). (*C*) Urethrogram after urethral stent is deployed.

SUMMARY

IR provides many options for both the diagnosis and the treatment of various urinary tract diseases in veterinary medicine. This technology has dramatically expanded therapeutic options for our patients over the past decade. Above are only a small handful of the most common procedures being performed in veterinary medicine to date, and this has become more popular in both academic and private practice settings in the last few years. These procedures are following the trend that has been occurring in human medicine over the past 25 years, and will likely continue.

It is highly recommended that operators get proper training before considering most of the procedures described because the learning curve is steep, and complications should be avoided whenever possible. Training laboratories are regularly available to perfect these types of skills.

REFERENCES

1. Berent A. New techniques on the horizon: interventional radiology and interventional endoscopy of the urinary tract ('endourology'). J Feline Med Surg 2014; 16(1):51–65.
2. Berent A. Ureteral obstructions in dogs and cats: a review of traditional and new interventional diagnostic and therapeutic options. J Vet Emerg Crit Care 2011; 21(2):86–103.
3. Adams LG, Goldman CK. Extracorporeal shock wave lithotripsy. In: Polzin DJ, Bartges JB, editors. Nephrology and urology of small animals. Ames (IA): Blackwell Publishing; 2011. p. 340–8.
4. Adams LG. Nephroliths and ureteroliths: a new stone age. N Z Vet J 2013;61:1–5.
5. Block G, Adams LG, Widmer WR, et al. Use of extracorporeal shock wave lithotripsy for treatment of nephrolithiasis and ureterolithiasis in five dogs. J Am Vet Med Assoc 1996;208:531–6.
6. Donner GS, Ellison GW. Percutaneous nephrolithotomy in the dog: an experimental study. Vet Surg 1987;16:411–7.
7. Berent A, Weisse C, Bagley D, et al. Endoscopic nephrolithotomy for the treatment of complicated nephrolithiasis in dogs and cats [Abstract]. San Antonio (TX): American College of Veterinary Surgeons; 2013.
8. Berent A, Weisse C, Bagley D, et al. Renal sparing treatment for idiopathic renal hematuria (IRH): endoscopic-guided sclerotherapy. J Am Vet Med Assoc 2013; 242(11):1556–63.
9. Berent A, Weisse C, Bagley D. Ureteral stenting for benign feline ureteral obstructions: technical and clinical outcomes in 79 ureters (2006-2010). J Am Vet Med Assoc 2014;244:559–76.
10. Berent A, Weisse C, Bagley D, et al. The use of a subcutaneous ureteral bypass device for the treatment of feline ureteral obstructions. Seville (Spain): ECVIM; 2011.
11. Zaid M, Berent A, Weisse C, et al. Feline ureteral strictures: 10 cases (2007-2009). J Vet Intern Med 2011;25(2):222–9.
12. Steinhaus J, Berent A, Weisse C, et al. Presence of circumcaval ureters and ureteral obstructions in cats. J Vet Intern Med 2015;29(1):63–70.
13. Horowitz C, Berent A, Weisse C, et al. Predictors of outcome for cats with ureteral obstructions after interventional management using ureteral stents or a subcutaneous ureteral bypass device. J Feline Med Surg 2013;15(12):1052–62.
14. Nicoli S, Morello E, Martano M, et al. Double-J ureteral stenting in nine cats with ureteral obstruction. Vet J 2012;194(1):60–5.
15. Lam N, Berent A, Weisse C, et al. Ureteral stenting for congenital ureteral strictures in a dog. J Am Vet Med Assoc 2012;240(8):983–90.
16. Kuntz J, Berent A, Weisse C, et al. Double pigtail ureteral stenting and renal pelvic lavage for renal-sparing treatment of pyonephrosis in dogs: 13 cases (2008-2012). J Am Vet Med Assoc 2015;246(2):216–25.
17. Pavia P, Berent A, Weisse C, et al. Canine ureteral stenting for benign ureteral obstruction in dogs. San Diego (CA): Abstract ACVS; 2014.
18. Berent A, Weisse C, Beal M, et al. Use of indwelling, double-pigtail stents for treatment of malignant ureteral obstruction in dogs: 12 cases (2006-2009). J Am Vet Med Assoc 2011;238(8):1017–25.
19. Weisse C, Berent A. Percutaneous fluoroscopically-assisted perineal approach for rigid cystoscopy in 9 male dogs. Barcelona (Spain): ECVS; 2012.

20. Berent A, Weisse C, Todd K, et al. Use of locking-loop pigtail nephrostomy catheters in dogs and cats: 20 cases (2004-2009). J Am Vet Med Assoc 2012;241: 348–57.

21. Vachon C, Defrages A, Berent A, et al. Passive ureteral dilation and ureteroscopy following ureteral stent placement in normal dogs. J Vet Intern Med 2014;28: 1073.

22. Berent A. Interventional urology: endourology in small animal veterinary medicine. Vet Clin North Am Small Anim Pract 2015;45(4):825–55.

23. Berent AC. Advances in urinary tract endoscopy. Vet Clin North Am Small Anim Pract 2016;46(1):113–35.

24. Gookin JL, Stone EA, Spaulding KA, et al. Unilateral nephrectomy in dogs with renal disease: 30 cases (1985-1994). J Am Vet Med Assoc 1996;208:2020–6.

25. King M, Waldron D, Barber D, et al. Effect of nephrotomy on renal function and morphology in normal cats. Vet Surg 2006;35(8):749–58.

26. Ross SJ, Osborne CA, Lekcharoensuk C, et al. A case-control study of the effects of nephrolithiasis in cats with chronic kidney disease. J Am Vet Med Assoc 2007; 230:1854–9.

27. Adams LG, Williams JC Jr, McAteer JA, et al. In vitro evaluation of canine and feline urolith fragility by shock wave lithotripsy. Am J Vet Res 2005;66:1651–4.

28. Chen KK, Chen MT, Yeh SH, et al. Radionuclide renal function study in various surgical treatments of upper urinary stones. Zhonghua Yi Xue Za Zhi (Taipei) 1992;49(5):319–27.

29. Reis LO, Zani EL, Ikari O, et al. Extracorporeal lithotripsy in children—the efficacy and long-term evaluation of renal parenchyma damage by DMSA-99mTc scintigraphy. Actas Urol Esp 2010;34(1):78–81 [in Spanish].

30. Hubert KC, Palmar JS. Passive dilation by ureteral stenting before ureteroscopy: eliminating the need for active dilation. J Urol 2005;174(3):1079–80.

31. Daugherty MA, Adams LG, Baird DK, et al. Acute pancreatitis in two dogs associated with shock wave lithotripsy [abstract]. J Vet Intern Med 2004;18:441.

32. Vaughan DE, Sweet RE, Gillenwater JY. Unilateral ureteral occlusion: pattern of nephron repair and compensatory response. J Urol 1973;109:979.

33. Meretyk S, Gofrit ON, Gafni O, et al. Complete staghorn calculi: random prospective comparison between extracorporeal shock wave lithotripsy monotherapy and combined with percutaneous nephrostolithotomy. J Urol 1997;157:780–6.

34. Al-Hunayan A, Khalil M, Hassabo M, et al. Management of solitary renal pelvic stone: laparoscopic retroperitoneal pyelolithotomy versus percutaneous nephrolithotomy. J Endourol 2011;25(6):975–8.

35. Tawfiek ER, Bagley DH. Ureteroscopic evaluation and treatment of chronic unilateral hematuria. J Urol 1998;160:700–2.

36. Bagley DH, Allen J. Flexible ureteropyeloscopy in the diagnosis of benign essential hematuria. J Urol 1990;143:549–53.

37. Villanueva S, Carreño JE, Salazar L. Human mesenchymal stem cells derived from adipose tissue reduce functional and tissue damage in a rat model of chronic renal failure. Clin Sci (Lond) 2013;125(4):199–210.

38. Kyles A, Hardie E, Wooden E, et al. Management and outcome of cats with ureteral calculi: 153 cases (1984–2002). J Am Vet Med Assoc 2005;226(6):937–44.

39. Roberts S, Aronson L, Brown D. Postoperative mortality in cats after ureterolithotomy. Vet Surg 2011;40:438–43.

40. Snyder DM, Steffey MA, Mehler SJ, et al. Diagnosis and surgical management of ureteral calculi in dogs: 16 cases (1990-2003). N Z Vet J 2004;53(1):19–25.

41. Kerr WS. Effect of complete ureteral obstruction for one week on kidney function. J Appl Physiol 1954;6:762.

42. Goldin AR. Percutaneous ureteral splinting. Urology 1977;10(2):165.

43. D'Anjou MA, Gedard A, Dunn M. Clinical significance of renal pelvic dilation on ultrasound in dogs and cats. Vet Radiol Ultrasound 2011;52(1):88–94.

44. Adin C, Herrgesell E, Nyland T, et al. Antegrade pyelography for suspected ureteral obstruction in cats: 11 cases (1995-2011). J Am Vet Med Assoc 2003; 222(11):1576–81.

45. Carr A, Wisner E, Westropp J, et al. Feline obstructive ureterolithiasis: utility of computed tomography and ultrasound in clinical decision making [Abstract]. American College of Veterinary Radiology and Ultrasound; 2012.

46. Hecht S, Lawson S, Lane I, et al. 99mTc-DTPA diuretic renal scintigraphy in cats with nephroureterolithiasis. J Feline Med Surg 2010;12:423–30.

47. Nyland TG, Fisher PE, Doverspike M, et al. Diagnosis of urinary tract obstruction in dogs using duplex Doppler ultrasonography. Vet Radiol Ultrasound 1993;34: 348–52.

48. Zimskind PD. Clinical use of long-term indwelling silicone rubber ureteral splints inserted cystoscopically. J Urol 1967;97:840.

49. Uthappa MC. Retrograde or antegrade double-pigtail stent placement for malignant ureteric obstruction? Clin Radiol 2005;60:608.

50. Lennon GM. Double pigtail ureteric stent versus percutaneous nephrostomy: effects on stone transit and ureteric motility. Eur Urol 1997;31(1):24.

51. Mustafa M. The role of stenting in relieving loin pain following ureteroscopic stone therapy for persisting renal colic with hydronephrosis. Int Urol Nephrol 2007; 39(1):91.

52. Yossepowitch O. Predicting the success of retrograde stenting for managing ureteral obstruction. J Urol 2001;166:1746.

53. Smith JD, Stone EA, Gilson SD. Placement of a permanent cystostomy catheter to relieve urine outflow obstruction in dogs with transitional cell carcinoma. J Am Vet Med Assoc 1995;206:496.

54. Stiffler KS, McCrackin Stevenson MA, Cornell KK, et al. Clinical use of low-profile cystostomy tubes in four dogs and a cat. J Am Vet Med Assoc 2003;223(3):325.

55. Beck AL, Grierson JM, Ogden DM, et al. Outcome of and complications associated with tube cystostomy in dogs and cats: 76 cases (1995-2006). J Am Vet Med Assoc 2007;230:1184.

56. Holmes ES, Weisse C, Berent AC. Use of fluoroscopically guided percutaneous antegrade urethral catheterization for the treatment of urethral obstruction in male cats: 9 cases (2000-2009). J Am Vet Med Assoc 2012;241(5):603–7.

57. Meige F, Sarrau S, Autefage A. Management of traumatic urethral rupture in 11 cats using primary alignment with a urethral catheter. Vet Comp Orthop Traumatol 2008;21:76–84.

58. Blackburn AL, Berent AC, Weisse CW, et al. Evaluation of outcome following urethral stent placement for the treatment of obstructive carcinoma of the urethra in dogs: 42 cases (2004-2008). J Am Vet Med Assoc 2013;242(1):59–68.

59. McMillan SK, Knapp DW, Ramos-Vara JA, et al. Outcome of urethral stent placement for management of urethral obstruction secondary to transitional cell carcinoma in dogs: 19 cases (2007-2010. J Am Vet Med Assoc 2012;241(12): 1627–32.

60. Hill TL, Berent AC, Weisse CW. Evaluation of urethral stent placement for benign urethral obstructions in dogs. J Vet Intern Med 2014;28:1384–90.

61. Brace MA, Weisse C, Berent A. Preliminary experience with stenting for management of non-urolith urethral obstruction in eight cats. Vet Surg 2014;43:199–208.

62. Knapp DW, Glickman NW, Widmer WR, et al. Cisplatin versus cisplatin with piroxicam in a canine model of human invasive urinary bladder cancer. Cancer Chemother Pharmacol 2000;46(3):221.

63. Norris AM, Laing EJ, Valli VEO, et al. Canine bladder and urethral tumors: a retrospective study of 115 cases (1980-1985). J Vet Intern Med 1992;16:145.

64. Liptak JM, Brutscher SP, Monnet E, et al. Transurethral resection in the management of urethral and prostatic neoplasia in 6 dogs. Vet Surg 2004;33:505.

65. Fries CL, Binnington AG, Valli VE, et al. Enterocystoplasty with cystectomy and subtotal intracapsular prostatectomy in the male dogs. Vet Surg 1991;20(2):104.

66. Stone EA, Withrow SJ, Page RL, et al. Ureterocolonic anastomosis in ten dogs with transitional cell carcinoma. Vet Surg 1998;17:147.

Index

Note: Page numbers of article titles are in **boldface** type.

A

Abdomen cancer
    CT for surgical planning in, 507
    CT in staging of, 506–507
Ablation
    IO in, 558–559
Abscess(es)
    pancreatic
        ultrasound appearance of, 472
Antegrade urethral catheterization, 590–591

B

Balloon dilation
    in IR, 546–548
Benign ureteral obstruction
    IR for, 577–587
        canine ureteral stenting, 583–584
        feline ureteral stenting, 580–583
        percutaneous nephrostomy tube placement, 577–578
        subcutaneous ureteral bypass device in cats, 578–580
        traditional ureteral surgery, 577
Bicipital tenosynovitis
    MRI of, 426–428
Bile duct
    normal ultrasound appearance of, 455
Biliary disease
    ultrasound appearance of, 461–465
Biliary tract
    inflammation of
        CT and MRI of, 488–490
    neoplasia of
        CT and MRI of, 485–487
Biopsy
    in IR, 543

C

Cancer
    diagnosis of
        PET/CT in, 520–522
    staging of

http://dx.doi.org/10.1016/S0195-5616(16)00028-0
0195-5616/16/$ – see front matter © 2016 Elsevier Inc. All rights reserved.
vetsmall.theclinics.com

Printed and bound by CPI Group (UK) Ltd, Croydon, CR0 4YY

03/10/2024

01040398-0010